LIMBIC SYSTEM MECHANISMS and AUTONOMIC FUNCTION

Proceedings of a Brain Research Symposium

Held at Massey College of the University of Toronto

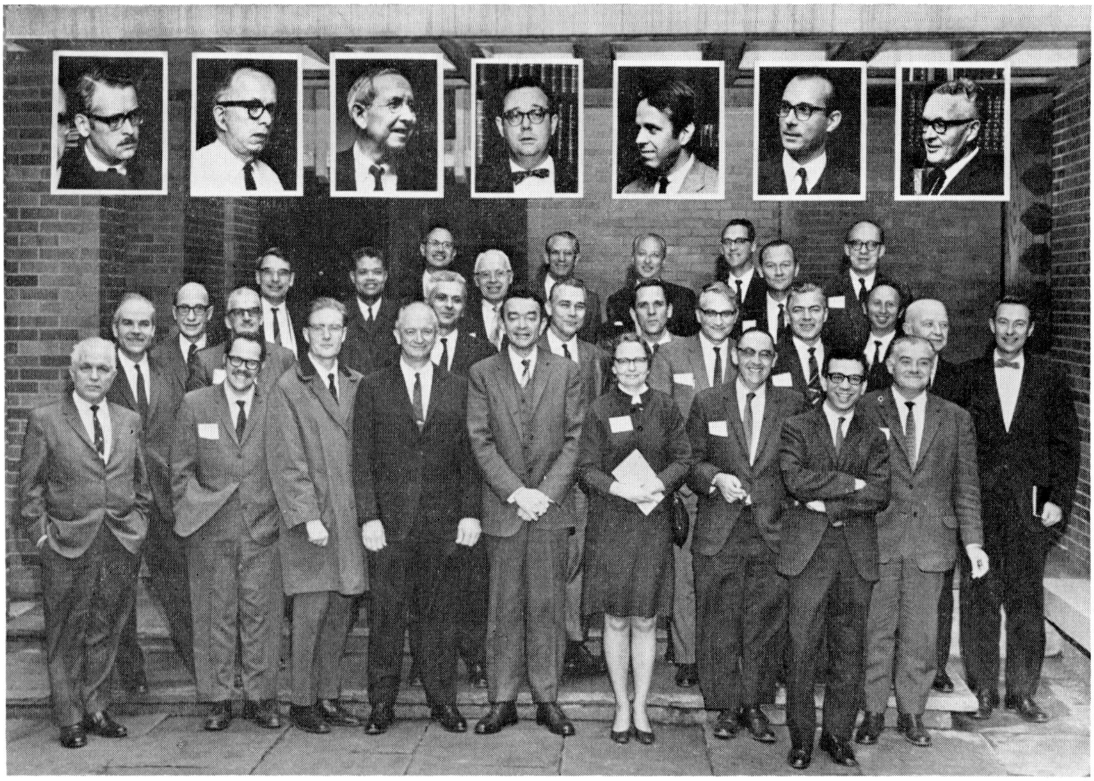

BRAIN RESEARCH SYMPOSIUM

Front row: Hoff, Hoffer, Marczynski, Lindsley, Hockman, Hall, Lacey, Calaresu, Dell. *Second row:* Gloor, Jasper, Haist, Hugelin, Wolf, Mauck, Sigg, Andy, Abrahams, Yakovlev, Livingston. *Third row:* Scott, Ling, Schallek, Green, Kalow, Talesnik, Mogenson, Nauta, Stevenson. *Inserts:* Kalant, Snider, MacLean, Killam, Reis, Hornykiewicz, French.

LIMBIC SYSTEM MECHANISMS and AUTONOMIC FUNCTION

Edited by

CHARLES H. HOCKMAN
Associate Professor of Pharmacology
University of Toronto
Toronto, Canada

In preliminary consultation with
KENNETH E. LIVINGSTON
Associate Professor of Pharmacology and Surgery
University of Toronto
Toronto, Canada

With a Foreword by

Giuseppe Moruzzi
Istituto di Fisiologia dell' Universita
e Laboratorio di Neurofisiologia del C.N.R.
Pisa, Italy

CHARLES C THOMAS · PUBLISHER
Springfield · Illinois · U.S.A.

Published and Distributed Throughout the World by
CHARLES C THOMAS • PUBLISHER
BANNERSTONE HOUSE
301–327 East Lawrence Avenue, Springfield, Illinois, U.S.A.
NATCHEZ PLANTATION HOUSE
735 North Atlantic Boulevard, Fort Lauderdale, Florida, U.S.A.

ISBN: 0–398–02315–8

Library of Congress Catalog Card Number: 77–175077

With THOMAS BOOKS *careful attention is given to all details of manufacturing and design. It is the Publisher's desire to present books that are satisfactory as to their physical qualities and artistic possibilities and appropriate for their particular use.* THOMAS BOOKS *will be true to those laws of quality that assure a good name and good will.*

Printed in the United States of America
K-8

Participants and Guests

Vivian C. Abrahams, *Department of Physiology, Queen's University at Kingston, Ontario, Canada*

Orlando J. Andy, *Department of Neurosurgery, University of Mississippi School of Medicine, Jackson, Mississippi*

John V. Basmajian,* *Department of Anatomy, Queen's University at Kingston, Ontario, Canada*

Franco R. Calaresu, *Department of Physiology, University of Western Ontario, London, Canada*

Donald R. Crapper, *Department of Physiology, University of Toronto, Toronto, Ontario, Canada*

Paul Dell, *Laboratoire de Neurophysiologie, C.N.R.S., Marseille, France*

John D. French, *Brain Research Institute, University of California, Los Angeles*

Pierre Gloor, *Montreal Neurological Institute and McGill University, Montreal, Canada*

Harold D. Green, *Department of Physiology, Bowman Gray School of Medicine of Wake Forest College,* Winston-Salem, North Carolina

Reginald E. Haist, *Department of Physiology, University of Toronto, Ontario, Canada*

Elizabeth Hall, *Department of Anatomy, University of Ottawa,* Ontario, Canada

Charles H. Hockman, *Department of Pharmacology, University of Toronto, Ontario, Canada*

Barry J. Hoffer, *Laboratory of Neuropharmacology, National Institute of Mental Health, Bethesda, Maryland*

Ebbe Curtis Hoff, *Departments of Physiology and Psychiatry, Medical College of Virginia, Richmond*

Oleh Hornykiewicz, *Department of Pharmacology, University of Toronto, Ontario, Canada*

Andre Hugelin, *Laboratoire de Physiologie, Universite de Paris, France*

Herbert H. Jasper, *Department of Physiology, University of Montreal, Quebec, Canada*

Harold Kalant, *Department of Pharmacology, University of Toronto, Ontario, Canada*

Werner Kalow, *Department of Pharmacology, University of Toronto, Ontario, Canada*

Keith F. Killam, Jr., *Department of Pharmacology, University of California, Davis*

John I. Lacey, *Department of Psychophysiology-Neurophysiology, The Fels Research Institute, Yellow Springs, Ohio*

Donald B. Lindsley, *Departments of Psychology and Physiology, University of California, Los Angeles, California*

George M. Ling, *Department of Pharmacology, University of Ottawa, Ontario, Canada*

Kenneth E. Livingston, *Departments of Pharmacology and Neurosurgery, University of Toronto, Ontario, Canada*

Edward Llewellyn-Thomas, *Departments of Biomedical Engineering and Pharmacology, University of Toronto, Ontario, Canada*

Paul D. MacLean, *Section on Limbic Integration and Behavior, National Institute of Mental Health, Bethesda, Maryland*

Taddeus J. Marczynski, *Department of Pharmacology, College of Medicine, University of Illinois, Chicago, Illinois*

H. Page Mauck, Jr., *Department of Medicine, Medical College of Virginia, Richmond*

Gordon Mogenson, *Departments of Psychology and Physiology, University of Western Ontario, London, Canada*

* Now at Emory University Regional Rehabilitation Research and Training Center, Atlanta, Georgia.

John T. Murphy,* *Department of Neurobiology, University of New York at Buffalo*
Walle J. H. Nauta, *Department of Psychology, Massachusetts Institute of Technology, Cambridge*
James W. Pearce, *Department of Physiology, University of Toronto, Ontario, Canada*
Donald J. Reis, *Department of Neurology, Cornell University Medical School, New York, New York*
William B. Schallek, *Department of Neuropharmacology, Hoffman La Roche, Inc., Nutley, New Jersey*
John W. Scott, *Department of Physiology, University of Toronto, Ontario, Canada*
Edward A. Sellers, *Department of Pharmacology, University of Toronto, Ontario, Canada*
Ernest B. Sigg, *Department of Neuropharmacology, Hoffman-La Roche, Inc., Nutley, New Jersey*
Harley S. Smyth, *Department of Surgery, University of Toronto, Ontario, Canada*
Ray S. Snider, *The Center for Brain Research, University of Rochester, Rochester, New York*
James A. F. Stevenson,† *Department of Physiology, University of Western Ontario, London, Canada*
Jaime Talesnik,‡ *Department of Experimental Medicine, University of Chile, South America*
Stewart Wolf,§ *Oklahoma Medical Research Foundation*
Paul I. Yakovlev,|| *Department of Anatomy, Harvard Medical School, Cambridge, Massachusetts*

* Now at Department of Physiology, University of Toronto, Ontario, Canada.
† Deceased. July 23rd., 1971.
‡ Now at Department of Pharmacology, University of Toronto, Ontario, Canada.
§ Now at The Marine Biomedical Institute, Galveston, Texas.
|| Now at E. E. Southard Unit, E. K. Shriver Research Center, Walter E. Fernald State School, Waverly, Massachusetts.

To Professor J. A. F. Stevenson,
A Friend

His untimely death is a
Great loss to neuroscience.
He not only did much to live up to his reputation
As a scholar,
But more than lived up to his reputation
As a man.

Foreword

THE SYMPOSIUM held at Massey College of the University of Toronto was wider in scope than one might expect from the title of this book. Although there was particular emphasis on the limbic system, the participants approached the problem of autonomic regulation from a physiological standpoint, without anatomical limitations. The title of the introductory report (Hoff), "Higher Cerebral Regulation of Autonomic Function," might well summarize such a line of attack. This was not the only approach, however, and the problem of the inter-relations between autonomic and somatic influences of the central nervous system was another important subject of study, both in the reports and in the extensive discussions.

It is perhaps advisable while reading this important book to keep in mind the two main lines of endeavor: (a) the analysis of the hypothalamic effects on visceral organs, the *restricted integration,* which is concerned only with autonomic activities and (b) the study of the responses involving both the somatic and autonomic activities, the *generalized integration.*

A short review of the development of hypothalamic physiology may perhaps be useful as an introduction to this book, since it epitomizes a trend which is clearly present in the study of cerebral regulation of visceral organs.

The classical experiments of Karplus and Kreidl had been carried out originally under anesthesia and later in curarized cats *; and this fact explains why the motor effects had not been observed. The autonomic effects produced by hypothalamic stimulation under these experimental conditions—pupillary dilation, retraction of the nictating membranes, increase in arterial blood pressure—were in fact only fragments of a broader response which was missed by the earlier investigators. This fact was responsible for the wrong impression that Karplus and Kreidl's hypothalamic centers were exclusively concerned with the control of sympathetic activities. There is little doubt, moreover, that the general title given by the Austrian physiologists to a series of seven papers published between 1909 and 1927—*Gehirn und Sympathicus*—contributed to this impression. Their pioneer studies became rightly famous and were extensively quoted and also, as a consequence of that, the hypothesis of the *restricted integration* remained unchallenged for several years.

The second major step was made when Hess † started his experiments of

* *Pfluegers Arch, 129:*138–144, 1909; *171:*192–200, 1918; *215:*667–682, 1927.

† Hess, W. R.; *Ber Ges Physiol, 42:*554–555, 1927; *Helv Physiol Pharmacol Acta, 2:*137–147, 1944.

electrical stimulation in the freely moving, unanesthetized cat. With a magnificent series of studies covering a period of about forty years—from 1925 to 1968—he showed that as a result of localized electrical stimulations, one obtained fully integrated responses reproducing the behavior of fear, rage or sleep. This led to the major discovery that several instinctive behaviors described by ethologists could be reproduced by well-localized hypothalamic stimulations. What matters from our point of view is that both motoneurons and preganglionic nerve cells of the autonomic nervous system—the final common paths of the somatic and visceral systems—were driven in a fully integrated way by localized diencephalic stimulations. It became clear then that the time honored distinction between somatic and vegetative neurons was impossible at hypothalamic levels, since the centers for higher integration played on the great keyboard of the motoneurons and the autonomic neurons' on the brain stem and the spinal cord. Thus the hypothalamus brought together "from separate organs an animal possessing solidarity, an individual." The quotation from Sherrington * appears to be particularly appropriate after Hess' discoveries, since the concept of integration—originally formulated for spinal motoneurons—could be extended to neural activities influencing also the autonomic sphere.

The third step was made when the hypothalamic stimulations were applied not in a "vacuum" environment, to use Konorski's † expression, but in the presence of an appropriate stimulus-object or with suitable conditioning procedures. This demonstrated convincingly that hypothalamic stimulation produced not only specific behaviors but also elicited the corresponding drives (hunger or thirst) or emotions (fear and anger).

The study of *restricted integration*—based on the quantitative analysis of one or a few autonomic responses and on the investigation of their anatomical and pharmacological correlates—is still a very important field of investigation. The importance of this approach is shown by several reports presented at the Toronto Symposium. The reader will be informed about recent studies concerning the anatomical correlations between the limbic system on the one side and the brain stem, the hypothalamus and the cerebral cortex on the other side (Nauta); the amygdaloid projections upon ventromedial hypothalamic neurons (Gloor *et al.*; Murphy *et al.*); and the exteroceptive inputs to limbic cortex (MacLean). He will also find an extensive report of the pharmacological aspects of limbic function (Killam) as well as reviews of the septal (Andy *et al.*) and cerebellar (Snider; Hoffer *et al.*) influences on autonomic activities. Along this line of endeavor, we may also quote the report on the supramedullary modulation of autonomic reflexes (Hockman *et al.*). It is mainly concerned with the central regula-

* Sherrington, C. S.: *The Integrative Action of the Nervous System.* New York, Charles Scribner & Sons, 1906, see p. 2.

† Konorski, J.: *Acta Biol Exp, 27:*265–267, 1967. This article may also be consulted for pertinent literature.

tion of the cardiac component of the baroceptive reflexes, a new phenomenon which may be observed only when the brain is intact.

The approach of the *generalized integration* was also represented at the Toronto Symposium. The studies (Dell) on the hypnogenic effects of the baroceptive volleys, relayed by the nucleus of the solitary tract, are excellent examples of this line of attack. If one leaves aside the changes of the cerebral cortical activity, which may be detected in the EEG or by single unit recording, sleep appears as a highly integrated pattern of behavior, due to stereotyped discharges of final common paths of both the somatic and the autonomic nervous systems: the motoneurons and the preganglionic nerve cells of the brain stem and spinal cord. Sleep behavior may be triggered by several inputs, and one of the most powerful among them is represented by baroceptive volleys coursing along Cyon's and Hering's nerves. The term "buffer nerves" implied the concept of a restricted integration, one mainly concerned with the regulation of blood flow and respiration. A shift to the physiology of the generalized integration appeared as a serious possibility almost twenty years ago, when Dell (1954) demonstrated that the sleep-like syndrome described by Koch (1932), following a strong rise in pressure within one isolated carotid sinus, could be reproduced when all accompanying changes of systemic circulation, lung ventilation and adrenaline discharges were abolished by spinal cord section at C_1.

Of course, the main problem is to see whether these effects were present also when stimulation of the baroceptors was within the normal ranges of blood pressure and could be demonstrated for the tonic discharge of the neurons of the solitary tract. Dell's observation, reported at this Symposium, that increased firing of neurons lying at the level of the neucleus of the solitary tract occurs during *spontaneous* sleep and that the discharge disappears during arousal would appear to give a positive answer to this basic question.

The deactivating influence of the baroceptive volleys, acting through neurons of the lower brain stem might have important psychophysiological implications which have been developed at this Symposium in a report mainly devoted to human studies. The author (Lacey) was concerned with the puzzling observation that heart rate decreases during attention. These parasympathetic-like effects occur paradoxically while pupils and electrodermal responses show sympathetic like effects. The author's explanation fits very closely with Dell's conception of baroceptive control, when he states that "the cardiovascular system has controlling effects on brain functions which are mediated by visceral afferent feedback mechanisms." This stimulating hypothesis implies that the tonic activity of the hypnogenic neurons of the solitary tract is critically maintained by the tonic flow of the baroceptive barrage existing for normal ranges of blood pressure. Obviously, only animal experimentation might provide an answer to this important question.

Finally in a report devoted to bodily changes during arousal, attention and emotion (Hugelin), a distinction is made between the intensive and the selective aspects of attention. The intensive dimension of attention corresponds to what is usually designated as arousal and can be explained by purely reticular mechanisms. On the other hand, "during selection of information, neural events, specific to this type of behavior, take place together with reticular discharge." The typical arousal is always characterized by an increase in heart rate and of the psychogalvanic response—that is, by ergotropic effects.

A good test of the importance of a Symposium is whether data or hypotheses presented at the meeting give rise to fundamental problems and eventually to new experimental approaches. This is likely to be the outcome of the Toronto meeting, not only for the participants but also for the readers of this book.

Pisa, Italy GIUSEPPE MORUZZI

Introduction

All of us who shared the warmth and friendship afforded by this Symposium will long cherish memories of the convivial atmosphere of Massey College nestled, as it is, in the heart of Toronto, yet untouched by the hustle and bustle of the big city. We shall also long remember the cordial welcome accorded us by its Master, Professor Robertson Davies, noted Canadian writer and humorist.

It was in this delightful setting that we met and talked to one another over a three-day period about the way the brain regulates visceral activities. These discussions ranged over a wide variety of topics, encompassing the role of the limbic system in the regulation of autonomic effector activity no less than its role in the processing of information and emotion. While some topics seem to have been given prominence by virtue of the titles of contributed papers, this impression is soon dispelled by the breadth of the discussions. Furthermore, Professor Moruzzi, in his Foreword, adds an important note of historical perspective in drawing attention to the development of hypothalamic physiology.

Equally important should be the reminder that eventually each investigator must attempt to fit his pieces into the puzzle that is life—always a most difficult if not impossible undertaking!

I should like to express my gratitude to Doctors Kenneth E. Livingston and John W. Scott for their invaluable assistance in the organization of the Symposium. I should also like to thank Mr. Eugene Leblanc for serving as projectionist; Dr. Richard G. Perrin for giving invaluable aid in retranscribing the original material; and Miss Pat Arnold and the secretarial staff of the Department of Pharmacology for their assistance in typing manuscripts.

Over a period of many, many months, my wife, Mildred Adèle, acted as my secretary and proofreader without respite for social activities, and for this I am eternally grateful.

Charles H. Hockman

Acknowledgments

GRATITUDE is expressed to the Master and Staff of Massey College for their cordial hospitality and to the following organizations for their generous support:

Alcoholism and Drug Addiction Research Foundation of Ontario
Charles L. Gundy, Toronto
Denison Mines Limited, Toronto
Department of Pharmacology of the University of Toronto
Helen Scott Playfair Memorial Fund of the University of Toronto
Koffler Stores Limited, Toronto
Medical Research Council of Canada

Contents

SESSION IV

Chairman: John I. Lacey

SESSION V

Chairman: Donald B. Lindsley

SESSION VI

Chairman: Ebbe Curtis Hoff

LIMBIC SYSTEM MECHANISMS and AUTONOMIC FUNCTION

SESSION I

Chairman: **Kenneth E. Livingston**

Chapter 1

Higher Cerebral Regulation of Autonomic Function: A Historical Perspective

EBBE CURTIS HOFF

IN LOOKING at the historical development of our understanding of higher central nervous regulation of autonomic functions, it is appropriate to think of four significant components of this history. The first of these concerns some of the classical hypotheses and experimental testing of these hypotheses of cortical regulation of autonomic activity. Second, one may isolate briefly the concept that so-called autonomic and so-called somatic functions are interrelated at functional levels and in functional systems within the central nervous system. Third, it has been and still is of captivating interest to determine the extent to which there is specificity of autonomic functional control at upper neural levels. Finally, our concerns with the central regulation of autonomic function lead us inevitably to an ever-growing and always practical curiosity into the precise relationships between mental and emotional experiences and behavior on the one hand and neurophysiological action and neuropathological processes on the other. While it has not yet been possible to agree exactly upon a conformation between the mechanisms of the brain and the mechanisms, so-called, of the mind in a single pattern and although older investigations of the effects of psychosurgical procedures and, more recently, of the action of psychopharmacological agents have done much to narrow the knowledge gap between psychological and neurophysiological functions, nevertheless, these issues remain widely exposed to research for the future.

The student of literature on central regulation of autonomic function is aware that the concept that metabolic, secretory, cardiovascular and other visceral activities are integrated at various levels of the central nervous system, including the cerebral cortex, rests upon an enormous literature extending now over a period of more than a hundred years. It was Hughlings Jackson [20] who set forth the general idea in its earliest clearly enunciated form. Jackson voiced the conviction that not only movements in the ordinary sense of the word—that is to say, voluntary movements of the body—are represented in the cerebrum but the movements of arteries and viscera are represented as well. Jackson comprehended that the highest processes are the most multifold and complex of sensory motor functions and that they represent, or re-represent, all lower nervous centers and thus also the organism as a whole. As early as 1869, Hughlings Jackson explicitly asserted that one must add to the constitution of the units of the cerebrum, nerve fibers to the heart, blood vessels and viscera, and he conceived the units of the cerebral hemisphere as representing potentially the entirety of the body processes —voluntary movements as well as activity of involuntary structures. He thus claimed that the highest nervous processes are potentially the whole organism. He arrived at this conclusion partly by reasoning that since emotional phenomena are on their physical side widespread agitations of the limbs, viscera and circulatory organs, there must, therefore, be representation of these parts in the highest centers. However, he was not limited to this reasoning but also emphasized that gross disease as, for instance, tumors of the "organ of the mind," as he called it, produced muscular as well as circulatory and other visceral symptoms.

Since Hughlings Jackson made an exploration of epilepsy a rich source of his observations and conclusions, it is not surprising that he recognized particular significance on the autonomic events of the epileptic seizure and these he took to be a striking demonstration of the truth of his hypothesis that the highest nervous centers represent all lower nervous arrangements and thus the whole body.

Jackson was not without forerunners in his comprehensive and holistic concept of the coordinating action of the central nervous system. Thus Cawadias [2] has quoted a passage from Bordeu, an eighteenth century clinician and representative of the School of Montpellier, who asserted that "functions first begin in the brain, which is divided into as many components as there are organs." Related ideas were expressed by the Russian physiologist, Setschenow, whose physiological concepts not only formed a base upon which Pavlov initiated his investigations but also provided an appreciation that involuntary functions may be coordinated at cortical levels. In his early postgraduate years, Setschenow worked in the laboratories of Helmoltz, DuBois-Reymond and Ludwig. Setschenow was singularly influenced by Ludwig and in the latter's laboratory had an opportunity to develop his interest in the nervous system, particularly nervous control of visceral function. Ludwig's influence is reflected in one of Setschenow's first studies which he saw as an attempt to delineate a physiological basis of psychic processes. These ideas were novel and daring and suffered censorship, but they were finally published in 1863 under a less startling title of "Reflex Action of the Brain." [26] Briefly, he taught that all activity of the brain and spinal cord can be expressed in movement or action of one sort or another and that such activity can be seen as an adjustment within the brain between the incoming sensory stimuli and muscular responses. Not only are voluntary movements mediated by such "reflexes" traversing the cortex, but involuntary visceral events are coordinated within the cerebral cortex as well.

Evidence for the concept of higher central neural regulation of visceral function derived from clinical studies such as those of Hughlings Jackson and a long series of clinical observers since then [16] have been reinforced by many investigations using methods of electrical stimulation and observations of the effects of lesions in the brain. Stimulation studies suffer from the inherent limitation of all such experiments conducted under more or less artificial laboratory conditions. Mechanisms of function seen in an experimental biological preparation do not necessarily fit perfectly with spontaneous activity in an intact animal or man. The validity of concepts derived from stimulation experiments is dependent upon the accuracy and completeness with which the experiment can be realistically compared with actual physiological responses. In the case of observations of lesions of the brain, deficits and functional abnormalities observed to be associated with lesions do not establish that physiological processes are limited to the areas of the lesion associated with disturbances of function.

Within a very few years of Hughlings Jackson's brilliant observations, experimental evidence for higher regulation of cardiovascular activity began to be sought in animals by measurement of heart rate and arterial blood pressure changes evoked by electrical stimulation of exposed cortical surfaces. Manifestly, this experimental approach, together with the study of the effects of cerebral resections, has provided an enormous body of evidence. These approaches are, as implied, vulnerable to the criticism that electrical stimulation imposes upon the brain an unphysiological task or even a biophysical abnormality and that deficits due to clinical or experimental lesions do not sufficiently localize or define normal functions. Also, as may be inferred, failure to elicit autonomic deficiencies by cortical ablations does not necessarily exclude the cortex from jurisdiction over these functions in the intact organism.

Many investigators, notably in Russia, have explored the problem by extension of the techniques of Pavlov and have established conditional reflexes in which a variety of visceral responses—cardiovascular, gastrointestinal, renal, endocrine and exocrine—have been temporarily linked with higher brain function. These studies offer evidence in the intact, unanesthetized animal of a broad potential control by the cortex and related levels of the central nervous system over autonomic as well as skeletal functions.

To allude briefly to the enormous literature on electrical stimulation, it may be recalled that the announcement in 1870 by Fritsch and Hitzig [11] that skeletal movements can be evoked in animals by appropriate electrical excitation of frontal regions of the contralateral cerebral hemisphere almost at once directed attention to localizing investigations by the technique of stimulation of currently accessible cerebral surfaces. Many experimenters began to explore the dorsolateral surfaces of the hemisphere in an effort to show that changes in the activity of the viscera can also be inaugurated by stimulation. Thus, the first direct observations that modification of autonomic function can originate from experimental electrical stimulation of the cortex were made by Schiff [25] and Danilewsky [6] in 1875. These investigators measured changes in heart rate as well as blood pressure from a variety of higher cerebral loci in young dogs.

These and many subsequent studies of the effects of cerebral stimulation upon systemic arterial blood pressure, heart rate and other autonomic functions established by the third decade of this century evidence from which it could be inferred that the highest levels of the central nervous system may play a part in the regulation of cardiovascular and other autonomic functions. This inference was reinforced by observations by Goldstein [13] of vasomotor and other autonomic disturbances following brain damage in patients and also localized lesions in experimental animals. However, the role of higher cerebral levels in the regulation of autonomic activity was by no means fully established, widely accepted or even well understood. Many of the experiments were very little known and many were criticized as being imperfectly controlled. Thus, in 1929, Bard [1] expressed a general skepticism in his statement that "many of the effects which were produced are to be accounted for on the basis of spread of strong stimulating currents to subcortical regions or to the production of cortical epilepsy in which a widespread and unphysiological discharge occurs." Nor was Bard alone or the first in questioning the significance of the stimulation studies. François-Franck[10] in 1887 had asserted that the blood pressure and heart rate changes resulting from cortical stimulation were secondary manifestations of generalized epileptic discharges. By others, the responses were ascribed not only to current spread to other areas but also to stimulation of the meninges of the brain which were observed by Danilewsky[6] to give pressor responses on direct stimulation. Hughlings Jackson's concept that "movements of the arteries and viscera" as well as "voluntary movements of the body" are represented in the cerebrum —a concept that commends itself to an evolutionary view of central nervous system development—seemed to have fared badly during the first half century following its enunciation. More obvious manifestations of cerebral activity held the center of the stage. Also, it is important to remember that there existed severe technical limitations in measuring not only systemic arterial blood pressure and heart rate but also in assessing other end effects of autonomic action. Furthermore, the techniques of electrical and other stimulation were imperfectly developed as also were stereotaxic methods as well as telemetric imposition of stimuli. Another serious deterrent was the great sensitivity of cerebrally invoked autonomic changes to anesthetics. This latter greater sensitivity of cerebrogenic autonomic responses to drugs has in part led to an opening up of studies of the action of psychoactive drugs on emotional aspects of the central nervous system and promises to be an important investigative area for the future. It is still of current historical interest that when Sherrington[27] began to concentrate on the integrative action of the central nervous system, he chose for his own studies the skeletal muscular reflex rather than the systemic blood pressure response as an end effect because of his conviction that the latter was not adequately reproducible quantitatively. How different might have been the history of psychiatry had Sherrington turned the searchlight of his magnificent intellect upon central autonomic mechanisms!

In the early 1930's Fulton[12] and his coworkers began to explore the mechanisms of central regulation of the autonomic nervous system at the cortical level. Fulton strongly emphasized that at all central nervous levels, including the highest, there seems to be a coordination of autonomic with somatic function. Evidence for this coordination was sought at isocortical, limbic, diencephalic and lower levels.

A wide variety of autonomic actions have been explored: circulation in special areas such as the kidney[17] and other visceral organs, salivary secretion,[29] cardiac dynamics and arrhythmias, endocrine activity, sexual functions and many others. Gradually a more and more integrative concept of levels of function and control systems is being worked out. Sensory as well as descending mechanisms are being explored. Significantly, pharmacological aspects of limbic system function are being subject to expert scrutiny.

Green and Hoff[14,15] and others in the 1930's worked on the crucial objective of determining whether the vasomotor and other autonomic phenomena evoked by application of electrical stimuli to the central nervous system were actually due to stimulation of neuronal elements locally. The techniques of proof of those days have been refined and it can now be asserted from well-designed experiments that stimulus input can be limited to circumscribed loci within the brain and that the effects are not invariably or inevitably the results of wide current spread and of generalized seizure activity.

These lines of evidence by Green and Hoff have been confirmed by Kaada [21] in monkeys, cats and dogs in the cingulate, insular, orbital and pyriform regions, and further refinements have been reported by Wall and Pribam.[31] The fact that central neural tissue is the essential recipient of the stimulation has been demonstrated by Chapman, Livingston and Livingston [3] in patients and in animals by Mettler, Hamilton, Allen, Woodbury and Mettler.[24] A further confirmation of the cortical origin of vasomotor responses evoked by electrical stimulation of cortical areas is provided (in studies of Hoff, Langford, Vester, Beckner, and Thomas) [18] by the *facilitation* of these responses (rise of blood pressure and renal vasoconstriction) by the technique of topical application of strychnine sulfate (2% solution) to excitable loci. Strychnine alone, under these conditions, caused no change and when applied to silent parietal areas from which blood pressure responses could not be evoked, by itself, yielded no responses from any cortical pressor locus. Also, application of 2% strychnine to a cortical point rendered unresponsive by dibucaine, topically applied, did not restore the excitability of the locus or result in any change in the pressor response from the symmetrically placed locus on the opposite hemisphere. Thus, in this concentration, strychninization exerted its facilitating effect by action upon the cortical gray matter at the site of application and was effective upon cortical neurones which yield autonomic responses to electrical stimulation.

With regard to the attribution by François-Franck [10] of the vasomotor responses to epileptiform seizures, later workers have shown that while blood pressure changes associated with epileptiform discharges of central origin can be induced by maximal stimuli, nevertheless, it is always possible to demonstrate specific alterations of blood pressure of brief duration using strengths of stimuli which produce no skeletal movements or seizure activity in noncurarized animals or animals not injected with Flaxedil®.

Just as somatic movements elicited from stimulation of limbic and hypothalamic regions are rather more massive and generalized and not so discrete as are responses from isocortical motor areas, so a similar differentiation may be proposed for autonomic functions. Thus, in acute stimulation experiments, pressor pathways from the isocortex may be distinguished from others enhancing adrenal medullary activity.[8] These investigators obtained transient pressor responses as well as increased adrenal medullary activity from stimulation of loci on the anterior sigmoid gyri and of corticofugal fibers in the internal capsule of cats. It was possible to separate, by changing electrode positions, the activation of fibers mainly responsible for blood pressure rise from fibers influencing the adrenal medulla. This can be interpreted to mean that vasomotor and adrenal secretory fibers from the isocortex may be mediated by discrete pathways and suggests a degree of selective control at that level. It would, therefore, appear that this upper governing mechanism is not served by pathways permitting only a diffuse, massive activation of all autonomic neurons at lower levels (in contradistinction to the conclusions of Crouch and Thompson).[4,5] The idea that considerable selectivity of response may be possible also for hypothalamic levels has been shown in cats by Folkow and von Euler,[9] who evoked secretion of epinephrine and norepinephrine in varying proportions according to the location of the stimulus in the diencephalon. From this, they inferred that epinephrine- and norepinephrine-producing cells are innervated or can be innervated by nerve fibers with different hypothalamic representation. These questions of specificity of autonomic control systems in the upper levels of the brain are by no means fully answered and provide rich opportunity for future research in the intact functioning organism. Kell and Hoff[23] have unmasked profound cerebrogenic cardiovagal responses in cordotomized cats (C3) and in our laboratory we are now studying conditioned cardiac slowing in animals.

The interrelations between autonomic and somatic control mechanisms must be highly complicated and there must be exquisitely balanced inhibitory and excitatory mechanisms by which visceral and secretory responses are adjusted to the total needs of the individual. Our insight into these mechanisms can be heightened most adequately by using, in an interrelated fashion, all of the techniques at our disposal and by extending our study to finest brain details. For other studies of the discreteness and specificity of higher central regulation of autonomic mechanisms, we may turn to those of Houssay and Molinelli,[19] Wall and Davis,[30] Delgado,[7] Kaada, Pribram and Epstein[22] and a number of others. Exact anatomical-physiological relationships in the central nervous system haves been delineated by Nauta, Andy, Gloor and Snider in this monograph. The action of visceral afferents in the autonomic control systems has been explored by Dell, Hockman and others. Of profound significance are the implications of microelectrode findings on exteroceptive inputs into the limbic system by Maclean.

This volume includes papers by Lacey and Hugelin as well as Killam which have important implications in the issue of the relationship between mental and emotional experience and behavior on the one hand and neurophysiological action on the other. Throughout this monograph we hope to pose some of the older psychosomatic problems in new terms so that we need no longer have to conclude, as Sherrington[28] was compelled to do, that the liaisons between psychological and physical was an insoluble mystery. Sherrington indeed asked, "What right have we to conjoin mental experience with physiological?" To Sherrington a mere juxtaposition of the two sets of happenings proclaimed their disparity. On the one side, there were changing electrical potentials with thermal and chemical action making a physiological entity held together by energy relations; on the other, a suite of mental experience. He did not doubt the latter was an activity but questioned what relation, if any, did it stand to neural energy. As for Sherrington, what little he claimed to know about the "how" of the one did not, speaking for him personally, even begin to help him toward the "how" of the other. The two, for all that he was able to see or do, seemed to remain disparate and disconnected. With characteristically sensitive insight, Sherrington presented the essential elements of the mystery as he saw them in 1933. Although our ignorance still may tempt us to despair in this problem, we may assure ourselves that man's progressing curiosity will direct him to seek and construct new and more comprehensive syntheses in which he will better see his so-called psychological and so-called physiological natures welded into a unity. It may be that we shall never be able to answer some of the older psychosomatic questions in the ways in which they have been asked and probably what we must do is to ask quite new questions and see how far they will lead us. Herein lies, in my view, one of the most exciting aspects of this remarkable subject.

REFERENCES

1. Bard, P.: The central representation of the sympathetic system. *Arch. Neurol. Psychiat., 22:*230, 1929.
2. Cawadias, A. P.: Theophile de Bordeu; an eighteenth century pioneer in endocrinology. *Proc. Roy. Soc. Med., 43:*93, 1950.
3. Chapman, W. P., Livingston, R. B., and Livingston, K. E.: Frontal lobectomy and electrical stimulation of orbital surface of frontal lobes; effect on respiration and on blood pressure in man. *Arch. Neurol. Psychiat., 62:*701, 1949.
4. Crouch, R. L., and Thompson, K.: Autonomic responses elicited by stimulating the frontal region of the cerebral cortex of the cat. *Anat. Rec., 64 (Suppl. 3)*: 11, 1936.
5. Crouch, R. L., and Thompson, J. K.: Autonomic functions of the cerebral cortex. *J. Nerv. Ment. Dis., 89:*328, 1939.
6. Danilewsky, B.: Experimentelle Beitrage zur Physiologie des Gehirns. *Arch. Ges. Physiol., 11:*128, 1875.
7. Delgado, J. M. R.: Circulatory effects of cortical stimulation. *Physiol. Rev. 40 (Suppl. 4)*:146, 1960.
8. Ferguson, R. W., Folkow, B., Mitts, M. G., and Hoff, E. C.: Effect of cortical stimulation upon epinephrine activity. *J. Neurophysiol., 20:*329, 1957.
9. Folkow, B., and von Euler, U. S.: Selective activation of noradrenaline and adrenaline producing cells in cat's adrenal gland by hypothalamic stimulation. *Circ. Res., 2:*191, 1954.
10. François-Franck, C. E.: *Leçons sur les fonctions motrices du cerveau (reactions volontaires et organiques) et sur l'epilepsie cerebrale.* Paris, O. Doin, 1887.
11. Fritsch, G., and Hitzig, E.: Ueber die elektrische Erregbarkeit des Grosshirns. *Arch. Anat. Physiol., 37:*300, 1870.
12. Fulton, J. F.: Limbic system: Autonomic and somatic functions. In Fulton, J. F.: *A Textbook of Physiology,* 17th ed. Philadelphia, Saunders, 1955, pp. 255–264.
13. Goldstein, K.: Ueber korperliche Storungen bei Hirnverletzten. II. Mitteilung: Ueber Storungen der Vasomotilitat des Pulses, des Blutbildes, des Blutdruckes, der Temperatur bei Hirnverletzten. *Munchen Med. Wschr., 65:*65,104, 1918.
14. Green, H. D., and Hoff, E. C.: Effects of faradic stimulation of cerebral cortex on limb and renal volumes in the cat and monkey. *Amer. J. Physiol., 118:*641, 1937.
15. Hoff, E. C., and Green, H. D.: Cardiovascular reactions induced by electrical stimulation of the cerebral cortex. *Amer. J. Physiol., 117:*411, 1936.
16. Hoff, E. C., Kell, J. F., Jr., and Carroll, M. N., Jr.: Effects of cortical stimulation and lesions on cardiovascular function. *Physiol. Rev., 43 (1)*:68, 1963.
17. Hoff, E. C., Kell, J. F., Jr., Hastings, N., Sholes, D. M., and Gray, E. H.: Vasomotor, cellular and functional changes produced in kidney by brain stimulation. *J. Neurophysiol., 14:*317, 1951.
18. Hoff, E. C., Langford, H. G., Vester, J. W., Beckner, W. W., and Thomas, P. R.: Strychnine facilitation of pressor responses evoked from cerebral cortex. *J. Neurophysiol., 14:*167, 1951.
19. Houssay, B.-A., and Molinelli, E.-A.: Centre adrenalino-secreteur hypothalamique. *Compt. Rend. Soc. Biol., 93:*1454, 1925.
20. Jackson, J. H.: *Clinical and Physiological Researches on the Nervous System. I. On the Anatomical and Physiological Localization of Movements in the Brain.* London, Low, Churchill, 1875. (Reprinted: *Selected Writings of John Hughlings Jackson.* London, Hodder & Stoughton, 1931, vol. 1, pp. 37–76.
21. Kaada, B. R.: Somato-motor, autonomic and electrocorticographic responses to electri-

cal stimulation of "rhinencephalic" and other structures in primates, cat and dog (Study of responses from limbic, subcallosal, orbito-insular, piriform and temporal cortex, hippocampus-fornix and amygdala). *Acta Physiol. Scand., 24 (Suppl. 83)*:1, 1931.
22. Kaada, B. R., Pribram, K. H., and Epstein, J. A.: Respiratory and vascular responses in monkeys from temporal pole, insula, orbital surface and cingulate gyrus. A preliminary report. *J. Neurophysiol., 12:*347, 1949.
23. Kell, J. F., Jr., and Hoff, E. C.: Descending spinal pathways mediating pressor responses of cerebral origin. *J. Neurophysiol., 15:*299, 1952.
24. Mettler, C. C., Hamilton, W. F., Allen, L., Woodbury, R. A., and Mettler, F. A.: Influence of the cerebral cortex upon the cardiovascular system. *Anat. Rec. 64* (*Suppl.* 3):33, 1936.
25. Schiff, M.: Untersuchungen uber die motorischen Functionen des Grosshirns. *Arch. Exp. Path. Pharmakol., Naunyn-Schmiedeberg's, 3:*171, 1875. (Transl. by F. Borel, from *Lezioni sopra il sistema nervoso encefalico.* Florence, 1874.)
26. Setschenow, I.: Reflex action of the brain. *Med. Vestnik. (St. Petersb.) 3:*461,493, 1863.
27. Sherrington, C. S.: *The Integrative Action of the Nervous System.* London, Constable & Co., 1906.
28. Sherrington, C. S.: *The Brain and Its Mechanism.* Cambridge University Press, 1933.
29. Velo, A. G., and Hoff, E. C.: Salivary responses to cortical and sciatic stimulation. *Amer. J. Physiol., 200:*46, 1961.
30. Wall, P. D., and Davis, G. D.: Three cerebral cortical systems affecting autonomic function. *J. Neurophysiol., 14:*507, 1951.
31. Wall, P. D., and Pribram, K. H.: Trigeminal neurotomy and blood pressure responses from stimulation of lateral cerebral cortex of *Macaca mulatta. J. Neurophysiol., 13:*409, 1950.

DISCUSSION

Dr. Livingston: In the preceding presentation Ebbe remarked that we are living examples of the fact that the brain is there, but that we have shrouded it in mystery because we simply don't understand it. I think probably his historical comments about Sherrington, in a sense, bewailing some of the thinking that Jackson had projected that might have led us more directly to a solution of some of these problems. There is much to be said about these ideas.

Dr. Hoff: I would just make one comment on that. If you look at the history of the nineteenth century, especially the second half of the nineteenth century, you find that men like Jackson and others were always running up against the strong views that one should not think about brain function in terms of intellectual or emotional processes. When Hughlings Jackson used terms like "the organ of the mind," he was subject to serious criticism. Part of the trouble of the history of psychosomatics is that we have not been nearly careful enough in the design of our studies.

Dr. Livingston: You have been awfully kind in suggesting that it ended with the end of the nineteenth century. I'm afraid a lot of this still persists—at least beyond the middle of the twentieth century.

Dr. Reis: I have always wondered if part of the problem in England wasn't due to the vivisection rules which prohibited the kind of experiments performed by Sherrington on higher level function. Do you believe that a lot of English neurophysiology was attracted to the spinal cord, nerve and muscle because of such governmental restraints?

Dr. Hoff: I don't doubt that this is true and, as I mentioned, if you anesthetize an animal deeply, say with ether or one of the barbiturates, you are likely to knock out upper cerebral autonomic responses. I don't know what Schiff did to his animals. He probably immobilized them with curare. You are quite right; it was difficult, and I think it was very remarkable what some of the early workers were able to do, especially in view of the "vivisection" restrictions. Sherrington himself was hampered by governmental restrictions while I was there.

Dr. Yakovlev: In the evolution of the concepts of brain functions, each generation elaborates its own, what may be called "establishment" of ideas. Each generation carries the seeds of dissent, and even protest against the "established" notions, and sets up a new "establishment" of notions of what the "reality" is. Such are the dynamics of progress. So it was with the concept of "functional levels." The concept of functional levels rising in tiers in a vertical superposition of "lower," "middle" and "higher" levels, was mid-Victorian representation of realities modeled in terms (that is, in language) of the age of *industrial* revolution. The higher levels "control" the lower ones, and when the higher levels are abrogated in some way, the lower levels are "released" and "escape the control"—a revolution! * The *technological* revolution of our time has radically changed the "geometry" of our representation of the organization of the brain. This organization is no longer represented in terms of vertical levels and of controls of the lower by higher "centers" but rather in terms of "pacemakers" in the open-ended, self-regulating action system which is represented as being organized from within out, rather than from below up. It is no longer a "vertical" system, but a "spherical" system of concentric layers or "spheres of activity. We speak generally of the brain as consisting of (a) a *central core* ("reticular activating system" of Moruzzi and Magoun; "centrencephalic system" of Penfield and Jasper; "endophylactic trophotropic system" of W. R. Hess), (b) and *intermediate layer* (the "extrapyramidal" system in a broad sense, the "intermediate neuropil" of Herrick; the "dynamogenic ergotropic and ereismokinetic" systems of Hess, in brief, the "limbic system" of this conference subject), and (c) the *superficial layer* (the "superficial neuropil" of Herrick, the system of "cortical analyzers" in Pavlov's sense). In this connection the analogy with Freud's metaphoric "strata" of the "mental apparatus" is intellectually entertaining and illustrates well this spherical "establishment" of ideas.* New ideas need new terms which are not always available in the language spoken by the established generation—hence the new "lingo" of technical terms and definitions. One may cite here the history of terms like "voluntary" and "involuntary" movements, still in everyday clinical usage. Three centuries ago, Thomas Willis had a new notion, revolutionary for his time, that brain "controls" the voluntary and the cerebellum the involuntary movements. The idea was new and the way of the language of the time and so was couched in language of the Aquinian "establishment" of ideas. Willis extrapolated the terms from the context of the scholastic concept of "liber arbiter" and of moral responsibility and used them in the context of a new idea for which there was no other language. In the context of the Aquinian idea, the definition is clear; man is not responsible for the beating of his

* See writings of Herbert Spencer on society and of John Hughlings Jackson on evolution and dissolution of functions.

* See Freud's article "Psychoanalysis" in *Encyclopaedia Britannica,* 14th ed., Vol. 18, 1929, and also Magoun's article in Sol Tax's *Evolution After Darwin,* Vol. II, 1960.

heart or for the churning of his guts, but he is responsible for the acts of his "will." We are still bogged down when defining physiologically the involuntary movements such as heartbeat and churning of guts, and those movements which consummate energy and produce work outside the body (for example, project man to the moon—"voluntary" movements). How to define these two "categories" of movements, empirically so clearly distinct, is still a rhetorical question.

Dr. Hoff: Wouldn't you agree, Paul, that you can criticize that idea—that geography—as well as you can the vertical?

Dr. Yakovlev: The present generation proceeds vigorously building their own intellectual "establishment" too, and that is—I think—as it must be.

Dr. Lindsley: Ebbe has already mentioned Sechenov and Hughlings Jackson and the resistance they met in aligning the mind and the brain, but certainly Sechenov suffered the consequences of his thoughts along the line of conative and inhibitory concepts and, as a matter of fact, lost his position in the university because of the conflict of his ideas with those of church and state, in terms of his rather forward-looking views. Despite the fact that he was working on the frog, he was really talking about the human mind and behavior much of the time.

Dr. Hoff: It is interesting that he taught in a women's college. It could be that he found more happy acceptance among the women students than he might have done otherwise.

Dr. MacLean: Ebbe, you ought to mention the difficulties in exposing the brain in what we call Karplus and Kreidl's "hanging" brain preparation. I have a recollection that Karplus and Kreidl give Bechterev the credit for being the first to stimulate the brain stem and to elicit the autonomic responses. I went back and reviewed those papers some time ago, and I couldn't find that reference.

Dr. Hoff: I have some references here which I'll give you on the early work of Bechterev if that will help you. I don't know about that particular point. I do know that when Sechenov came to Ludwig's laboratory, he was measuring blood pressure. It was the general view, apparently, that there were not many supramedullary control mechanisms for the autonomic. Ludwig's blood pressure manometer very much excited Sechenov, but I don't know just exactly what Bechterev did, except that he did stimulate up around the optic thalamus. Harold, do you remember Bechterev going into the medulla? I believe he did.

Dr. Green: No, I don't know Ebbe.

Dr. Hoff: Bechterev did elicit blood pressure changes in the globus pallidus, all around the internal capsule, caudate nucleus and from the cortex. He did cut the vagus and abolish the heart rate slowing.

Dr. Nauta: I'm not too well informed about the history, as Dr. Hoff outlined it, but I wondered if, in Sherrington's time, any observations were made concerning temporal lobe epilepsy. Psychomotor epilepsy must really have changed the concept about "brain and mind." That was quite revolutionary compared with Sherrington's time. I wonder if you have any information about the first inklings that temporal lobe pathology could cause these tremendous changes in mood and behavioral attitudes. I don't know what the time disparity was.

Dr. Gloor: It seems that it preceded Sherrington considerably. It was Hughlings Jackson, in the 1870's who described these fits and actually attributed their origin to the temporal lobe, but he did not call the area of their presumed origin "amygdaloid nucleus," he called it the "sphenoidal lobe"—that is, the uncus and the underlying gray matter.

Dr. Nauta: It is, of course, possible that these things may take a long time to become established, and I just wondered if some of the older points of view were not simply brushed aside by the "mental establishment" of the time, as really completely abstruse, having really no relation to the brain.

Dr. Livingston: Was the quotation that you made from Sherrington a direct one? Did he suggest that you would get into a lot of trouble if you pursued autonomic investigation but that it, nonetheless, would be a good idea?

Dr. Hoff: No, but he talked to me many times about central autonomic study. I believe that he thought that in the manner he had studied integrative action of the nervous system one could do this also in the area of autonomic function. He believed, I think, that one could demonstrate physiological principles and processes which were comparable. I think he did believe that there was a totality of functions and processes. My own idea from Sherrington's informal remarks was that he believed that integration is a function of the neuron, and I think this was a way of saying that the whole nervous system functions with the whole body together.

Dr. Livingston: Your comments about the confusion as to the visceral responses that were obtained at least implies that there is much more specificity in terms of this control than we are now aware of. It seems an interesting contrast to what we have experienced with the investigation of pain. It took us so long to get off the assumption that pain was a "specific" sensation. Now that we are looking at visceral mechanisms of control, it seems to me that we are similarly restricting our view.

Dr. Lindsley: I might mention, that for those of us who, unlike Paul Yakovlev, do not read Russian, Chernigovskiy's book which we translated, and which is now published in English, does contain a lot of documentary evidence. It is called *Interoceptors.* It contains a wealth of information about Pavlov's early experiments and the subsequent studies which were continued in those laboratories in Leningrad by his successors, especially Bykov and Chernigovskiy, including cortical representation of visceral function, and so on.

Dr. Reis: I wonder if Dr. Gloor would comment about Walter Hess, who, at this time, was showing so much about the relationship between autonomic responses evoked by brain stimulation and integrated patterns of behavior. He must have started in the early 1920's. Did he have any influence at all on Sherrington? Was Sherrington aware of Hess and his work?

Dr. Hoff: I'm sure he was, but I don't know the answer to that.

Dr. Gloor: I don't know about the relationship between Hess and Sherrington and in what way they may have influenced each other. Hess's work started in the 1920's; I don't know how much he owes to Sherrington. When Hess refers to the older literature, he mostly mentions Karplus and Kreidl, the people whose work suggested to him that the exploration of the hypothalamus and its relations to autonomic function would be a worthwhile undertaking.

Dr. Reis: Was not Hess originally a cardiovascular physiologist?

Dr. Gloor: Hess started his career as an opthalmologist. He was always proud to say that being an opthalmologist, he didn't need a stereotaxic instrument; as an eye surgeon he had learned to be precise at aiming at small targets.

Dr. Livingston: If you go back to the

model that Ebbe suggested, and that is the way our own bodies function, you must certainly assume that there is a great deal of flexibility in this apparatus. You don't turn it all on or it all off at once, by any means, and it is surprising that we haven't been able to define that more.

Dr. Hoff: That's right. To look at a human being function, you know that he is experiencing most delicate and complex inhibitory excitatory action.

Dr. Livingston: Why is it so hard to pick up?

Dr. Hoff: Maybe there is something distorting in the way we are eliciting responses. Electrical stimuli, for example, may distort function severely.

Dr. Livingston: Is the assumption that there is a close correlation between visceral activity and emotion and behavior, one that is generally accepted? We talk about the visceral correlates of behavior quite glibly. If this correlation is as precise as we think it is, then we must be looking at a system which is, in fact, the analogue of other behavioral activities. But is not this where our thinking breaks down? We don't quite accept that.

Dr. Hoff: Yes, here our thinking breaks down.

Dr. Nauta: I want to comment on Dr. Hoff's last point. I remember from a period in the late 1940's when I was fortunate enough to be in Zurich, an idea that Hess brought up and that I would very much like to hear you reflect upon. Hess' point of departure was his observation that stimulation in the caudal hypothalamus could elicit virtually a complete mobilization of the orthosympathetic nervous system; he eventually called that area the ergotropic zone of the hypothalamus. Cats stimulated in this hypothalamic zone would present all the signs of intense emotional excitement, including pupillodilation, pilo-erection and agitated pacing. The question is, is such an animal really angry or otherwise agitated, or is it simply exhibiting the peripheral manifestations of an emotion? Being the naturalist he really was, Hess had noticed something that seemed to argue against "real" anger or other emotional feelings underlying the overt behavior—namely, that such animals would be ready and eager to drink milk offered no more than a few minutes after the end of a stimulation episode. In contrast to this, a cat that has been confronted with the real-life situation of having to defend itself against a barking dog is usually unable to take any milk for a period of half an hour or longer. In my discussions with Hess I was swayed toward the view that hypothalamic stimulation elicits only the outward manifestations, the concomitants rather than the real emotion.

I don't know if Hess at present would still see it in the same way, for in the meantime, findings have been reported from Flynn's laboratory which suggest that the issue may be a very complex one. In the experiments in question, cats being stimulated in the hypothalamus were presented with a live laboratory rat. Most domestic cats are not very eager to attack a rat; they just pay it some scornful attention and don't move in for the kill. However, cats being stimulated in the hypothalamus were found to be very much more likely to lunge and deal with the rat as if it were a mouse. This seems to indicate that hypothalamic stimulation may do more than produce the visceral and somatic external manifestations of emotion. In the experiments here mentioned it appears to have swung the behavioral propensity of the cat from one of avoidance to one of predatory approach.

Dr. Gloor: I'd like perhaps just to fill in a few things about Hess' attitude to this. To him, the animal which is stimulated in the posterior hypothalamus displays a form of angry behavior which is true rage. The argument which he uses in support of this view, is that the animal will, for instance, attack the experimenter, that it will display a well-directed attack. In other words, it will display angry behavior exactly as it would in a natural situation. The fact that the rage apparently decays so rapidly after brain stimulation is, I think, merely a function of the intensity of the emotion that has been aroused. Normal cats are not too easily aroused to a high-pitched emotional state, as anyone who owns a cat knows. It is easy to arouse a cat to anger, it may spit and hiss, but this normal rage will immediately quieten down, when the offending stimulus is removed and the cat will be ready to be petted, and it may even purr immediately after the display of angry behavior. There is usually only an extremely short aftereffect of this behavior, but I think that the duration of the aftereffect reflects the intensity of the stimulus. Certainly if the cat has been cornered by a dog the emotional state is not quite that short lived.

Dr. Lacey: I like your phrase, Walle, ". . . swung the behavioral propensity." It reminds me of Marranon's studies on the administration of exogenous Adrenalin.® This produced the so-called cold emotions. The subject would say, "Well, I feel *as though* I should be afraid, or I feel *as though* I should be angry." Then, like the cat, if you presented the human subject, after an Adrenalin injection, with an appropriate situation, then he said, "I'm angry" or "I am afraid." This experiment has been revived recently by Schachter, a social psychologist. He was able to show that the effects of administration of Adrenalin depended upon the social context of the cues which the human subjects were able to pick up. This enabled them to organize their perceptions of their internal state. I will report some findings with, I think, the same import stimulation of the mesencephalic reticular system had no effect on heart rate during intertrial periods in the cat reaction-time experiments when the animal engaged in the actual business of a reaction-time trial; however, the stimulation facilitated and magnified the typical cardiac deceleration seen during the foreperiod of the trial.

Dr. Nauta: It is really a very interesting finding that the administration of exogenous Adrenalin does so little to change the behavioral state. It suggests that the organism constantly needs perceptual or even conceptual corollaries to his internal state and in the absence of such matching cannot formulate a behavioral program.

Dr. Lindsley: Walle raised a very important question certainly with respect to human emotions; the pervasiveness of the affective aspect of emotion has always been one of the things that impresses us. But when you're stimulating, say in the ventromedial hypothalamus, as Egger and Flynn, and others have done, the reactions rarely outlast the stimulation. When you think of this in terms of the James-Lange theory, this concept is somehow documented or reinforced by the higher level influences of the social situation and the continuing feedback centrally, perhaps also by memory, and the basis for anger, fear and other emotions.

Dr. Reis: We have been doing some experiments to determine if any enduring effects can be produced by evoking rage by hypothalamic stimulation in cats over many days using the rat-killing behavior described by Flynn as the behavioral endpoint. It is of interest that rage evoked from the hypothalamus over several days has little effect on behavior except during the stimulation. In contrast when rage is produced by amygdala stimulation some changes in behavior occur. Over the course of many hours these animals will attack a rat during the interstimulation period and may show behavioral recruitment. It would thus appear that evoking behavior by brain stimulation from "higher levels" can produce more enduring effects than by stimulating at lower way stations such as the hypothalamus.

Dr. Nauta: Could we suggest that this may be a general characteristic of what we, with great difficulty, call "higher levels"? In any case, the findings in Sherringtonian experiments involving truncation of the brain at various levels would seem to suggest that only the forebrain—perhaps in particular the cerebral hemisphere—appears capable of sustaining long-term behavioral programs. Lower levels such as the rhombencephalon would seem largely to lack such "stability in time"; instead, these more caudal levels appear to function in a more short-term manner, dealing with exigencies in a janitorial rather than strategic fashion.

Dr. Abrahams: Coming back to stimulation of the hypothalamus, you can actually separate the autonomic effects from the behavioral effects very well on a temporal basis. So if you work at just about threshold, measuring things like blood flow, these come on instantaneously, they're fully developed in two or three seconds. At this stage, you look at the cat and see there is some pupillary dilatation, and it may be fifteen or twenty seconds before the cat goes mad. By that time the autonomic nervous system has swung completely back.

Dr. Killam: Let's look at the other side of the coin, particularly with the work that Olds was involved in, and that is the pleasurable aspect of stimulation, as we've been talking about the defensive aspects of stimulation. If you assess performance in terms of things that sustain the response, you almost get the impression that you are skirting around feedback loops which will shut one system on or one system off. So that an animal to receive shock in the hypothalamus will press itself to death rather than eat or drink. This is the part of the thing where you normally have feedback systems which will shock this or control that. There is some recent work in which people have used dual stimulation, asking to discriminate what is an Sd or an S△, and they play the game as to whether the animal can now shut this thing off. There are very interesting relationships to Old's original work as to the shape of the curve on which the reinforcement occurs, the intensity of the currents involved, and the like. Thus you have a duality: the defensive system in the first case and positive reinforcement in the second.

Dr. Lindsley: There's a real contrast, I think, between some of this self-stimulation work where an animal's operant behavior may stop very appropriately when it doesn't get reinforced, and a monkey that has been deprived of light will continue to press for light stimulation for as long as sixteen weeks, despite the fact that he gets an immediate reinforcement of one second of light for each lever press. This response does not extinguish very readily when the animal has been deprived of light stimulation over a period of time.

Dr. Mogenson: Mr. Chairman, in all these experiments that we have been discussing, I think that the important thing is the persistence of the system and, of course, this is what Masserman suggested. It indicates that the autonomic effects are not gradations of emotional behavior because in several experiments by Flynn and others, and in the type of work done by Olds, I think that the critical thing in the persistence of this somatomotor behavior is an interaction between the appropriate sensory input and the activation of the system. I believe that in Dr. Lindsley's example of light being able to reduce these somatomotor effects, we are dealing with the production of a very weak type of behavior. There is now a good deal of evidence to show that if you take a system that controls water intake, or a system that controls food intake, and combine these with appropriate afferent inputs, you can produce a very strong effect. In fact, we have done some experiments in which activation of the central system was self-stimulation for drinking, and if water was available at the same time to provide the appropriate afferent input, appropriate for the activation of the central mechanism, the rate at which the animal self-stimulated itself was greatly enhanced. If additional inputs were added, the response was even further enhanced, and the somatomotor effects were much, much stronger. The point I'm making is that in both cases of *fear-like* or *rage-like* behavior of Olds and Milner, the critical thing appears to be the appropriate afferent input, and I suspect the maximum discharge is producing some sort of central event in the hypothalamus without any appropriate afferent input. Place the rat in a situation which contains something for it to attack, and you change the behavior very much.

Dr. Andy: We've made some observations on the behavior of these cats, from time to time, and I am intrigued with the way you could get an animal to make a directed attack during hypothalamic stimulation. On the one hand, a situation exists in which they hiss and open their mouth and reach a point of opening and closing automatically. You can put your finger right into their mouth as they open it, and they won't clamp down; they won't attack. On the other hand, you may have just the opposite. The stimulation that produces the attack and directed response appears to be one which starts with a low threshold and slowly builds up over a period of time. You may visualize an integration of brain activity taking place in which the entire brain is getting into the act, so to speak. With a suddenly applied threshold stimulus, which is not attained gradually, the animal is not given a chance to integrate the activity. The reaction is more automatic: open the mouth, close it, et cetera, repeatedly.

Dr. Abrahams: I wonder if we don't have someone who is knowledgeable in the history of physiology, so he can tell us how this situation relates to the chronic decorticate cat. When the chronic decorticate cat attacks, is it a meaningful attack? Is it a well-directed attack?

Dr. Nauta: I think that, as Burn described it under these conditions, it is extremely poor. Rioch did a great deal of later work on the problem of decorticate behavior. He once told me the thing that impressed him most about the decorticate cat by drawing a comparison between two situations: You have on your lap a perfectly healthy young kitten; you stroke its fur, and after a few strokes, it goes into contortions of delight and begins to claw—it is in seventh heaven. If right in the middle of this situation you suddenly decide to become mean, and you suddenly pinch its tail, it can, in a split second, change its attitude and become a little hellion, hissing, spitting and all these things, really with lightning speed. Now the decorticate cat apparently takes very much longer stroking in order to show anything like the clawing movements, and once in this state, you have to pinch its tail repeatedly and very hard to bring it to the opposite situation.

So that Rioch's point draws our attention to the relationship of neocortical circuitry in this whole realm of not only emotion but of the autonomic nervous system playing the role of, shall we say, an accelerating mechanism and enabling the animal to change attitudes at a much greater speed than is possible without it. I don't think that the decorticate cat is a dangerous animal to work with, because its information about localization is too imprecise.

Chapter 2

The Central Visceromotor System: A General Survey

Walle J. H. Nauta

Up to the present time, the existence of a visceromotor system central to the preganglionic motor neurons has been very largely a physiological concept that appears to have originated shortly after the middle of the nineteenth century with Flourens' notion of a respiratory "noeud vital" in the medulla oblongata, Schiff's identification of a medullary "vasoconstrictor center" and Claude Bernard's medullary "pîqure glycosurique." Only half a century later was the hypothalamus identified as a major visceromotor territory, largely by the fundamental studies of Karplus and Kreidl.[9] The central visceromotor system thus became visualized, as it still is today, as consisting essentially of the hypothalamus and the neural links connecting the latter with the preganglionic motor neurons. In the intervening sixty years, a great store of anatomical and physiological information with respect to the hypothalamus has accumulated, but the anatomical picture of the mesencephalic, bulbar and spinal intermediaries of the central visceromotor system has remained so rudimentary that little more than a few general statements can be made about these levels between the hypothalamus and the preganglionic motor neurons.

The account to follow is intended to serve as a general overview of the anatomical organization of the central visceromotor system. It must be emphasized that it is based largely upon observations made in the course of studies conducted by conventional neuroanatomical methods, in particular Golgi and fiber-degeneration techniques. Explorations by fundamentally different methods, histochemical techniques in particular, may eventually lead to modifications of the present concepts regarding the organization of the central visceromotor system.

DESCENDING NEURAL PATHWAYS OF THE CENTRAL VISCEROMOTOR SYSTEM

Clinical experience as well as physiological observations[13] indicate that the functional connections linking the hypothalamus with the preganglionic motor neurons are spread widely over the cross section of the midbrain and rhombencephalon. The results of experimental studies by axon-degeneration methods suggest that these conduction lines are interrupted by synaptic junctions at several points along their descent. Contrary to earlier descriptions,[3] such experimental studies have failed to demonstrate direct hypothalamic efferents extending caudalward beyond the mesencephalic tegmentum and circumaqueductal grey substance.[8,17]

Descending Connections of the Hypothalamus

The neural conduction routes descending from the hypothalamus have been found to follow two major trajectories. Foremost among these connections is a descending component of the medial forebrain bundle which originates chiefly in the lateral hypothalamic zone and can be subdivided into a medial division distributed largely to paramedian mesencephalic cell groups, and a lateral component that traces a wide path through the adjoining, more lateral region of the mesencephalic tegmentum approximately corresponding to the zone indicated by Taber [28] as the subcuneiform area.[17] A second conduction route leading caudalward from the hypothalamus is provided by descending constituents of the dorsal longitudinal fasciculus of Schütz which appear to originate in more medial hypothalamic cell groups and are distributed over the ventral half of the central grey substance of the midbrain. Both the dorsal longitudinal fasciculus of Schütz and the medial subdivision of the medial forebrain bundle connect the hypothalamus with a paramedian region of the midbrain composed of the central grey substance and several tegmental cell groups including the large and complex raphe nucleus (nucleus centralis tegmenti superior) of Bechterew and two circumscript round cell groups, the nuclei tegmenti dorsalis and ventralis of Gudden near the pontomesencephalic border. The efferent connection of the hypothalamus with this paramedian mesencephalic territory (the "limbic midbrain area")[17] is reciprocated by at least two circumscript fiber systems: the ascending component of Schütz's bundle and the mammillary peduncle. The "limbic midbrain area" thus can be considered to represent, in part at least, the caudal pole of a hypothalamo-mesencephalic circuit. It is very likely, however, that the descending components of this circuit are also involved in the transmission of hypothalamic discharge to the preganglionic motor neurons. Morest [15] has traced fiber degeneration elicited by lesions placed caudally in the central grey substance caudalward through the periventricular grey matter of the fourth ventricle as far as the medulla oblongata; the ultimate synaptic distribution of this periventricular fiber system remains to be determined. A further possible pathway for the transmission of hypothalamic impulses to the motoneuronal level would seem to be provided by the central tegmental radiation of Weisschedel, a diffuse and radially disposed fiber system linking the central grey substance with a large cross-sectional area of the mesencephalic tegmentum.

The foregoing account can be summarized by the statement that the currently available data suggest the existence of two major pathways descending from the hypothalamus, one of which directly involves a wide region of the midbrain tegmentum, whereas the other follows a trajectory confined to the central grey substance. There almost certainly exist numerous cross-links between the two conduction channels, both in the form of long dendrites extending in both directions across the border between the tegmentum and central grey substance and in the form of axonal connections between these two major subdivisions of the mesencephalon. Neither of the two descending hypothalamic pathways appears to extend beyond the caudal border of the midbrain, and it therefore seems likely from the current anatomical data that the impulse transmission from the hypothalamus to the motoneuronal level largely, if not indeed entirely, depends on conduction systems originating in the mesencephalon.

Descending Connections from the Mesencephalon and Rhombencephalon

It is fair to say that beyond the descending hypothalamic efferents the trail of the central visceromotor pathways becomes very largely lost. With the exception of the periventricular fibers traced to the medulla oblongata by Morest—a conduction pathway which likely represents only a relatively small component of the visceromotor system—no single anatomical structure in the midbrain or rhombencephalon can be identified with any certainty as a link in the chain of conduction toward the preganglionic motor neurons. It seems certain that the pathways in question follow a wide course through the brain stem reticular formation, and in view of the latter's known characteristics,[25] it appears likely that the downward conduction involves numerous synaptic junctions. This notion is borne out by observations made in experimental studies of fiber systems descending to the spinal cord from the brain stem. According to our observations, and in confirmation of previous reports by Kuypers *et al.*[12] and Nyberg-Hansen,[20] the massive fiber degeneration elicited in the reticular fiber systems by lesions in the mesencephalic tegmentum rapidly diminishes in volume as it descends; in the cat and monkey even the longest of the mesencephalic reticular fibers appear not to extend caudally beyond the medulla oblongata. Lesions in the pontine and medullary reticular formation, by contrast, lead to reticulospinal fiber degeneration that extends throughout the length of the spinal cord and is the more massive the farther caudal the lesion is located. Considered together, these observations suggest that the preganglionic visceral motor neurons of the spinal cord may be accessible to the neural efflux of the hypothalamus only (or nearly so) by way of *successive* synaptic articulations at mesencephalic and rhombencephalic levels.

Findings such as those mentioned above, although suggesting a highly complex neural organization, are still quite general and leave some elementary questions unanswered. It is, for example, uncertain whether and to what extent even neurons of the rhombencephalic tegmentum have direct synaptic connections with the preganglionic motor neurons of the spinal cord. By analogy with the somatic motor system, it would seem possible and even likely that rhombencephalic neurons affect the final common path neurons of the visceral nervous system largely by way of spinal interneurons. The existence of such "visceral interneurons" (that is, propriospinal neurons having efferent connections with visceral motor neurons) in the spinal cord is all the more likely as it appears from recent evidence [26] (Petras, personal communication) that no dorsal root fibers terminate within the clusters of preganglionic visceral motor neurons, an observation suggesting that spinal autonomic reflex arcs may have no monosynaptic components. The results of a recent series of experiments in the cat (Merrill and Nauta, unpublished) in which the vagus nerve was cut central to the nodose ganglion suggest the same conclusion with respect to the parasympathetic vagus neurons: in all cases examined, the Fink-Heimer stain failed to reveal any fiber degeneration within the borders of the dorsal motor nucleus of the vagus. It must be stressed that such negative findings do not preclude the possibility that some at least of the primary sensory fibers synapse with dendrites extending beyond the cytoarchitectonic limits of the motoneuronal cell groups. Extremely laborious histological procedures would be required to identify such axodendritic relationships.[5] At the least, however, the evidence here mentioned suggests a marked difference between visceral and somatic motoneuronal cell groups in the sense that in the mammalian spinal cord at least, the latter are indeed invaded (and known to be synaptically contacted) by primary sensory fibers.

SEQUENTIAL "LEVELS" IN THE CENTRAL VISCEROMOTOR SYSTEM

All of the sparse and largely circumstantial evidence reviewed above is compatible with a morphological notion of the visceral nervous system as organized essentially in the form of serially connected levels. In the terms of this formulation, the "ground floor" of the central visceromotor organization could be thought to consist of a local motor apparatus composed of preganglionic motor neurons and their associated interneurons. Descending upon this most distal level of the central visceromotor apparatus is a complex longitudinal conduction system, the synaptic fractionation of which allows three serially connected rostrocaudal subdivisions to be distinguished: hypothalamic, mesencephalic and rhombencephalic. Each of these large "blocks" in the central visceromotor system must be assumed to be a highly complex neural organization in its own right, encompassing numerous specific functional subsystems. It seems probable, moreover, that each is supplied by its own characteristic afferent input systems, besides receiving information from functional realms common to all levels. It is, for example, likely from Morest's[16] findings that the viscerosensory information received by the nucleus of the solitary tract via vagal and glossopharyngeal afferents is distributed primarily to the rhombencephalic level. Fibers of the so-called spinothalamic tract probably are distributed to both rhombencephalic and mesencephalic levels, and all levels may be affected by the neural efflux from one or another region of the neocortex.

ASCENDING CONNECTIONS IN THE CENTRAL VISCEROMOTOR SYSTEM

The more or less local nature of some of these afferent relationships naturally does not imply confinement of the information in question to the level or levels upon which it impinges, for there is ample evidence that the various levels are interconnected by ascending fiber systems no less closely than by descending "visceromotor pathways." The anatomical evidence concerning such ascending connections is not entirely equivocal. The results of studies by fiber-degeneration methods[19] suggest that—much like the descending pathway—ascending impulse conduction (very largely at least) sequentially involves rhombencephalic, mesencephalic and hypothalamic levels. In particular, such experimental studies have failed to demonstrate ascending fiber systems that reach the hypothalamus from levels below the mesencephalon. Those that thus far have been demonstrated by fiber degeneration methods all appear to originate in the paramedian region of the mesencephalon as components of the mammillary peduncle and the dorsal longitudinal fasciculus of Schütz. Very recently, however, evidence of a quite substantial fiber system ascending to the hypothalamus through more lateral zones of the mesencephalic tegmentum has been encountered in this laboratory (Graybiel, unpublished); the origin of this connection has not yet been determined.

In conflict with the notion that the origin of ascending afferents to the hypothalamus is confined to the mesencephalon, one Golgi study at least [25] has revealed a rhombencephalic neuron having an ascending axon that extends with some of its ramifications into the hypothalamus. One possible explanation of this discrepancy would be that such long ascending afferents of the hypothalamus are relatively few and widely spaced and thus easily escape detection in anterograde-degeneration studies. Alternatively, the neurons in question could have chemical properties that render their axons resistant to demonstration by any of the current degeneration techniques. Observations in studies by histofluorescence methods,[2] for example, have suggested the presence of norepinephrin-containing neurons in the rhombencephalon that project directly to the hypothalamus and even beyond it to the cerebral cortex.

Once again, it must be emphasized that most of the central visceromotor circuitry will have to remain a matter of inference as long as the neural components intercalated between the hypothalamus and the preganglionic motor neurons remain as largely unidentified as they are at present. The existence of functionally specific systems in the organization would seem a virtual certainty, yet the anatomical identification of the corresponding neural continua so far has been hampered severely by the circumstance that they all form part of the brain stem reticular formation.

THE RETICULAR FORMATION

In brief, the reticular formation can be described as a massive but only vaguely delimited neural apparatus that extends throughout the length of the spinal cord and brain stem. It is composed of neurons having (a) long, rectilinear and sparsely arborizing dendrites subtending large and widely overlapping dendritic fields (a characteristic that has led to the term "isodendritic core" [24] as an alternative designation of the reticular formation); (b) heterogeneous afferent relationships; and (c) axons disposed so as to favor the formation of predominantly polysynaptic lines of conduction in both the ascending and descending direction. Neural tissue of this description is usually interpreted as "nonspecific," but it must be emphasized that this term can be applied with certainty only to the afferent characteristics of the formation. Naturally, the degree of functional specificity of any neural mechanism is determined not only by its input-properties but also by its intrinsic organization and its efferent relationships. The somatic motor neurons, for example, must be assumed to have extremely diverse afferent connections ranging from dorsal root to corticospinal fibers yet can hardly be considered nonspecific from a more general point of view. It would therefore seem profitable to attempt a functional characterization of the reticular formation in terms of its effector characteristics rather than its afferent relationships, even though the latter, perhaps more than any other peculiarity, identify the reticular formation as the most widely "open" system of the brain (that is, open to the greatest diversity of afferent channels) and thus distinguish it from other, more nearly unimodal ("closed line") neural mechanisms.

It is obviously impossible to characterize in a simple phrase the effector properties of a neural apparatus as vast and complex as the isodendritic core of the brain stem. Nevertheless, a major general function of the system appears to express itself in phenomena of adaptive stability or "posture." In the somatic sphere this property is manifested as somatic posture or *stability in space.* The analogous visceral expression of this general function is characterized by Cannon's term "homeostasis," or stability of the internal milieu. Finally, at the level of the cerebrum, the reticular formation appears to affect neural mechanisms involved in behavioral responsiveness (*alertness*), a function that could likewise be viewed as a form of stability. Needless to say, the term, "stability," as used in this account does not necessarily imply rigid maintenance of a particular unalterable functional set. The familiar diurnal, seasonal and other periodic fluctuations in all of the functional realms here mentioned are in all likelihood attributable to variations, largely of an intrinsic (metabolic?) nature, in the functional bias of the reticular formation. In a sense, the reticular formation thereby assumes the significance of an internal adjustment system of the brain itself.

It is important to note that the hypothalamus in its structural organization exhibits all of the essential features attributed to the reticular formation.[14] In fact, from an anatomical point of view, the hypothalamus appears to be a rostral extension of the midbrain reticular formation, in particular of the central grey substance and the ventromedial region of the mesencephalic tegmentum. In turn, this diencephalic extension of the mesencephalic reticular formation continues forward to form the preoptic and septal regions (rostral to this level the mammalian brain at least is composed of cortical formations which are structurally so unique as to require separate classification). The hypothalamus thus appears as a major component of a continuum of reticular (isodendritic) neural tissue that extends the brain stem reticular formation forward beyond the midbrain as far as the septal region.

Similarity of general organizational tissue properties does not imply functional or anatomical sameness throughout. The hypothalamus may be continuous, and reciprocally connected, with the rhombencephalic reticular formation by way of mesencephalic links, but it is nonetheless true that it, and not the rhombencephalon, receives direct projections from a variety of limbic forebrain structures, whereas the rhombencephalic reticular formation but not the hypothalamus is converged upon by a variety of afferents that include direct projections from the cerebellum, the sensorimotor cortex, the superior colliculus, the spinal cord, the vestibular nuclei and the nucleus of the solitary tract. The efferent associations of the hypothalamus, moreover, include the important hypothalamohypophyseal connection, a relationship not shared by any other part of the brain.

However, it is perhaps the most distinctive peculiarity of the hypothalamus that it appears to be the only major expanse of the reticular core of the brain stem that can be identified almost categorically with the visceral and endocrine effector systems. Even though the hypothalamus has been shown to have some of its effects in the realm of somatic motor function,[11] it appears to lie outside the path of the great efferent fiber systems of the sensorimotor cortex, the corpus striatum and cerebellum. Below the hypothalamic level, this high degree of territorial privacy in the visceromotor system rapidly dwindles. At the level of the rhombencephalon in particular, nearly all subdivisions of the reticular formation are distribution zones of one or several fiber systems generally regarded as somatic in character. The medial, gigantocellular zone of the reticular formation of the medulla oblongata, for example, is such a distribution area for fibers from the cerebellar nucleus tecti, and the same region receives a substantial number of fibers from the "premotor" area 6 of the cerebral cortex. In the lateral, smaller-celled zone of the medullary reticular formation many fibers from the nucleus ruber and cortical area 4 terminate. It seems certain that there is, at this level at least, a considerable regional overlap between the somatic and visceral motor systems. Whether this overlap is really only regional or, conversely, extends to single neurons is a matter of conjecture. Observations such as those reported at this conference by Snider, however, suggest that cerebellar impulse efflux has access to one or other link in the central visceromotor pathways, and a fairly extensive literature, reviewed by Kennard,[10] indicates that the same is true of the projections from the premotor cortex. As it appears that neither the cerebellum nor the premotor cortex has direct efferent connections with either the spinal cord or hypothalamus, it seems likely—though by no means certain—that such somatovisceral linkages are located at the level of either the rhombencephalon or mesencephalon, or both. In any event, the nature of these physiological observations indicates that the reticular formation, despite the heterogeneous afferentation of its constituent neurons, may subserve functions of marked qualitative and topographic specificity. In at least some of the functional aspects of the reticular formation the characteristic of afferent heterogeneity evidently serves purposes of convergent integration rather than diffuseness, an integration that appears to extend across the border between somatic and visceral effector categories.

NEURAL ASSOCIATIONS OF THE HYPOTHALAMUS

The fiber connections of the hypothalamus have recently been reviewed in detail elsewhere[18] and only a brief summary of the known associations of the hypothalamus with other parts of the brain will here be given. The most fundamental conclusions that have been suggested by the results of fiber-degeneration studies are (a) that the hypothalamus has its most massive extrinsic connections with the tegmentum and central grey substance of the midbrain and with limbic structures of the cerebral hemisphere and (b) that with the certain exception of efferents from the olfactory cortex, and the possible exception of some fibers from the retina, no specific sensory pathways have direct access to the hypothalamic mechanisms.

Hypothalamic Connections with the Mesencephalon

The relationships of the hypothalamus with the mesencephalon were already mentioned earlier in this account. Direct hypothalamic efferents have been found distributed over a large region of the midbrain tegmentum as well as over the ventral half of the central grey substance. Reciprocating projections to the hypothalamus from the central grey substance and from the medial tegmental nuclei of Bechterew and Gudden appear to close a hypothalamomesencephalic circuit. This mesencephalohypothalamic projection prominently involves the lateral hypothalamic region—largely by way of fibers of the mammillary peduncle that bypass the mammillary body, ascend in the medial forebrain bundle and in part extend forward as far as the medial zone of the septum—but also (by ascending components of the dorsal longitudinal fasciculus of Schütz) the medial and periventricular hypothalamic zones.

The circuitous hypothalamomesencephalic connection here outlined is doubtless an important conductor of impulses to and from the hypothalamus. Its probable role in the conduction of descending discharge from the hypothalamus was discussed earlier in this chapter. It is no less likely involved in the transmission of neural impulses ascending to the hypothalamus from rhombencephalic and spinal levels. Numerous fibers of the spinothalamic tract, for example, terminate in the circumaqueductal central grey substance along with fibers ascending from the reticular formation of the medulla oblongata. Morest's [16] findings suggest a similar distribution for some fibers ascending from the nucleus of the solitary tract. As even the most painstaking studies by the aid of fiber-degeneration techniques have failed to disclose direct projections from either the spinal cord or the medulla oblongata (but see earlier discussion of this matter), it seems likely that most at least of the visceroceptive and nociceptive information received at rhombencephalic and spinal levels can reach the hypothalamus only by way of mesencephalic way stations. It is logical, in view of the anatomical evidence, to suggest the "limbic midbrain area" (central grey substance and nuclei of Bechterew and Gudden) represents such an intermediary processing mechanism, but it appears likely that this paramedian midbrain region is not the only link in ascending conductions to the hypothalamus, especially in view of the recent evidence (mentioned earlier) of hypothalamic afferents that follow a more lateral trajectory through the mesencephalic tegmentum. Until further data become available, the present account of ascending conduction routes to the hypothalamus must therefore be considered provisional and incomplete.

Connections of the Hypothalamus with Limbic Forebrain Structures

Most typical perhaps among the extrinsic associations of the hypothalamus are its strong and in part reciprocal connections with the limbic system. The term, "limbic system," is derived from the name *great limbic lobe* originally used by Broca to designate the marginal region (the "hem") of the pallial mantle that encircles the hilus of the mammalian cerebral hemisphere as a somewhat protuberant ring. This "lobe" harbors a marked variety of neural structures, some of which are paleocortical in organization (the olfactory cortex of the piriform lobe and the cortical fields composing the hippocampal formation), others neocortical (the cingulate or limbic cortex), yet others noncortical (the amygdaloid complex). The use of a collective term to denote such an heterogeneous array of neural organizations has been severely criticized; yet some justification for a categoric denomination may be found in the clinical experience that most or all of the components of Broca's limbic lobe appear to share the characteristic of having a low seizure threshold and in the anatomical evidence that all have close relationships with the septo-preoptico-hypothalamic continuum. The term, "limbic system," has the merit of being noncommittal in the sense that it, unlike the earlier designation, *rhinencephalon*, does not allude to a dominant relationship to any particular sensory modality.

The most voluminous afferent connections of the hypothalamus with the limbic system originate from the hippocampal formation, the amygdaloid complex and the olfactory cortex. The hippocampohypothalamic connection is established by the fornix system. Approximately half of this massive fiber bundle distributes itself in the septal region which, in turn, originates a septohypothalamic fiber system that forms a large component of the medial forebrain bundle, a major longitudinal hypothalamic conduction system that extends caudally into the mesencephalon, largely by way of synaptically interposed neurons of the lateral hypothalamic region. The remaining half of the fornix system forms the compact columna fornicis which terminates chiefly in the anterior thalamic nuclei and in the mammillary body. From the latter structure arises the massive and compact bundle of Vicq d'Azyr which bifurcates into (a) the mammillothalamic tract distributed to the anterior thalamic nuclei and (b) the smaller mammillotegmental tract to the nuclei of Gudden in the paramedian region of the caudal midbrain. Both by direct fornix connections and by way of the mammillary body and mammillothalamic tract the hippocampus is linked to the anterior thalamic nuclei, a cell complex that in turn projects to the cingulate cortex, a cortical region thought to be connected by long association fibers to the parahippocampal cortices (presubiculum and entorhinal area) which have massive efferent connections with the hippocampus. This complex circuitous sequence of connections unites the hippocampus, mammillary body, thalamus and cingulate cortex into the so-called Papez circuit. This circuit is only one—and certainly a very composite—instance of the reciprocity which exists in the relationships between the limbic system and the hypothalamic region. A less complex "circuit" of this general nature may be closed by fibers ascending from the lateral hypothalamic region to the septum which is known to project in part at least to the hippocampus and thus completes a neural sequence: hippocampus—septal region—lateral hypothalamic nucleus—septal region—hippocampus.

The major direct afferent connection of the hypothalamus with the amygdaloid complex is established by the stria terminalis, a fiber system that, unlike the hippocampal afferents, appears to involve mostly the medial hypothalamic zone and consequently does not (or only minimally) contribute to the medial forebrain bundle. In recent studies by the Fink-Heimer methods three circumscript areas of stria terminalis distribution have been identified—namely, one in the anterior hypothalamic region, a second one in the so-called cell-poor zone surrounding the ventromedial nucleus and a third in the region of the ventral premammillary nucleus. A second major amygdalohypothalamic conduction route may be contained in the so-called ventral amygdalofugal pathways, a conduction system spreading widely in the forebrain and including a component that terminates in the lateral hypothalamus. Although apparently avoiding the medial hypothalamic zones, there is physiological evidence[7] that this ventral conduction route secondarily converges upon the ventromedial hypothalamic nucleus. It must be emphasized that it is not certain that this pathway actually originates in the amygdaloid complex proper and not in the overlying periamygdaloid region of the olfactory cortex.[23] The amygdalohypothalamic relationship, much like the hippocampal connections with the hypothalamus, is to some extent at least reciprocal, for both the stria terminalis and the ventral amygdalofugal pathway contain fibers of the opposite polarity.

All of the structures composing the limbic system are closely associated with the hypothalamus, but the relationship may not invariably be a reciprocal one. The results of a recent experimental study, for example, have raised some doubts as to whether the cingulate cortex has any direct efferent connections with the hypothalamus.[6] Although undoubtedly implicated in hypothalamic circuitry by virtue of its afferent relationship with the anterior thalamic nuclei, the cingulate cortex, according to the results of this study in the rat, projects to subcortical structures not known to be associated with the hypothalamus. This observation suggests the possibility that the primary influence of the cingulate cortex is upon functional realms other than the visceromotor system.

The Limbic Forebrain-Midbrain Circuit

The evidence summarized in the foregoing account implicates the hypothalamus in at least two complex neural circuits, one of which connects it reciprocally with major components of the limbic lobe, the other with the paramedian region of the mesencephalon. In a wider context, these two sets of associations could be thought to compose a large circuit that reciprocally links the limbic forebrain structures with the paramedian midbrain region. The hypothalamus—its lateral zone in particular—is synaptically intercalated in both the ascending and decending limbs of this larger "limbic forebrain-midbrain circuit."

Specific Sensory Connections of the Hypothalamus

The only sensorium having anatomically identifiable direct connections with the hypothalamus is the olfactory. The connection is established by fibers that originate in the piriform cortex and olfactory tubercle, join the medial forebrain bundle and thus in all likelihood are distributed mainly in the lateral hypothalamic region.

There are several reports of direct projections to the hypothalamus from the retina. Thus far, however, the evidence for such a direct visual connection has been rather equivocal. The well-known influence of the diurnal light-cycle upon gonadotrophic mechanisms in many vertebrate species appears to require some form of neural communication from the retina to the medial hypothalamic region, yet such impulse conduction could conceivably be mediated by intercalated cell groups such as the medial terminal nucleus of the accessory optic tract (nucleus opticus tegmenti), a circumscript cell group in the ventral tegmental region immediately adjoining the hypothalamus.

Connections with the Neocortex

Of all subdivisions of the neopallium, only the granular frontal cortex ("prefrontal cortex") is known to project directly to the hypothalamus. In the rhesus monkey, a major part of this substantial connection arises from the caudal half of the orbital surface, but frontohypothalamic fibers have been traced also from the convexity of the frontal lobe. It seems somewhat ironical that the granular frontal cortex on the basis of this projection to the hypothalamus could be considered part of the limbic system, a suggestion accentuated further by the massive direct associations of large areas of the prefrontal cortex with the cingulate cortex and presubiculum.

As the remainder of the neopallium appears to lack direct communication channels to the septohypothalamic continuum, it must be assumed that the neural efflux of the great sensory fields of the neocortex can affect the hypothalamic mechanism only indirectly by way of either (or both) higher-order connections of the neocortex with the limbic system, or neural links connecting the subcortical projections of these cortical fields with the hypothalamus. Recent findings in the monkey [21,22] suggest the prefrontal cortex, the inferior temporal region and the cingulate gyrus as major convergence areas in the sequential processing of sensory informations by the neocortex. All three of these regions have efferent connections with the limbic system: the prefrontal and cingulate fields by way of their close association with the hippocampal mechanism, the inferior temporal region in the form of a substantial projection to the amygdaloid complex. It is tempting in view of this evidence to consider the prefrontal, cingulate and inferior temporal regions as the origin of major links between the neocortex and limbic system, the prefrontal cortex moreover as the site of a neocortical mechanism directly affecting hypothalamic functions.

Elsewhere in this account, the hypothalamus was characterized as the only major subdivision of the brain stem that can be identified almost entirely with visceral (and the closely allied endocrine) effector mechanisms. This statement, however, requires some qualification, for the reason that clinical observations [1,4] and behavioral findings in animal experiments [27] suggest that the hypothalamus is implicated in the neural mechanisms governing the organism's behavioral attitudes. Such mechanisms, needless to say, are extremely complex, for they must encompass processes that integrate information from both external and internal environments received over quite literally all peripheral sensory systems and, moreover, by way of non-neural chemical transmissions from the blood plasma itself (for example, blood glucose; target-gland hormones) to more or less selectively receptive central neurons. In mammalian species, this integration must commonly comprise neural codes resulting from elaborate information processing by the cerebral neocortex. It would be naive, therefore, to ascribe the neural substrata of behavioral motivation to any one particular level of the central nervous organization. Nonetheless, the distribution of the sites at which electrical stimulation or tissue destruction have been found to cause marked biases in the organism's behavioral responses to his environments appears to outline, however vaguely, a neural mechanism centrally involved in processes underlying "moods" and, hence, vital drive states. This mechanism extends from the limbic structures of the cerebral hemisphere caudalward to the septo-preoptico-hypothalamic continuum and medial parts of the thalamus and beyond these into medial regions of the mesencephalon. In its apparent outline, this motivational mechanism largely corresponds to the complex system of neural connections reciprocally linking the limbic structures of the cerebral hemisphere with the paramedian mesencephalic region, a system of associations indicated in the foregoing account by the collective term, "limbic forebrain-midbrain circuit." The hypothalamus, preoptic region and septum are integral components of this mechanism in the sense that part at least of their neuronal population is intercalated in both the ascending and descending limbs of the limbic forebrain-midbrain circuit. The hypothalamus thus appears to be an essential link in the neural substratum of affect and motivation no less than it is an important component of the central visceral and endocrine effector mechanisms. In fact, in the light of this dual functional relationship it is possible to see the hypothalamus, together with the septum and the paramedian region of the mesencephalon, as forming that level of the brain at which the visceral and endocrine effector systems emerge as major efferent channels from a wider neural mechanism underlying the organism's affective involvement in his environments.

REFERENCES

1. Alpers, B. J.: Personality and emotional disorders associated with hypothalamic lesions. *Res. Publ. Ass. Res. Nerv. Ment. Dis., 20:*725, 1940.
2. Andén, N-E., Dahlström, A., Fuxe, K., Larsson, K., Olson, L., and Ungerstedt, U.: Ascending monoamine neurons to the telencephalon and diencephalon. *Acta. Physiol. Scand., 67:*313, 1966.
3. Beattie, J., Brow, G. R., and Long, C. N. H.: Physiological and anatomical evidence for the existence of nerve tracts connecting the hypothalamus with spinal sympathetic centers. *Proc. Roy. Soc.* [Biol] *106:*253, 1930.
4. Bellone, G. B., and Terzian, H.: Autonomic nervous system and mental pathology. In Von Monakow, K. H. (Ed.): *The Autonomic Nervous System. Akt. Fragen Psychiat. Neurol., 4:*139, 1966.
5. Blackstad, T. W.: Electron microscopy of Golgi preparations for the study of neuronal relations. In Nauta, W. J. H., and Ebbesson, S. O. E. (Eds.): *Contemporary Research Methods in Neuroanatomy.* Berlin, Springer Verlag, 1970, pp. 186–216.
6. Domesick, V. B.: Projections from the cingulate cortex in the rat. *Brain Res., 12:*296, 1969.
7. Dreifuss, J. J., and Murphy, J. T.: Contrasting effects of two identified amygdaloid efferent pathways on single hypothalamic neurons. *J. Neurophysiol., 31:*237, 1968.
8. Guillery, R. W.: Degeneration in the hypothalamic connexions of the albino rat. *J. Anat., 91:*91, 1957.
9. Karplus, J. P., and Kreidl, A.: Gehirn und Sympathicus. II Ein Sympathicus-Zentrum in Zwischenhirn. *Arch. Ges. Physiol., 135:*401, 1910.
10. Kennard, M. A.: Autonomic function. In Bucy, P. C. (Ed.): *The Precentral Motor Cortex.* Urbana, University of Illinois Press, 1944, pp. 294–306.
11. Koella, W. P.: Control of skeletal motor activity, with emphasis on the role of diencephalic mechanisms. In Haymaker, W., Anderson, E., and Nauta, W. J. H. (Eds.): *The Hypothalamus.* Springfield, Charles C Thomas, 1969, pp. 645–658.
12. Kuypers, H. G. J. M., Fleming, W. R., and Farinholt, J. W.: Subcorticospinal projections in the rhesus monkey. *J. Comp. Neurol., 118:*107, 1962.
13. Magoun, H. W., Ranson, S. W., and Hetherington, A.: Descending connections for the hypothalamus. *Arch. Neurol. Psychiat., 39:*1127, 1938.
14. Millhouse, O. E.: A Golgi study of the descending medial forebrain bundle. *Brain Res., 15:*341, 1969.
15. Morest, D. K.: Connexions of the dorsal tegmental nucleus in the rat and rabbit. *J. Anat., 95:*229, 1961.
16. Morest, D. K.: Experimental study of the projections of the nucleus of the tractus solitarius and the area postrema in the cat. *J. Comp. Neurol., 130:*227, 1967.
17. Nauta, W. J. H.: Hippocampal projections and related neural pathways to the midbrain in the cat. *Brain, 81:*319, 1958.
18. Nauta, W. J. H., and Haymaker, W.: Hypothalamic nuclei and fiber connections. In Haymaker, W., Anderson, E., and Nauta, W. J. H. (Eds.): *The Hypothalamus.* Springfield, Charles C Thomas, 1969, pp. 136–209.
19. Nauta, W. J. H., and Kuypers, H. G. J. M.: Some ascending pathways in the brain stem reticular formation of the cat. In

Jasper, H. H., Proctor, L. D., Knighton, R. S., Noshay, W. C., and Costello, R. T. (Eds.): *Reticular Formation of the Brain.* Boston-Toronto, Little Brown & Co., 1958, pp. 3–30.
20. Nyberg-Hansen, R.: Functional organization of descending supraspinal fibre systems to the spinal cord. Anatomical observations and physiological correlations. *Ergebn. Anat. Entwicklungsgesch, 39:*2,3, 1966.
21. Pandya, D. N., Hallet, M., and Mukherjee, S. K.: Intra- and inter-hemispheric connections of the neocortical auditory system in the rhesus monkey. *Brain Res., 14:*49, 1969.
22. Pandya, D. N., and Kuypers, H. G. J. M.: Cortico-cortical connections in the rhesus monkey. *Brain Res., 13:*13, 1969.
23. Powell, T. P. S., Cowan, W. M., and Raisman, G.: The central olfactory connexions. *J. Anat., 99:*791, 1965.
24. Ramón-Moliner, E., and Nauta, W. J. H.: The isodendritic core of the brain stem. *J. Comp. Neurol., 126:*311, 1966.
25. Scheibel, M. E., and Scheibel, A. B.: Structural substrates for integrative patterns in the brain stem reticular core. In Jasper, H. H., Proctor, L. D., Kington, R. S., Moshay, W. C., and Costello, R. T. (Eds.): *Reticular Formation of the Brain.* Boston-Toronto, Little Brown, 1958, pp. 31–55.
26. Shriver, J. E., Stein, B. M., and Carpenter, M. B.: Central projections of spinal dorsal roots in the monkey. *Amer. J. Anat., 123:*27 (two parts), 1968.
27. Valenstein, E. S. (Ed.): Biology of drives. *Neurosciences Research Program Bulletin, 6 (No. 1)*, 1968.
28. Taber, E.: The cytoarchitecture of the brainstem of the cat. *J. Comp. Neurol., 116:*27, 1961.

DISCUSSION

Dr. Schallek: Dr. Nauta, you will recall that in 1953, Brady and you described the hyperirritability of rats with lesions in the septal area of the brain. I wonder if you would give us your current views as to what causes the irritability with such forebrain lesions?

Dr. Nauta: I have always been afraid of that question. The explanation at the time, much in line with the traditional notion of "higher centers" inhibiting "lower centers," was that the hypothalamic mechanism is released from some restraining telencephalic influence, and I am afraid that I cannot go beyond that tautological statement.

Dr. Mogenson: The septal region and the cingulate region have similar effects on somatic motor behavior in animals running down alleys and engaged in other motor behavior. Findings of this sort would very much support the point you are making about the cingulate region not being primarily involved in autonomic functions. But they do have one function in common, that of inhibiting ongoing somatomotor behavior.

Dr. Nauta: This idea could, perhaps, be checked by examining the effects of bilateral ablation of the cingulate cortex upon, respectively, operant and autonomic responses to an avoidance situation. It would gain in likelihood if such an ablation were to abolish or impair the operant response (for example, bar pressing to avoid a noxious stimulus) while leaving the autonomic responses to the warning signal unchanged.

Dr. Mogenson: Well the medial thalamic region seems to do just this, doesn't it?

Dr. Nauta: I would think so—yes.

Dr. Reis: I think there are experiments by Garson in which he made lesions in the amygdala in the "flight area" and showed that the animal was unable to respond by flight to a stimulus. It is very interesting in that only this particular aspect of behavior was blocked.

Dr. Nauta: Dr. MacLean has reported somewhat similar findings in a study in which he implanted crystals of carbachol in the hippocampus of cats. These animals did show signs of agitation as the warning signal came on, but they seemed confused and unable to release the appropriate avoidance response.

Dr. MacLean: To go back to the cingulate again, I thought that you had shown that the so-called dorsal fornix projected to quite a different part of the midbrain from the regular fornix. Cragg has some findings which would go along with this from stimulation of the dorsal fornix and getting blood pressure changes. Do the recent findings of the people in your laboratory agree? Are these observations counter to what you originally observed yourself as far as the dorsal fornix is concerned?

Dr. Nauta: We have lately become very uncertain to what extent the cingulate cortex contributes fibers to the fornix dorsalis. In Domesick's study, degeneration in the dorsal fornix appeared to be related to lesions of the indusium griseum rather than retrosplenial granular cortex. A much more detailed study of this matter seems necessary than has been done thus far. Incidentally, it is virtually certain that the fornix longus contains fibers originating in the CA-1 sector of Ammon's horn and likely that it represents a major connection of the fornix system with the paramedian zone of the mesencephalon.

Dr. French: The Scheibels identified fibers from the reticular nucleus of the thalamus as a very important feedback mechanism, presumably for exerting inhibitory control over the mechanism for behavioral events. I think that Reis' work is related to this phenomenon physiologically. Do you see any corollary of such a thalamic feedback control mechanism in the hypothalamic-limbic system? It seems to me that you did point out some similarities between the somatically oriented system and perhaps one more viscerally oriented. Could you comment on these similarities?

Dr. Nauta: The cingulate cortex projects quite massively to the reticular nucleus of the thalamus but, so it seems, do all or most cortical regions. It is unfortunate that the reticular nucleus is so inaccessible to lesion experiments. The nucleus forms, so to speak, a shell around the thalamus. Most of the thalamocortical projections penetrate it and so do many corticothalamic pathways. Any lesion to the nucleus would affect such traversing fiber systems as much as it would interfere with the caudally oriented connections arising in the reticular nucleus itself. The functional significance of the reticular nucleus will therefore probably prove difficult to identify. But your suggestion, if I have understood it correctly, Dr. French, can be answered affirmatively in the sense that of all the telencephalic structures considered "limbic," only the cingulate cortex appears to project to the reticular nucleus of the thalamus.

Dr. French: Then do I understand that the reticular nucleus may show similar effects upon hypothalamic structures through its connections with the cingulate system?

Dr. Nauta: The Scheibel's findings would suggest the possibility that the reticular nucleus can modulate neuronal activity patterns in the anterior thalamic nuclei and thus affect the mechanisms of the cingulate and parahippocampal cortices. If not directly, the latter regions could influence hypothalamic structures indirectly via the hippocampus and fornix system.

Dr. Hockman: I should like to ask if you know of any link between the red nucleus and the limbic system? In stimulating this nucleus, we have elicited a host of visceromotor responses.

Dr. Nauta: No, I don't know of any link

between the limbic circuits and the red nucleus. The closest I can come is the fields of Forel which adjoin the red nucleus on the rostral side and receive, among other afferents, a projection from the mammillary body—the so-called mammillo-subthalamic bundle. It is, however, unknown to what extent, if any, the fields of Forel project to the red nucleus. Despite our ignorance concerning limbic afferents to the red nucleus, your finding that electrical stimulation of the nucleus elicits visceral effects ought not to be surprising. By way of the rubrobulbar connection, the red nucleus could be thought to affect the rhombencephalic reticular formation. All systems having such links with the reticular formation could be expected to be potential modulators of one or the other central autonomic regulation mechanism (see, for example, Hoff and Green's [1932] report of cardiovascular changes elicited by stimulation of the motor cortex). Later, Dr. Snider will tell us of autonomic effects observed in the course of cerebellar stimulation. Some of these may be mediated by the red nucleus.

Dr. Lacey: What sort of autonomic effects would you expect from the red nucleus, for example, in a chronic animal?

Dr. Hockman: We haven't worked with chronic animals. We have stimulated cats that have been immobilized with either gallamine or succinylcholine, and we have observed fairly pronounced increases in blood pressure and alterations in cardiac rate and rhythm. I should expect to see similar responsiveness in the freely moving animal.

Dr. Gloor: Are there fibers going to the red nucleus which might explain this? Fibers that are really not connected to the nucleus at all but just going through it?

Dr. Nauta: I don't know of any that do. The red nucleus seems to be a fairly "closed" territory in the sense that the great conduction pathways ascending and descending through the midbrain tend to circumvent rather than traverse it.

Dr. Lacey: This is a very important question for me, and I would like to pursue it. You say that there is no communication from the red nucleus to the reticular system. Did I understand you to say that this is simply mimicking the activity of the reticular stimulation, or what reason did you give?

Dr. Nauta: I only said that the red nucleus has descending efferents that distribute themselves in the rhombencephalic reticular formation. I could imagine, seeing how widely the neurons of the autonomic nervous system are distributed over the reticular formation, that just about any such fiber system could have some synaptic connections with neurons forming part of central autonomic circuits. The picture of such relationships, seen from the anatomical point of view, would suggest diffuseness, but we should be careful not to equate anatomical diffuseness with functional nonspecificity. From the anatomist's point of view, the entire central autonomic nervous system, from the hypothalamus on down, appears to be a wide open neuronal system in the sense that it can be entered over a great variety of local, ascending and descending conduction pathways. We may have to interpret the openness of the system as a reflection of the multitude of environmental and internal (including "motivational" and "motor") changes that necessitate some or other visceral and endocrine adjustments.

Dr. Livingston: Is it because the indicators are too gross to identify its selectivity—that the sophistication of your end-point is not sufficient to discriminate? The discrimination must be there.

Dr. Lacey: And it is. Discrimination and

specificity become clear if the correct behavioral circumstances are used. I will talk about this point later, but I must point out that there are many data that argue against the notion of diffuseness and lack of specificity.

Dr. Nauta: It would be folly to raise anatomical arguments against physiological findings. Moreover, I cannot find anything particularly disconcerting in the contrast between functional specificity and apparent anatomical diffuseness. The anatomist is at a disadvantage in this issue: human perception cannot cope with visual complexities such as offered by the neuronal arrangements of the brain stem reticular formation. Only rarely can a neuronal concatentation be made to stand out selectively and be traced through. The physiologist, by contrast, can record visceral and endocrine effects and correlate these with particular, more or less controlled, inputs.

Dr. Lacey: But it can be played upon by a variety of influences that will produce rather specific patterns of activity.

Dr. Livingston: But it may be necessary to use a more focal end-point, which we are not really yet able to do.

Dr. Lacey: I hate to impose on Don Reis, but he has some beautiful fractionations of effects on the carotid sinus reflex, for example, in which he can independently influence the systolic and diastolic pressures and the heart rate. Can you talk about that, Don?

Dr. Reis: I want to dodge discussing my own work on this for a minute to comment on some rather impressive evidence for fractionation of autonomic effects of the sympathetic division of the autonomic nervous system. The first clear evidence is the work of Neal Miller and his associates at the Rockefeller University, showing that in operant conditioning one can get very impressive differentiation of sympathetic vasomotor activity. For example, under the appropriate experimental conditions, one can obtain slow changes limited to one limb or one organ system independently of mean blood pressure. Secondly, there are studies by Feigl and also by Ueno and associates showing that punctate stimulation of the hypothalamus can produce changes in blood flow restricted to one organ. By moving the stimulating electrode less than one millimeter away in the hypothalamus, a new pattern of organ flow can emerge. I think that the evidence, even at that level, is that there are highly differentiated organ blood-flow patterns represented in the brain. Now one wonders if this patterning of organ blood flow evoked by brain stimulation does not represent the visceral component of specific behavioral patterns organized within that same area of the brain. In other words, the question is whether or not such stimulation brings into play different kinds of behavior in which by only isolating blood flow, one can miss the whole pattern of the animal's activity. This sort of analysis has been explored by Folkow and Rubenstein. Thus there are several converging lines of evidence that there is a viscerotopic organization within the brain.

Dr. Lacey: As Karl Pribram has said, "Give me the freedom of seven neurons and I will take you from any one place to any other place in the nervous system."

Dr. Nauta: Could I say that certain somatic motor neurons are estimated to have something in the order of eight thousand synapses on their membrane. Obviously, this multitude represents a tremendous convergence of afferents. Despite the anatomist's confusion in confronting such a convergence, the motor neuron seems by no means confused: its participation in the range of possible movements is evidently very precisely defined. There is no a priori reason to think that matters should be fundamentally different in the reticular formation. I would like to emphasize once more that terms such as "diffuse" or "nonspecific" refer to the *afferent* side of neural organizations. The effector side simply demands specificity or there would be no free-ranging organism alive today. To give an example: the central mechanisms governing blood pressure must be very precisely organized, yet be accessible to the neural signals emanating from peripheral monitor regions such as the carotid sinus, as well as to impulses signaling changes in the animal's behavioral set. Here, too, there must be neurons involved that are converged upon from many sides. The anatomical appearance of such an organization could seem to be diffuse, yet its effector manifestations are obviously very specific.

Dr. Lacey: Not only the effector specificity, but a more global behavioral specificity.

Dr. MacLean: To go back more specifically to the anatomy, Walle, would you comment on the recent findings of Shute and Lewis on the two ascending systems—the dorsal and ventral tegmental systems that they claim they have demonstrated with Koelle's cholinesterase stain? Then, of course, they have gone from the septum on up to the hippocampus too and studied the afferent systems that way.

Dr. Nauta: Histochemical techniques, such as those demonstrating cholinesterase and the histofluorescence methods for the demonstration of neuronal systems characterized by monoamine content, have considerably enriched the neuroanatomical technology. Observations such as those of Shute and Lewis, and Fuxe and his colleagues, deserve serious attention. For one thing, their methods demonstrate chemical specificity of particular systems or subsystems and can be traced out in anatomically intact brains. These histochemical techniques do not require the production of tissue defects, and investigators using these techniques are thus absolved of some perennial doubts that beset the users of degeneration methods, in particular the uncertainty as to whether the lesions sampled an adequately large region of the brain. Naturally, the histochemical methods likewise have some blind spots. One major worry should be the question whether these techniques can be relied upon to show the synaptic fractionation of polyneuronal conduction systems; in other words, whether perhaps connections that appear to be direct may not in fact be interrupted by synaptic junctions. In time, such questions will, we hope, be answered.

Dr. Reis: I wonder if I can ask a question relating to your first comments on the function of the hypothalamus. When a cat is acutely stimulated, as Bard and Cannon showed, the animals have spontaneous outbursts of sham rage. Acute decerebration at the midcollicular level, as Sherrington showed, results in a quiet animal as long as he is unperturbed. However, while the midcollicular decerebrated cat does not move spontaneously, similar autonomic and somatic components of sham rage can be evoked by intense noxious stimulation. This has raised the question in the minds of some as to whether the hypothalamus functions more as an energizer of certain activities of lower brain centers rather than serving as a seat for integrating behavior. I wonder if you have any thoughts on this, Dr. Nauta?

Dr. Nauta: Bard's findings, more than any other Sherringtonian observations, suggest the important assumption that behaviors directed toward remote (that is, non-body contact) goals are largely if not entirely governed by the forebrain. More caudal levels of the brain, as well as the spinal cord, are obviously involved in such behaviors, but their participation would seem to be more nearly janitorial than strategic or "policy-making," in the usual sense of these words. If the forebrain should indeed be the only level at which behavioral itineraries are written out in neural code, it is likely also to encompass the neurological substratum of those central states that, on the basis of outward and subjective manifestations, are called "motivational" or "drive states." Along with many others, I interpret the physiological and anatomical evidence that has accumulated since Bard's observations were reported as strong suggestions that the limbic ring of the cerebral hemisphere together with its main brain stem correspondent, the septohypothalamic continuum, are central components of the sensorimotor substratum underlying such behavioral states. This substratum must be accessible to all forms of information from both internal and external environments and exquisitely sensitive to all those features of this information that signal the existence of physiological needs and social-environmental threats or opportunities. The visceral and endocrine manifestations of hypothalamic function in the intact animal seem forever to reflect the fluctuations of this "central state" which in turn could be seen as the end-product of more or less elaborately processed informations from the animal's "total world." To this extent we could indeed consider the hypothalamus as an "energizer" of the neural mechanisms in more caudal parts of the brain. This formulation, however, cannot accommodate the subtle modulations that we must assume the hypothalamus to be able to impose upon the visceral and endocrine effector systems. However, instead of delivering this lengthy disquisition I should perhaps have returned the question to you, Dr. Reis, and have asked if the "energizer" notion appeals to you as a physiologist.

Dr. Reis: I am not sure of it as a universal, but in this particular aspect of behavior it is extremely interesting because it does set the key for the spontaneous outburst. Without the hypothalamus you have all the machinery for this sham rage behavior, but you don't have the spontaneous display.

SESSION II

Chairman: **Walle J. H. Nauta**

Chapter 3

Septal Influences on Autonomic Function

ORLANDO J. ANDY, KENTARO KOSHINO, STANLEY R. NELSON,
DAVID L. SPARKS, GLEN C. WARREN AND ALEX SANFORD

PREVIOUS STUDIES have implied that the septum contributes predominantly, if not exclusively, to the parasympathetic component of autonomic function.[5,8,10,11,14] In our earlier studies, the technique of electrically inducing discharges in the septum revealed that this region of the brain may contribute to either the parasympathetic or sympathetic divisions of autonomic function. Pressor responses were associated with fast frequencies and depressor responses with slow frequencies of the discharge as shown in Figures 3–1 and 3–2.[2] Since septal discharges propagate readily to the hypothalamus[13] and since arterial blood pressure changes associated with stimulation of the hypothalamus have been shown to be frequency-dependent,* it was postulated that septal effects were dependent upon the integrity of the hypothalamus. Consequently, the purpose of the experiments that I shall describe was to evaluate the effects of hypothalamic lesions upon arterial blood pressure changes associated with septal after-discharges.

METHODS

Forty-seven adult cats were utilized. The experiments were performed with the animals lying in a hammock. A 1% solution of lidocaine was used to anesthetize the tissues operated upon, and incisions were made after pain sensibility was abolished, as determined by the pinprick test. Succinylcholine chloride was used to immobilize the animals, and artificial respiration was maintained through a tracheostomy. Bipolar Hess electrodes, 1.5 mm apart with 1-mm bared tips, were lowered into the septum, hypothalamus and onto the motor cortex. Arterial pressure was recorded continuously through a polyethelene catheter leading from the femoral artery to a transducer and displayed on a Twin Viso Sanborn recorder. Heparin was administered to prevent blood clotting. Temperature was maintained at approximately 37 C. Electrical stimuli were delivered from a Grass square-wave stimulator and the parameters were 50 cps, 1 msec pulse width, in trains of one to five seconds with voltages sufficient to produce threshold after-discharges. EEG recordings were made on a Grass Electroencephalograph. The durations of discharges were determined from the end of the five-second stimulus to the point of transition from a sustained "tonic" or "clonic" discharge to that of the pre-discharge (control) or depressed EEG pattern. The frequency patterns of the after-discharges were corre-

* See the following references: 4, 6, 7, 10, 12, 14 and 15.

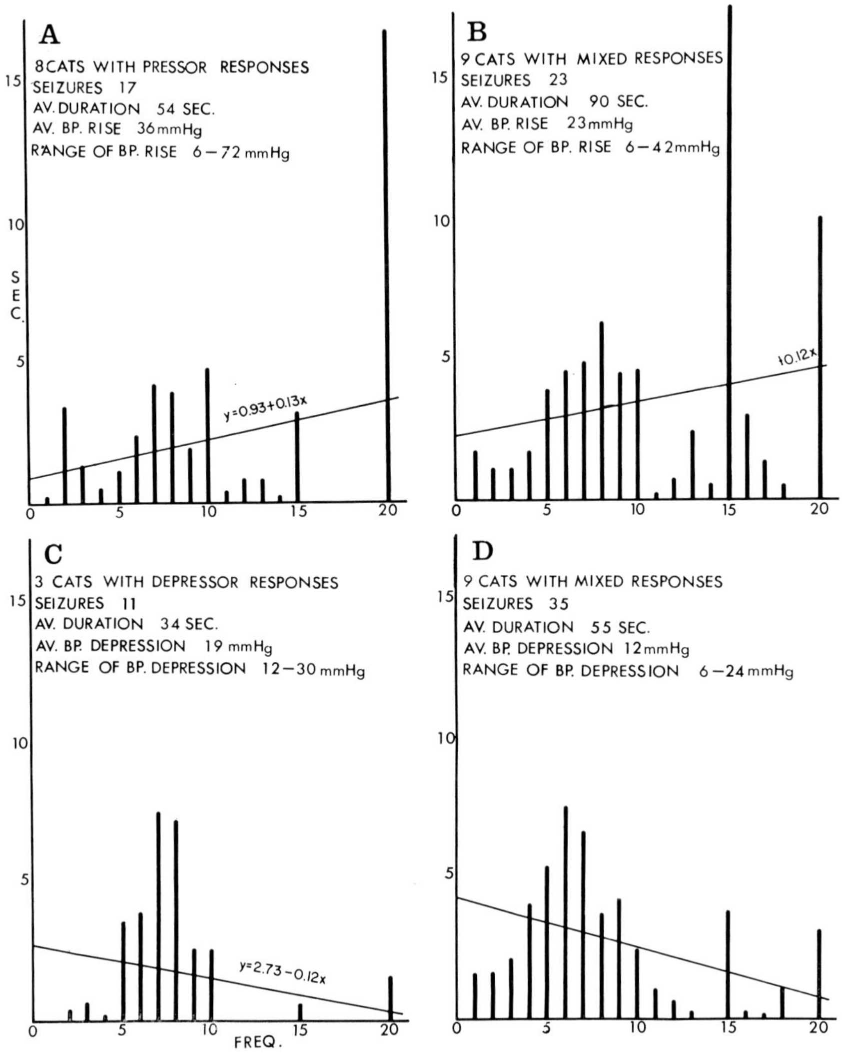

Figure 3–1. The average frequency pattern was prepared in graphic form. (*A*) In eight animals discharges were accompanied by only arterial pressure elevation, and (*C*) in three animals discharges were accompanied by only arterial pressure depression. Nine cats had mixed responses (*B, D*). Twenty-three discharges were associated exclusively with pressor responses (*B*), and 35 discharges were associated exclusively with depressor responses (*D*). Discharges accompanied by pressor and depressor changes during the course of the same discharge were not used for this analysis. In each insert, the abscissa represents frequency and the ordinate represents the average amounts of frequency according to total period of occurrence (in seconds) per discharge. Regression lines were drawn to facilitate comparisons (From Andy, O. J. *et al.*: *Electroenceph. Clin. Neurophysiol., 24*:357, 1968.)

lated with their accompanying arterial blood pressure responses. Arterial pressure changes of less than 6 mm Hg were not considered significant and were categorized in the unaltered "groups." Lesions in the hypothalamus were made through single or multiple electrodes with 1-mm bared tips. In thirty-nine animals, small

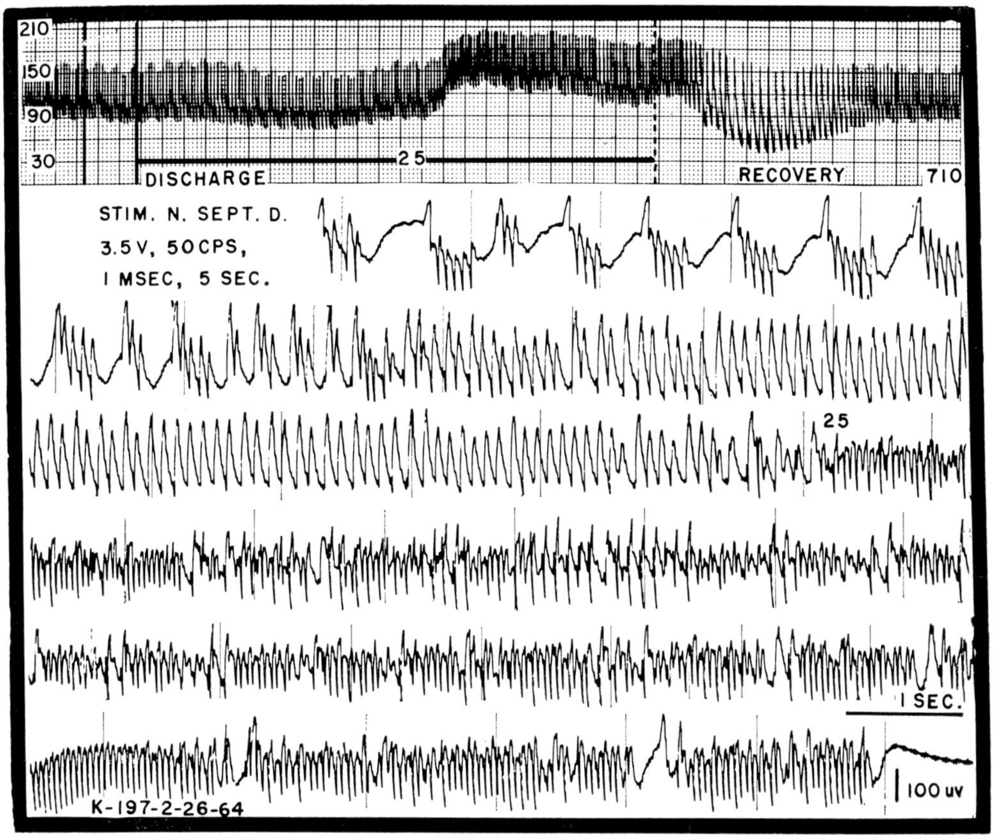

Figure 3–2. Arterial pressure changes during an after-discharge induced by stimulation of the dorsal septal nucleus. Electrographic recording was taken from the stimulated point. A 5-second period of stimulation is represented between the vertical bars. The horizontal bar corresponds to duration of the after-discharge. The vertical dotted line corresponds to termination of the electrographic discharge. Note the elevation of the pressure which was concomitant with the change from slow to fast frequencies, as indicated at the 25-second period in the insert and electrographic tracing, respectively. During the 9 cps frequency, there is a 12 mm Hg drop in arterial pressure before the pressor changes take place. Since the most prominent change is a rise in arterial pressure, this response is considered as predominantly pressor. (From Andy, O. J. *et. al.*: *Electroenceph. Clin. Neurophysiol.*, *24*:357, 1968.)

unilateral lesions (1 by 1 mm) were placed in the hypothalamus. In eight animals, large bilateral lesions (approximately 8 by 10 mm) were made with direct current (6 ma/15 sec). Before the placement of hypothalamic lesions, a minimum of five control discharges and simultaneous arterial pressure recordings were observed. Discharges were elicited after an interval of ten minutes to three hours following placement of the lesions. All experiments were terminated by an intravenously administered overdose of a barbiturate. The animals' brains were perfused with saline followed by a 10% formalin solution and serial histologic sections made in order to identify histologically the points of stimulation and recording. Anatomical designations were according to the atlas of Jasper and Ajmone-Marsan [9] for the hypothalamus and Andy and Stephan [3] for the septum.

RESULTS

Septal discharges propagated to the hypothalamus in all experiments. The propagated discharges tended to display frequency patterns similar to those occurring simultaneously in the septum. Arterial pressure depression was associated with

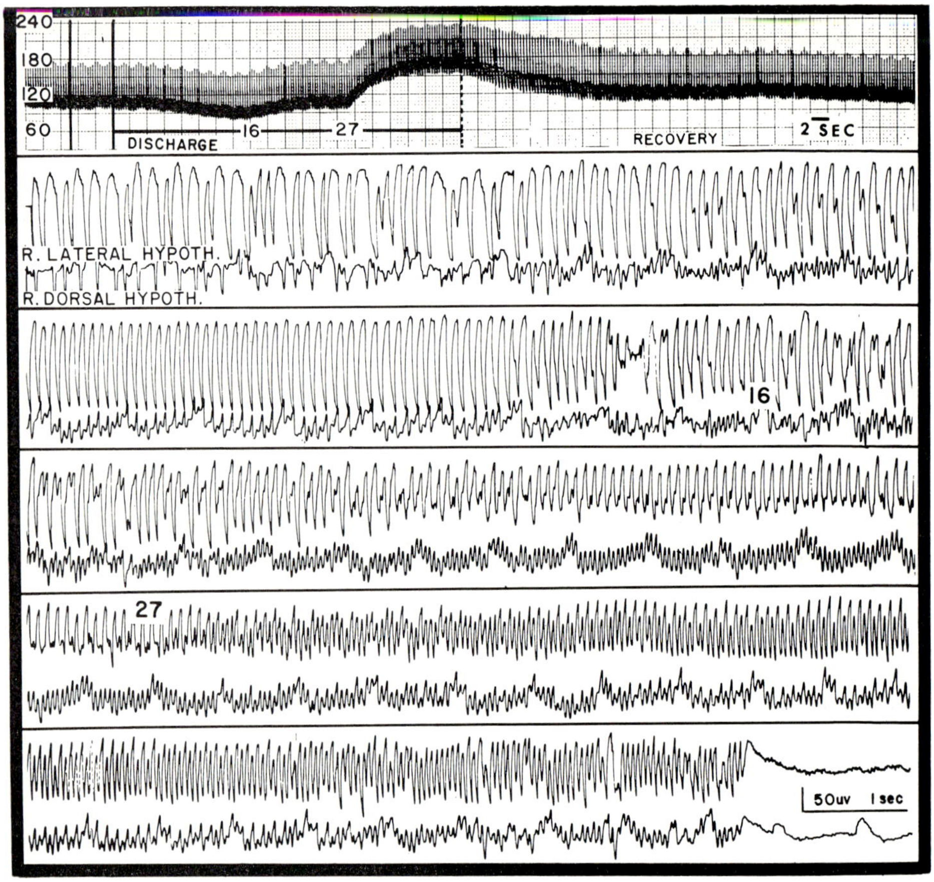

Figure 3–3. Simultaneous and continuous recording of arterial pressure and propagated after-discharge at two sites in the hypothalamus consequent to stimulation of the nucleus septalis dorsalis (2 v, 50 cps, 1 msec pulse, 5-second duration). Vertical bars in the arterial trace represent 5 seconds of applied electrical stimulation. Horizontal bar represents the duration of the after-discharge and the vertical interrupted bar represents the termination of the after-discharge following which is the recovery period. It is important to note that there is a sequential increment in arterial pressure associated with a sequential appearance of fast frequencies, first in the dorsal hypothalamus (at 16 seconds), and later in the right lateral hypothalamus (at 27 seconds). It is believed that this represents potentiation of a pressor response resulting from sequential recruitment of greater numbers of spacially separated hypothalamic elements by the fast frequency. Diagrammatic illustration of the two sites of hypothalamic recording is shown in Figure 3–4.

HYPOTHALAMIC SEQUENTIAL APPEARANCE OF FAST FREQUENCIES FROM SEPTUM DISCHARGE AND ARTERIAL PRESSOR RESPONSE

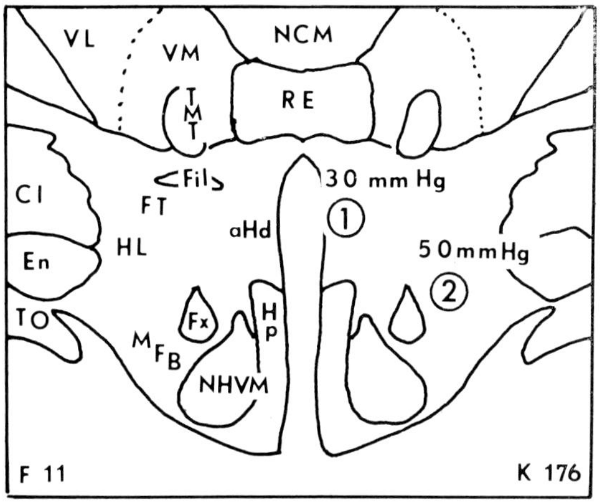

Figure 3–4. Hypothalamic sites which correspond with the EEG recordings illustrated in Figure 3–3. Right dorsal hypothalamus is encircled (*1*) and lateral hypothalamus is encircled (*2*). The degree of pressor response associated with the propagated discharge to each site is given above its respective locus. *Abbreviations:* VL (N. ventralis lateralis), VM (N. ventralis medialis), NCM (N. centralis medialis), RE (N. reuniens), TMT (tractum mammillo-thalamicus), CI (capsula interna), En (N. entopeduncularis), TO (tractus opticus), Fil (N. filiformis), HL (hypothalamus lateralis), FT (fasiculus thalamicus), Fx (fornix), MFB (median forebrain bundle), aHd (area hypothalamica dorsalis), Hp (hypothalamus posterior), NHVM (N. hypothalami centromedialis).

slow frequencies and elevation with fast frequencies. Discharges with frequencies predominantly above 10 cps tended to be associated with pressor responses and those with frequencies predominantly below 10 cps were associated with depressor responses. In one experiment, a sequential increment of pressure was associated with differential involvement of the hypothalamus as seen in Figure 3–3. It is noted that during the first sixteen seconds of the after-discharge, a slight depressor response occurred, associated with a dominant low-frequency pattern of less than 10 cps. Arterial pressure started to rise concomitantly with the appearance of propagated fast frequencies in the right dorsal hypothalamus at sixteen seconds (Figs. 3–3 and 3–4) and subsequently was greatly potentiated by fast frequencies (above 10 cps) appearing in the right lateral hypothalamus at twenty-seven seconds. The arterial blood pressure slowly returned to its resting level following the cessation of the after-discharge.

Abolishment of Blood Pressure Responses Following Hypothalamic Lesions

Following all hypothalamic lesions, the resting arterial blood pressure was not significantly altered (changes were less than 6 mm Hg).

Bilateral large lesions placed posteriorly in the medial-ventral hypothalamus abolished the pressor responses (average increase of 36 mm Hg, 3 exps). These lesions implicated the mammillary body and a region of the medial forebrain bundle as illustrated in Figure 3–5. Lesions implicating the region of the median forebrain bundle with minimal involvement of the mammillary body also abolished a pressor response associated with the septal after-discharge as seen in Figure 3–6. It should be stressed that large bilateral lesions in the anterior hypothalamus involving the ventromedial nucleus of the hypothalamus did not abolish the pressor responses associated with septal after-discharge.

Unilateral lesions placed posteriorly in the medial-ventral hypothalamus, in the region of the median forebrain bundle and mammillary body, also abolished the pressor response. This is shown by the solid circles in Figure 3–7. The arterial pressor response averaged 24 mm Hg before placement of the lesion. In contrast, there

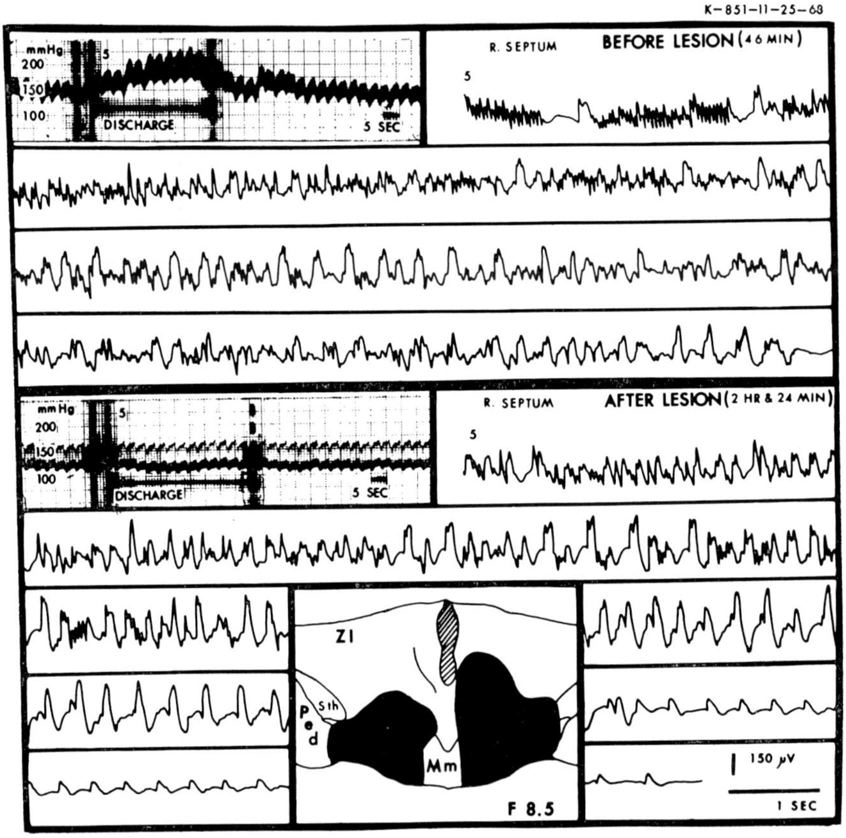

Figure 3–5. Arterial pressure and EEG recordings during septal after-discharges before and after placement of hypothalamic lesions, in upper and lower half of figure respectively. Pressor response associated with septal after-discharge illustrated in upper half of figure is completely abolished by bilateral lesions placed in the posterior medial hypothalamic area, as illustrated in lower half of figure. Insert in lower half of figure indicates lesion sites: F (frontal place), Ped (pedunculus cerebralis), S th (N. subthalamicus), Mm (corpus mammillare) and ZI (zona incerta).

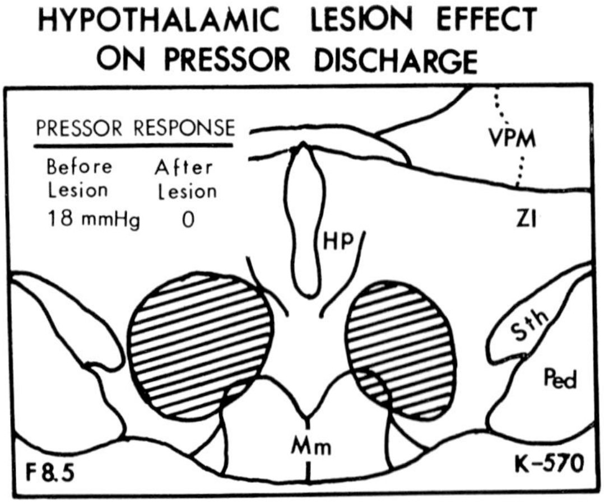

Figure 3–6. Pressor response associated with the septal after-discharge before the placement of the lesion is 18 mm Hg. Following placement of the lesion (oblique lined area) the pressor response is abolished. (See Fig. 3–4 for abbreviations.)

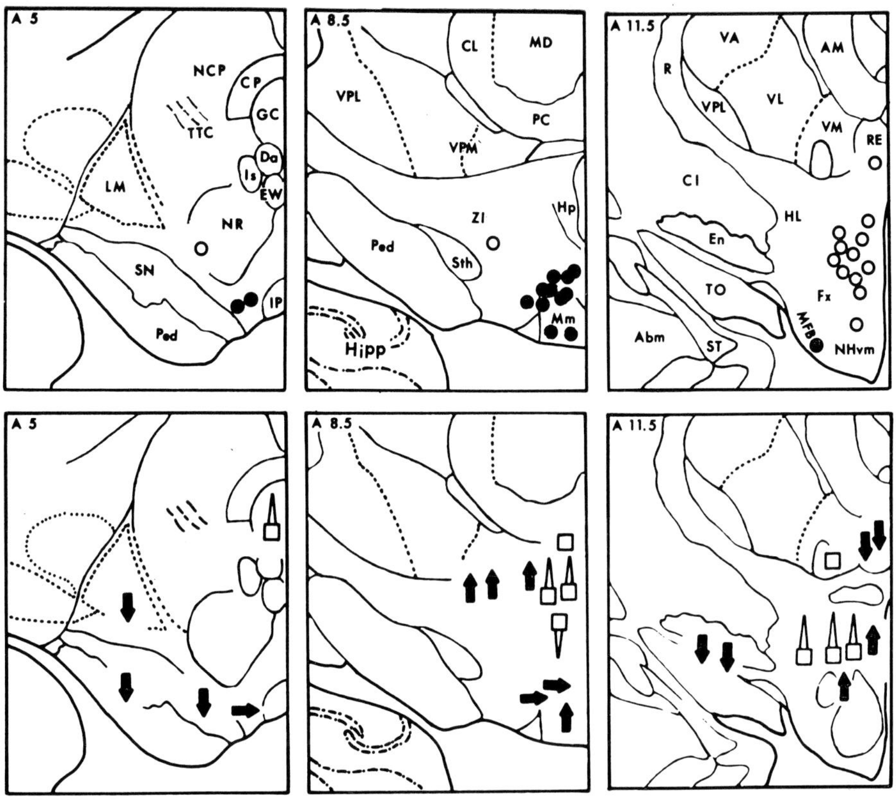

Figure 3–7. Unilateral hypothalamic lesion effects on arterial pressure during septal after-discharges. (*Upper half of the figure*) Open circles indicate lesion sites which did not abolish the pressor response, and solid circles indicate lesion sites which did abolish the pressor response. Note that lesions which abolish the pressor response are predominately located posteriorly in the ventromedial area in the region of the mammillary body, median forebrain bundle and lateral to the interpeduncular nucleus. (*Lower half of the figure*) Solid arrows pointing downward indicate lesion sites which did not abolish depressor responses occurring with a septal after-discharge; solid arrows pointing upward indicate lesion sites which reversed a depressor response to a pressor, and solid arrows horizontally oriented indicate lesion sites which abolished the depressor response. Note that the lesions which abolished the depressor response are located in the region of the mammillary body and lateral to the interpeduncular nucleus. It is of special interest that lesions which did not alter the depressor response are located outside the limits of the hypothalamus. In some instances, arterial pressures which were not altered during a septal after-discharge became pressor responses following the placement of lesions in the hypothalamus and the central gray (open squares with pyramids pointing upward). In only one instance, the lesion was followed by a depressor response (open square with pyramid pointing downward). The two instances in which the lesion did not alter the arterial pressure in this group were located outside the limits of the hypothalamus (open square without pyramid). (See Fig. 3–4 for the abbreviations.)

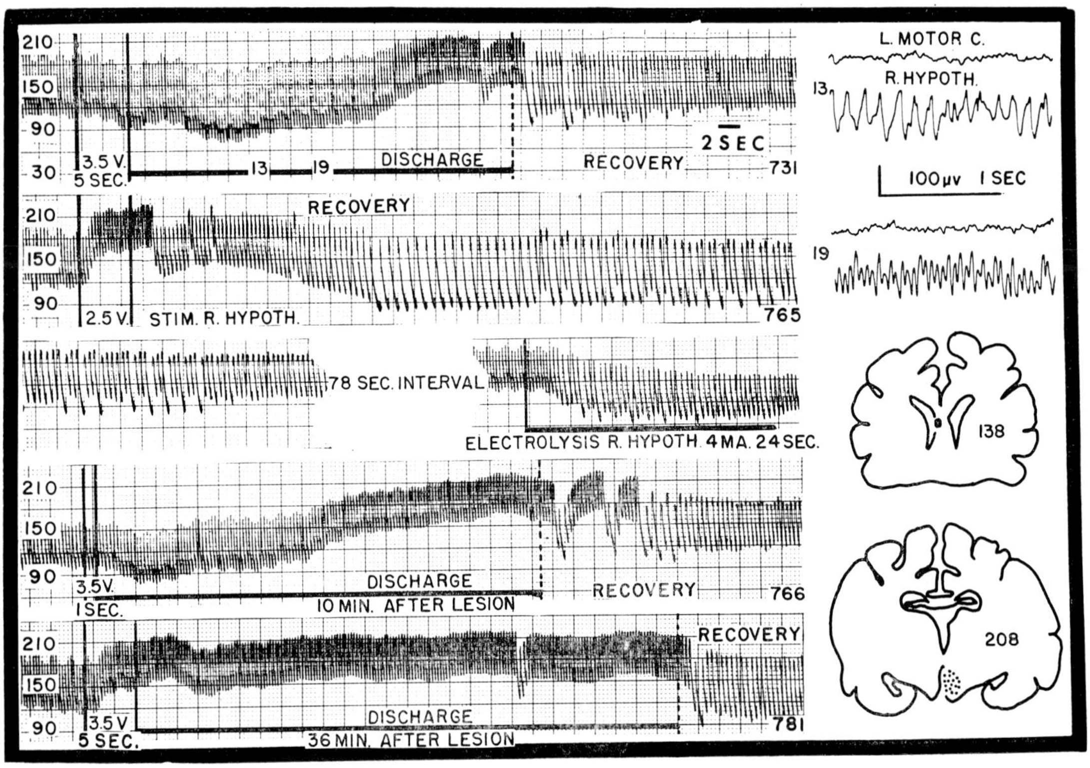

Figure 3–8. Arterial pressure changes associated with septal after-discharges (traces 1, 4 and 5). Trace 2 represents arterial response to direct stimulation of the hypothalamus at the site indicated in histology insert 208 (stippled area). The site of electrical stimulation was subsequently lesioned with an electrolytic current during which time a depressor response was obtained as illustrated in trace 3. Traces 4 and 5 represent pressure changes associated with discharges elicited after placement of a lesion in the hypothalamus. These should be compared with the control (trace 1). In relation to the discussion, note the similarities of the graphic pattern of the arterial pressor response between a directly applied stimulus to the hypothalamus as illustrated in trace 2 and the termination of a propagated discharge to the hypothalamus as illustrated in traces 1, 4 and 5. Histology insert 138 indicates the point stimulation (black dot) of which elicited the after-discharges.

were fourteen experiments in which unilateral lesions placed in the more anterior areas of the medial, dorsal and lateral hypothalamus which did not abolish the pressor responses, as indicated by the open circles in Figure 3–7. Lesions which did not abolish the pressor responses, in some instances, actually resulted in its potentiation. In Figure 3–8 note the progressively earlier development of a sustained pressor response with discharges elicited at ten and thirty-six minutes after placement of a hypothalamic lesion in comparison to the response before the lesion.

Abolishment of Depressor Responses Following Hypothalamic Lesions

In six experiments *bilateral* lesions which abolished the depressor response were located in the area similar to that which abolished the pressor responses, the posterior-medial-ventral hypothalamus.

The average decrease was 20 mm Hg before placement of the lesions.

Unilateral lesions which abolished the depressor response were also located posteriorly in the ventromedial part of the hypothalamus as illustrated by the solid arrows pointing sideways in Figure 3–7.

Reversal of Depressor Response Following Hypothalamic Lesions

In five experiments *bilateral* lesions located in the lateral hypothalamus reversed a depressor to a pressor response. The average decrease before the lesion was 18 mm Hg, and the average increase following the lesion was 20 mm Hg.

Unilateral lesions placed in the anterior, medial-dorsal, and lateral-dorsal areas of the hypothalamus reversed a depressor to a pressor response. A depressor response averaging 14 mm Hg became an average 31 mm Hg pressor response following the lesions as indicated by arrows pointing upward in Figure 3–7. Note in one experiment, a very small lesion which implicated less than one quarter of the total volume of one mammillary body also reversed a depressor to a pressor response as shown in Figure 3–7, A 8.5. Lesions which did not abolish or reverse a depressor response were not located in the hypothalamus. Arrows pointing downward in Figure 3–7 depict these responses.

Unilateral Hypothalamic Lesion Effects on Septal "Neutral Discharges" *

In nine experiments the septal after-discharges were not accompanied by changes in the resting arterial pressure before the placement of the hypothalamic lesions. After placement of the unilateral hypothalamic lesions, however, pressor responses averaging 21 mm Hg were elicited in six of the experiments. This is illustrated in Figure 3–7 by pyramids pointing upwards. The lesions that were followed by pressor responses were located in the posterodorsal hypothalamus and in the central gray. In one experiment, a depressor response of 10 mm Hg followed a lesion which was placed just ventral to the area responsible for the pressor response. This is shown in Figure 3–7 by pyramids pointing downwards. In two experiments, the lesions were located outside the limits of the hypothalamus and these did not alter the arterial pressure as indicated by squares in Figure 3–7.

CONCLUSIONS

The terminology "septal after-discharge" does not imply that the septum is involved to the exclusion of other limbic system structures.[1] The term identifies primarily the point of stimulation which results in a discharge which invariably implicates other limbic regions, the foremost being the hippocampus. Consequently, from these experiments we conclude that the limbic system participates as a whole in both parasympathetic and sympathetic modulation of autonomic activity, specifically, in relation to arterial blood pressure control mechanisms.

These studies indicate that limbic system influences on arterial pressure control mechanisms are dependent upon the integrity of the hypothalamus. Lesions in the postero-ventro-medial hypothalamus abolish both the pressor and depressor responses. It is suggested that the mammillotegmental system and median forebrain bundle (which are implicated by those lesions) serve as the major septohypothalamic pathways mediating the limbic in-

* "Neutral discharges" refer to a septal after-discharge which is not accompanied by a simultaneous change in arterial pressure.

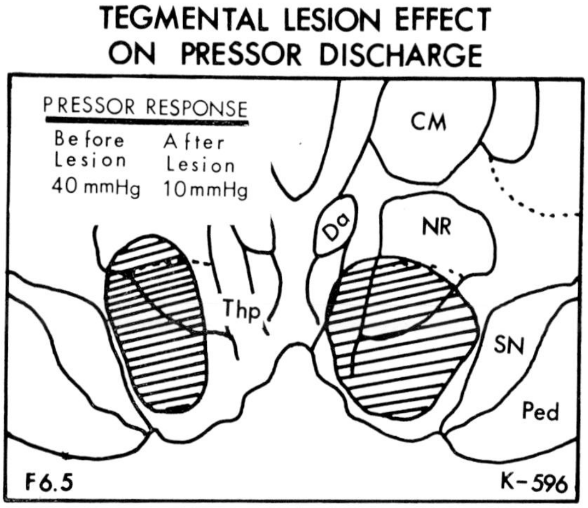

Figure 3–9. A pressor response of 40 mm Hg associated with the septal after-discharge is reduced to 10mm Hg following placement of lesions in the bilateral ventral tegmental area (oblique lined areas indicate lesion sites). *Abbreviations:* CM (N. centrum medianum), Da (N. of Darkschewitsch), NR (N. ruber), Ped (pedunculus cerebralis), SN (substantia nigra), and Thp (tractus habenulopeduncularis).

fluences on lower brain stem structures. This conclusion is also supported by the evidence that ventral tegmental lesions, lateral to the interpeduncular nucleus, markedly reduce arterial pressor responses associated with septal after-discharges as seen in Figure 3–9.

An intriguing and unexplained observation was the tendency for pressor mechanisms to prevail following anteromedial, dorsal and lateral hypothalamic lesions. This occurred even at the expense of depressor mechanisms (arterial depressor responses were changed to arterial pressor responses following hypothalamic lesions at those sites, but the opposite effect did not occur). One plausible explanation for this observation may be the following: biochemical and structural changes taking place in the peripheral zones of the lesion render the high-frequency responsive cells more excitable, whereas they raise the threshold of cells responsive to the lower frequencies. For purposes of this argument, it is being assumed that a propagated discharge to the hypothalamus possesses similar stimulation characteristics for evoking a hypothalamic pressor or depressor response as does directly applied electrical stimulation to the hypothalamus. This assumption is supported, in part, by observations such as illustrated in Figure 3–3 and by similarities in the graphic patterns of the pressor response obtained by direct stimulation of the hypothalamus and by propagated discharges to the hypothalamus as shown in Figure 3–8.

SUMMARY

1. The effect of hypothalamic lesions on arterial blood pressure changes associated with septal after-discharges was studied in adult cats that were immobilized with succinylcholine chloride.

2. The limbic system contributes to the modulation of both sympathetic and parasympathetic divisions of the autonomic nervous system, especially in relation to the regulation of arterial blood pressure.

3. Limbic system influences on arterial blood pressure control mechanisms are dependent upon the integrity of the hypothalamus.

4. Lesions involving the mammillotegmental and median forebrain bundle systems abolish both pressor and depressor responses associated with septal after-discharges.

5. Lesions in other parts of the hypothalamus tend to facilitate pressor responses, even at the expense of depressor responses.

REFERENCES

1. Andy, O. J., and Koshino, K.: Duration and frequency pattern of the after-discharge from septum and amygdala. *Electroenceph. Clin. Neurophysiol., 22:*167, 1967.
2. Andy, O. J., Koshino, K., Nelson, S. R., Gibbs, J. T., and Sparks, D. L.: Septum after-discharges and associated arterial pressure responses. *Electroenceph. Clin. Neurophysiol., 24:*357, 1968.
3. Andy, O. J., and Stephan, H.: *Septum of the Cat.* Springfield, Charles C Thomas, 1964.
4. Berry C., McKinley, W., and Hodes, R.: Reversals of blood pressure responses caused by changes in frequency of brain stem stimulation. *Amer. J. Physiol., 135:*338, 1942.
5. Covian, M. R., Antune-Rodriques, J., and O'Flaherty, J. J.: Effects of stimulation of the septal area upon blood pressure and respiration in the cat. *J. Neurophysiol., 27:*394, 1964.
6. Folkow, B., and Rubinstein, E. H.: Cardiovascular effects of acute and chronic stimulation of the hypothalamic defence area in the rat. *Acta Physiol., Scand., 68:*48, 1966.
7. Hare, K., and Geohegan, W. A.: Influence of frequency of stimulus upon response to hypothalamic stimulation. *J. Neurophysiol., 4:*266, 1941.
8. Hess, W. R.: *The Functional Organization of the Diencephalon.* New York, Grune & Stratton, 1958.
9. Jasper, H. H., and Ajmone-Marsan, C.: *A Stereotaxic Atlas of the Diencephalon of the Cat.* Ottawa, Ontario, National Research Council of Canada, 1954.
10. Kabat, H., Magoun, H. W., and Ranson, S. W.: Electrical stimulation of points in the forebrain and midbrain. The resultant alterations in blood pressure. *Arch. Neurol. Psychiat., 34:*931, 1935.
11. Kurotsu, T., Sakai, A., Megawa, A., and Ban, T.: The changes in blood pressure and gastric motility induced by electrical stimulation in the preoptic and septal areas. *Med. J. Osaka Univ., 9:*201, 1958.
12. Mauck, H. P., and Hockman, C. H.: Central nervous system mechanisms mediating cardiac rate and rhythm. *Amer. Heart J., 74:*96, 1967.
13. Niemer, W. T., Powell, E. W., and Goodfellow, E. F.: The subcortex and hypothalamic after-discharge in the cat. *Electroenceph. Clin. Neurophysiol., 12:*345, 1960.
14. Ranson, S. W., Kabat, H., and Magoun, H. W.: Autonomic response to electrical stimulation of hypothalamus, preoptic region and septum. *Arch. Neurol. Psychiat., 33:*467, 1935.
15. Torri, S., and Kawamura, H.: Effects of amygdaloid stimulation on blood pressure and electrical activity of hippocampus. *Jap. J. Physiol., 10:*374, 1960.

DISCUSSION

Dr. Killam: Is there a possibility that during the postictal period you are in fact having a temporary functional ablation, so that you are, in effect, flipping over from a parasympathetic to a sympathetic type of response by simple inhibition?

Dr. Andy: After the termination or before?

Dr. Killam: During the postictal period.

Dr. Andy: (Note Figure 3–10.) This is a stimulation. This is a discharge, and this is postictal. This is what you are asking about down here. At this point, the sympathetic, if you want, is no longer playing a part, and I believe that what we have is an unopposed parasympathetic activity. This is also supported by the fact that vagotomy eliminates it.

Dr. Lacey: Do you think that there are theoretical grounds for drawing theoretical conclusions from the frequency requirements of the direction of the blood pressure response? It reminds me of some of the old peripheral nerve studies—stimulating the mixed nerve like the sciatic. If you want to produce a blood pressure decrease, you stimuate with pulses with a

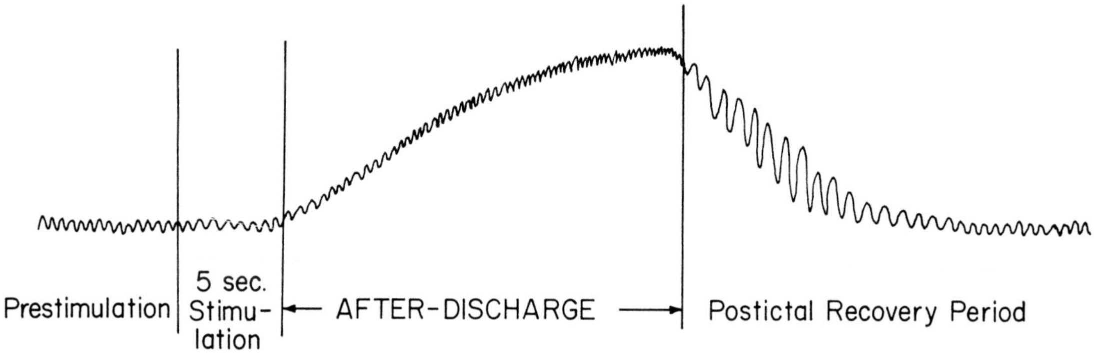

Figure 3–10. Blackboard drawing. The interval between the vertical bars on the left represents a 5-second period of stimulation, followed by a pressor response with an associated fast pulse change. This pressor response is associated with a high-frequency discharge pattern. The postictal recovery period contains a relatively very slow pulse rate with a pulse pattern consistent with vagal-like effects.

wide pulse width, while if you want to produce a blood pressure increase by selective activation of the fibers of a mixed nerve, you go to fast pulses. The same thing is true of central stimulation. If you get a spontaneously recurring different temporal pattern of stimulation induced during discharge periods—does that analogy strike you as relevant?

Dr. Andy: Yes. In fact, it was that information which attracted me to this problem. Not only can one get variation in blood pressure according to different peripheral stimulus frequencies but also to different stimulus frequencies within the hypothalamus itself.

Dr. Lacey: Here you have naturally occurring changes. Could you not influence the frequency with stimulus parameters?

Dr. Andy: No.

Dr. Lacey: You just took the naturally occurring variation in frequency of discharge and correlated it with blood pressure?

Dr. Andy: Now, just let me bring out one other point. We have resected the hippocampus, and in the majority of those, we have a slower frequency band than in the intact hippocampal animal; however, in spite of that, we still get high pressor responses.

Dr. Lacey: Does the same frequency relationship hold?

Dr. Andy: Yes, this is the same frequency relationship; however, the low-frequency stimulations in the hippocampectomized animals will give you a rise, whereas in an animal with an intact hippocampus, the lower frequencies may not. It doesn't always occur. For example, we will have some animals which have rates of perhaps 10/sec in the intact condition, and during that time the blood pressure will go down. Now in the hippocampectomized animal, you can have a 10/sec activity during which time the blood pressure will rise.

Dr. MacLean: Does the discharge last as long, Orlando, in the hippocampal ablated animal?

Dr. Andy: Yes, it may be. In general, though, it is likely to be shorter. At times, it seems that the pressure changes are discharge-duration dependent, but that is not true either, because, as you notice in the mammillary-lesioned animal and ventral tegmental-lesioned animal, the discharges last much longer.

Dr. Lacey: I want to go back to my question. Do you draw any theory as to which mechanism is involved from the frequency dependence?

Dr. Andy: This is a question that I had hoped someone else would answer for me. I just feel that we have a cell that we know (as has been demonstrated) can discharge at various frequencies. You may have some that discharge up to 20/sec, while others discharge at a lower frequency. This cell that discharges at 20/sec must have some meaning in terms of its frequency, and I just wonder whether the frequency in this situation may actually determine whether or not there is a final block or facilitation of sympathetic activity.

Dr. Lacey: Then one must turn to microelectrode studies which show a frequency dependency of the actual cell itself.

Dr. Andy: Yes.

Dr. Lacey: And this implies different pathways of communication?

Dr. Andy: No, not necessarily. It may go through the same system and the same pathways, if we are dealing with the same cell. This is, of course, all hypothetical.

Dr. Abrahams: Well, if you look at Eccles and Anderson's paper, you may get a very brief facilitation or prolonged inhibition from thalamic cells in response to cortical stimulation. You can overcome the prolonged inhibition that you get from single shock by a repeated stimulus that sets up the EPSP. So here is part of the answer for the question of changes in the response when you change frequencies.

Dr. Andy: You actually can have a block with increased frequencies.

Dr. Abrahams: Also if you stimulate elsewhere, you may get a very brief facilitation followed by a very prolonged depression which, in effect, holds that cell off the line for some time. On the other hand, if you put in a train of pulses, you build up facilitation, so that the cells discharge instead of being inhibited.

Dr. Lacey: What are the possibilities remaining for this phenomenon being dependent on selective activation of different neurons in different pathways as is true of peripheral nerves?

Dr. Andy: Well, I can visualize a "parasympathetic" cell activated by slow frequencies and a "sympathetic" cell by high frequencies. That just doesn't fit with the information that is available. Our thinking is to eliminate that at least for the present, or as far as this particuar system is concerned.

Dr. Lacey: I am opposed to eliminating it.

Dr. Andy: Well, it may not be. There may be several mechanisms operating.

Dr. Abrahams: What expectation do you really have that you can get an increase in blood pressure from the sympathetics and a fall from the parasympathetics? I think that this is what you said—a fall from the parasympathetics.

Dr. Andy: There is some evidence that others have had in terms of a fall in blood pressure, in which——

Dr. Abrahams: No. I am thinking of the sort of work in which you increase regional blood flow and so on, and really look at what happens when you have a change in blood pressure. For example, you can get sympathetic activation of cholinergic vasomotor fibers, but if you get no concomitant cardiovascular changes, then you get a fall in blood pressure. It isn't a parasympathetic effect, but it is a fall in blood pressure. The other thing that happens is that you get a suspension of baroreceptor reflexes in the intact preparation under certain conditions. If that system isn't operating, then you get a peculiar picture of cardiovascular activation. The thing that you showed with rebound bradycardia, I

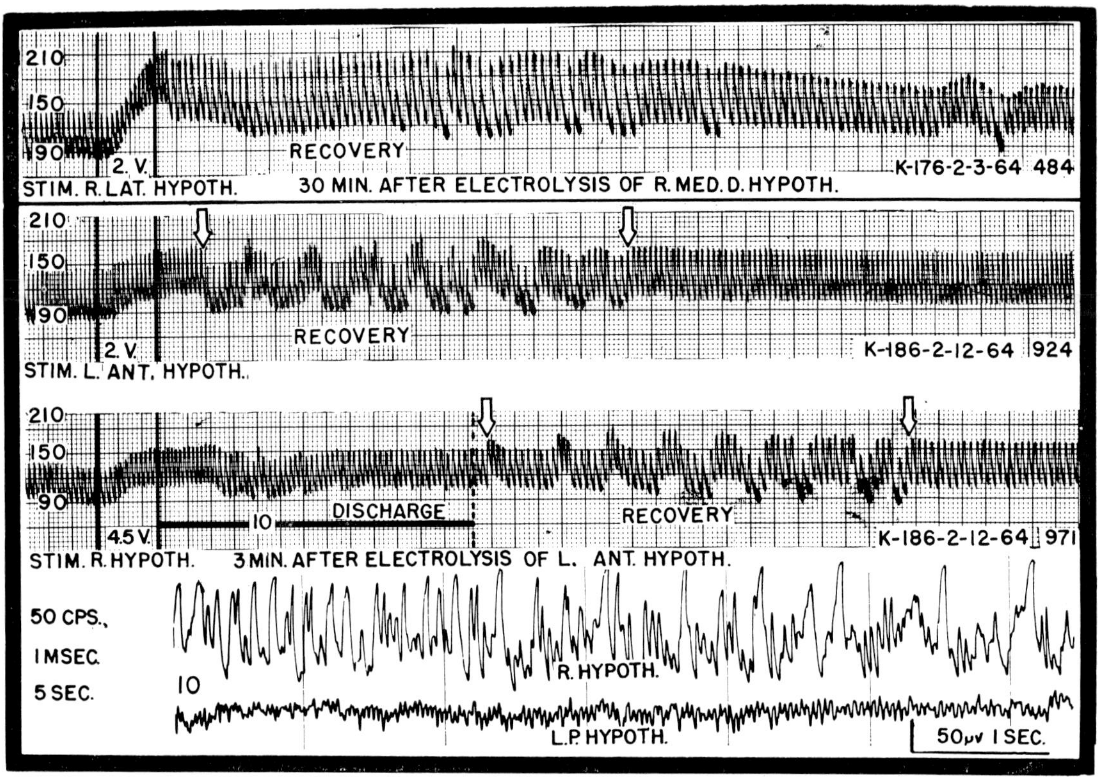

Figure 3–11. This figure compares the effects of an after-discharge in the hypothalamus with those of direct electrical stimulation of the hypothalamus. The upper trace demonstrates a pressor response to direct electrical stimulation of the right lateral hypothalamus. The interval between the vertical bars represents 5 seconds of electrical stimulation. Note the increased pulse pressure and slowing of the heart during the recovery period. The second tracing illustrates a pressor response resulting from direct electrical stimulation in the left anterior hypothalamus for 5 seconds. Note the poststimulus recovery period which is characterized by the oscillation pattern of arterial pressure and the slowed heart rate (between the arrows). The third tracing shows an after-discharge induced by a 5-second stimulation of the right hypothalamus. Note that the recovery period following the after-discharge is very similar to the oscillating pattern illustrated in the second tracing which was obtained by direct electrical stimulation without an after-discharge. In relation to arterial pressure, this suggests that an after-discharge in the hypothalamus possesses stimulation properties similar to those which are associated with a directly applied electrical stimulus. Electrographic tracing corresponds to the 10-second period of the arterial pressure recording as illustrated in the third tracing.

would guess is almost certainly explained by the fact that you hit a spot where you suspended baroreceptor buffer reflexes during the period of stimulation. You stopped the electrical stimulation, and then you get a very dramatic slowing of the heart which goes on for some time.

Dr. Andy: I would visualize that as a contest between the sympathetic and parasympathetic activity. As I see it, during this period I visualize the sympathetic activity outspacing the parasympathetic, and now the sympathetic drops off because the stimulation of the hypothalamus is no longer there.

Dr. Hoffer: What is the effect of atropine on the depressor response?

Dr. Andy: I said that atropine abolishes it.

Dr. Gloor: I wish to make just one brief comment about this question of why one could obtain different effects by changing the frequency of discharge. In our own studies in the amygdalohypothalamic system, we observed with Drs. Murphy and Dreifuss that with repetitive stimulation one may activate many hypothalamic cells, if the amygdaloid nucleus is stimulated repetitively up to a rate of about 8 to 10/sec. However, if one stimulates at a faster rate than that, most of the hypothalamic cells just stop responding. What the mechanism of this differential effect is we do not know, but certainly going beyond 10/sec just shuts many of the cells right off. If we assume that such a cell would be involved in mediating blood pressure responses, one could expect that with stimuli up to 10/sec, the blood pressure response would go in one direction and beyond 10/sec the response would go in the opposite direction, because rapid stimulation eliminated the contribution of the neurons mediating the first type of response. This may be one part of the mechanism explaining these dual effects.

Dr. Andy: I have a few illustrations that may be of interest in response to some of these questions. As some of you know, it is very difficult to get an after-discharge from the hypothalamus. Note Figure 3–11, which was taken from the cat again. In this instance, we have two areas in which we are interested: the left side of the hypothalamus and the right side. We stimulated the right side, and at the beginning of the stimulation, we get a pressor response and at the end of stimulation, we get an oscillation and a recovery period. There is no discharge in this instance. Stimulation of the left anterior hypothalamus (tracing 2) also produced a pressor response with arterial pressure oscillation during the poststimulus recovery period. We then made a lesion at this site

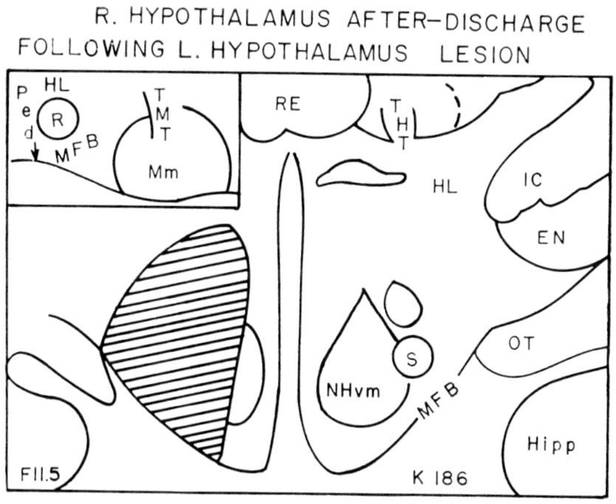

Figure 3–12. The insert in the left upper trace illustrates the area of recording in the left posterior hypothalamus from which the electroencephalographic tracing in Figure 3–11 was taken. The diagonal lines indicate the location and size of the lesion in the left hypothalamus. The locus of electrical stimulation (circled s) of the right hypothalamus, 3 minutes after the lesion, which resulted in the arterial pressure changes in Figure 3–11, trace 3.

(left anterior hypothalamus). Three minutes after making the lesion (tracing 3), we stimulated the opposite side of the hypothalamus at approximately the same level as for the first tracing, and this is the effect of stimulating the opposite side: a pressor response. Then we have a discharge that lasts up to that point. We see that during the discharge the pressor response is maintained. After the termination of the discharge, we have a similar pattern as we have in the poststimulation period up here (tracing 2). Here again, I look upon this as a discharge which is simulating a directly applied stimulus. Let us look at Figure 3–12 and see where this is located. This is the lesion. This is the stimulus site. Recording from the lateral hypothalamus posterior to this level shows the fast frequency discharges.

Dr. Reis: Do you assume that the after-discharges are arising from cells in the septum, or are they merely reflecting projected activity coming from remote areas such as the amygdala or hippocampus?

Dr. Andy: The beauty of this particular technique is that it doesn't allow me to say that this is coming from the septum. Recording in other places reveals that apparently the hippocampus is firing and so is the amygdala. So I look upon this as a system. When I stimulate the septum, I am not only activating cells in the septum but activating hippocampal cells and amygdaloid cells, and probably others. I look upon this as being a septal system because it is the septum that is doing the pacing so to speak. It is the conductor in this situation.

Dr. MacLean: With regard to Donald's statement, I doubt that one would get an after-discharge in the amygdala if it did not have related cortex to reverberate with. Herbert, do you have any comments to make on whether one could get an after-

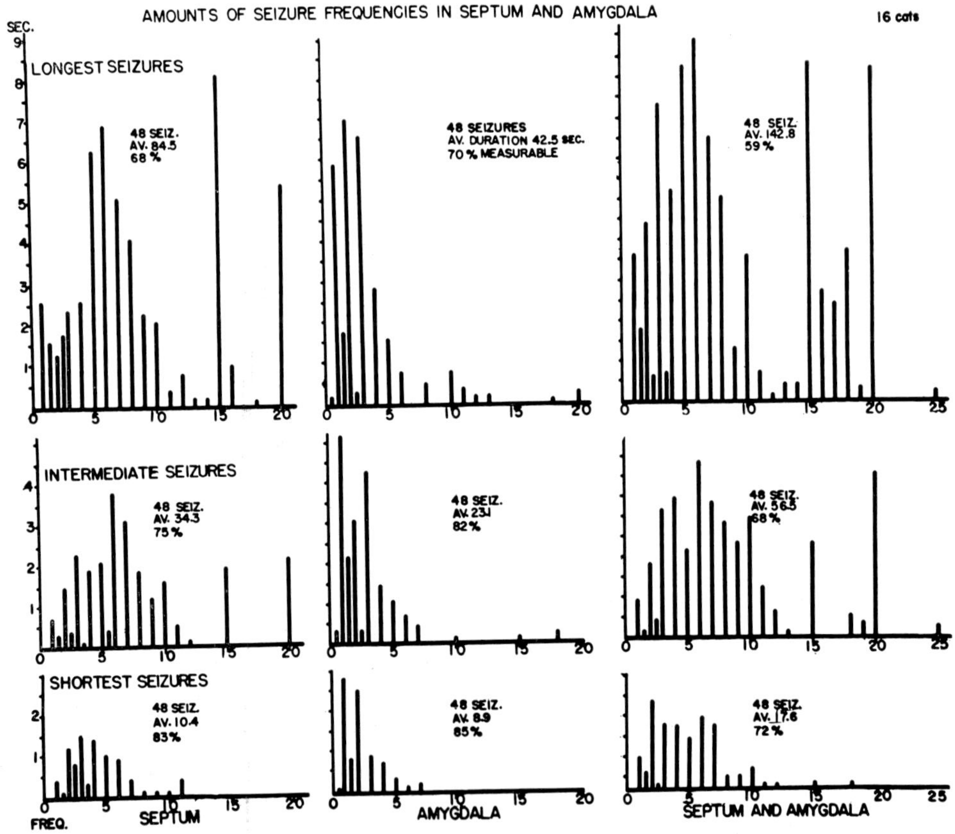

Figure 3–13. This figure illustrates the frequency spectra for the average septal, amygdaloid and combined septo-amygdaloid discharges in the cat. Frequencies are along the abscissa, and the amounts at a given frequency are expressed in seconds on the ordinate. Note that with each set of analysis, there were 48 seizures. The average duration and the percent measurable frequency is given in each set. The group on the left represents the septum, the middle group, the amygdala and the right group, the septum and amygdala combined. (From Andy, O. J., and Koshino, K.: Duration and frequency patterns of the after-discharge from the septum and amygdala. *Electroenceph. Clin. Neurophysiol., 22:* 167, 1967.)

discharge from just stimulating within the nuclear structures themselves without related cortical areas?

Dr. Jasper: If you stimulate within the amygdala, you get local after-discharges there, some conducted to the hippocampus, which cannot be seen on the inferior temporal region.

Dr. MacLean: The question is whether within the nucleus itself one can elicit after-discharges without getting reverberation from the related cortex. That is the question I am raising.

Dr. Andy: In view of local stereotaxic stimulation, you can even have a discharge within the hippocampus. It is very localized and does not propagate. In these instances, there is no propagation to the motor cortex. It is confined, in general, to the limbic structures. With respect to

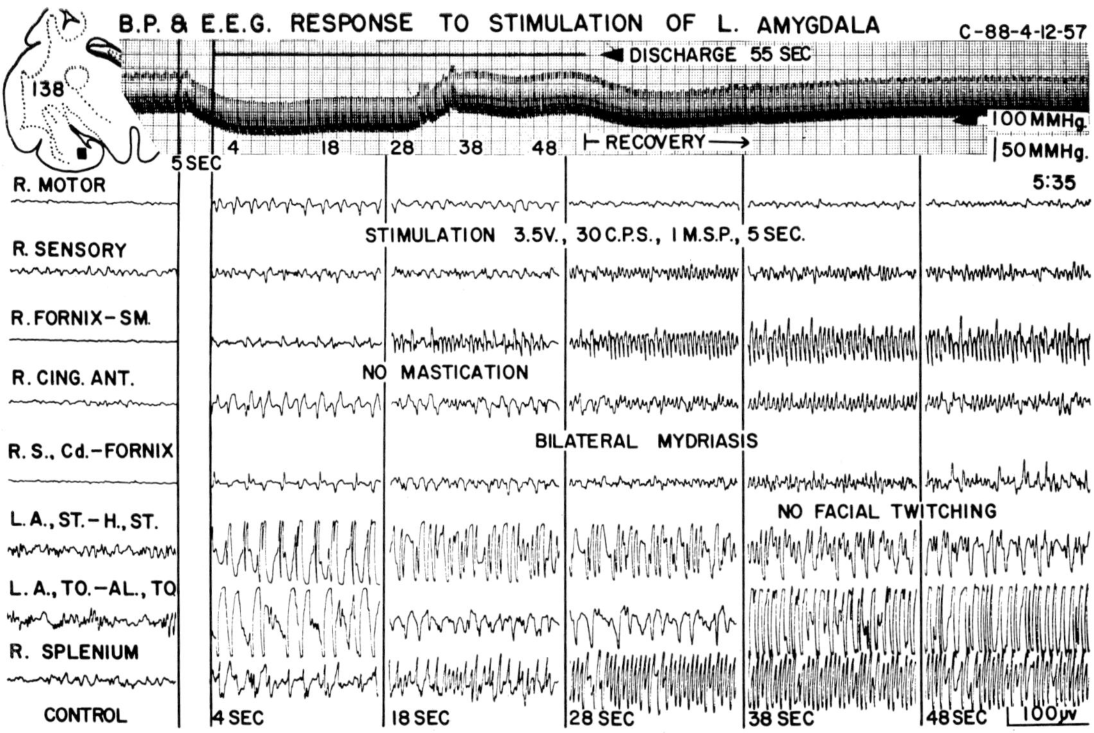

Figure 3–14. Simultaneous arterial pressure and electroencephalographic recordings before, during and after stimulation of the left amygdala (insert 138, black square). The vertical bars in the blood pressure tracing represent the 5-second period of stimulation, and the horizontal bar represents the duration of the 55-second discharge which corresponds to the blood pressure changes. Excerpts of the electroencephalographic patterns are illustrated at five specific points in time in relation to the blood pressure, as indicated by the numbers 4- 18- 19- 38- and 48-second periods during the after-discharge. Note that the pressor response which develops at the 28-second period of the after-discharge corresponds to the development of fast frequencies in the fornix-hippocampal system. *Abbreviations:* A. (amygdala), AL (ansa lenticularis), Cd. (nucleus caudatus), CING. ANT. (anterior cingulate gyrus), H. (hippocampus), L. (left), R. (right), S. (septum), SM. (stria medularis), Splenium (gyrus), ST. (stria terminalis), TO. (tractus opticus). (From Andy, O. J. *et al.:* Blood pressure alternations secondary to amygdaloid and periamygdaloid after-discharges. *J. Neurophysiol.*, 22:51, 1959.)

amygdaloid stimulation, I think that Dr. Reis has seen the same thing. You get ipsilateral facial movements many times during the course of the discharge, and in spite of the fact that the same discharge will propagate to the opposite amygdala, you will not have any facial movements on that side.

Figure 3–13 is an analysis of discharge frequencies in an attempt to relate septal amygdaloid interaction during the period of the discharge. This is a frequency analysis of the septal discharge (left column of graph). We see three modes in this instance: 5 to 7, 15 and 20. This is in contrast to the amygdaloid frequency distribution during the period of discharge. We see that it is definitely in the lower range (central graphs). Studies that we have done prior to this analysis in the amygdala, in relation to blood pressure changes during the discharge from that structure, revealed primarily a blood pressure depression, although we did have instances in which there was a blood pressure elevation. This is a combined discharge evoked from the septum and the amygdala simultaneously (right column of graph). The frequency distribution in this instance shows more or less potentiation of all three

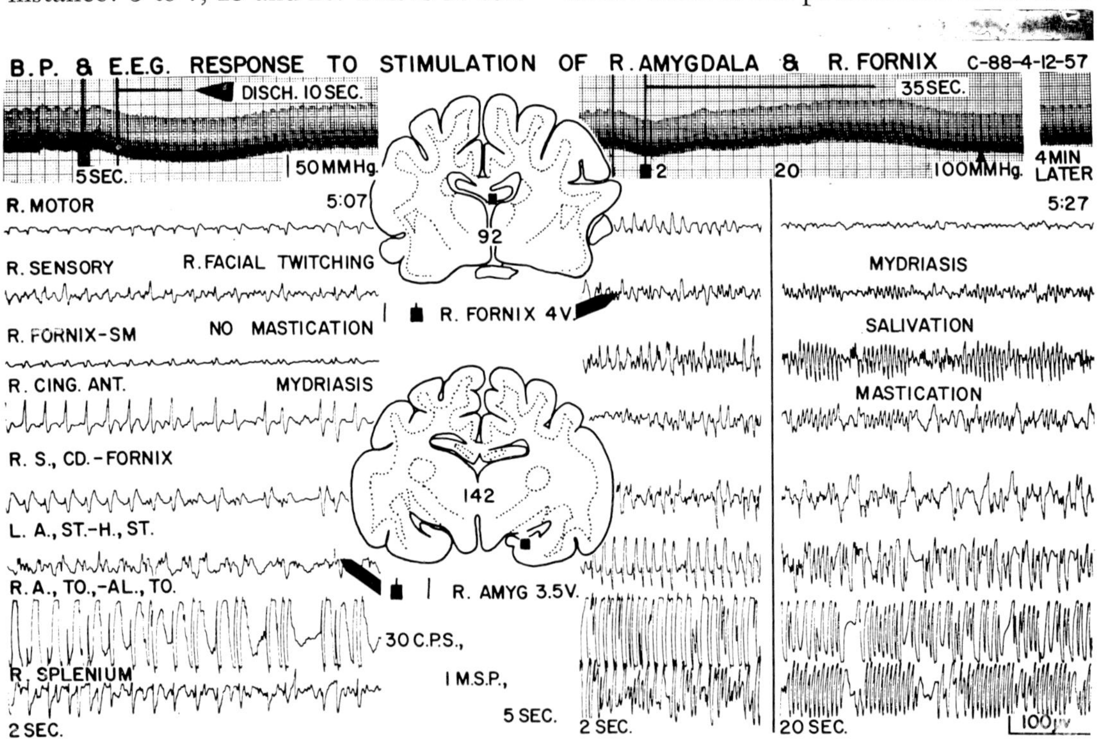

Figure 3–15. The blood pressure and electrical recordings in the left half of the figure were made after stimulation of the right amygdala (insert 142, black square). The recordings in the right half of the illustration were taken after stimulation of the right fornix (insert 93, black square). It should be noted that the depressor response which is associated with the slow frequency discharge resulting from stimulation of the amygdala in the left half of the figure and the pressor response associated with the fast frequency discharge associated with electrical stimulation of the fornix, right half of the figure. (From Andy, O. J. *et al.*: Blood pressure alternations secondary to amygdaloid and periamygdaloid after-discharges. *J. Neurophysiol.*, *22*:51, 1959.)

major components. Let's look at Figure 3–14. This is the amygdaloid discharge. During the course of this early period of discharge, we see a relatively low frequency being displayed at 4 seconds. This corresponds to this EEG, and at 18 seconds which corresponds with this period, we see a slight elevation now taking place. When this other system comes into play with the faster frequencies, we see a pressor response occurring. At the onset of recovery, there is a rebound downward depression and then back to normal. We felt this was a discharge which, from the amygdala, actually ended up by activating the hippocampal-septal-fornix system at this point (at 28 seconds) so we have fast frequencies coming into play.

Figure 3–15 illustrates a separation of those two systems. A stimulation of the amygdala in which there was no activation of this other system, and this is a stimulation of the fimbria at this point (upper histologic insert) showing the discharge frequency pattern that we saw in that other stimulation in the same animal. There is no question that we have an interplay here of systems. It is possible that during the slow frequency part of the discharge, immediately after stimulation, the amygdala may be coming into play more than the hippocampal system. But with repeated observation and experience, I don't believe that is really the explanation for the immediate depressor effects following stimulation. I feel that there is something else—the effect of the stimulus itself. It is just like throwing in an "atomic bomb" into a system and temporarily paralyzing it.

Dr. French: I have a comment regarding Orlando's very nice demonstration that these structures have a good deal to do with autonomic regulation. Neurosurgeons are quite aware that in operating in the preoptic area or regions near the anterior hypothalamus, the perforating vessels supplying regions concerned with these mechanisms can very easily be put into a spasm, and autonomic manifestations such as a precipitous rise in blood pressure can result. Also, there is evidence to suggest that after-discharge, such as that which he has used here so effectively, may be a physiological mechanism in controlling bodily function. The experimental and clinical data appear to me to be compatible in this connection.

Chapter 4

Anatomical and Physiological Characteristics of the Two Amygdaloid Projection Systems to the Ventromedial Hypothalamus

PIERRE GLOOR, JOHN T. MURPHY AND JEAN-JACQUES DREIFUSS

WHEN, EONS AGO, the first vertebrates climbed out of the water onto dry land, they presumably carried with them a set of sensory systems and their related central nervous system representations that had been adapted to aquatic life. This included among others, an olfactory placode located in a shallow pit above the upper lip. This placode was connected to an olfactory bulb giving origin to an afferent projection system which ended in an undifferentiated region of the ventrolateral forebrain where its terminations overlapped with that of other ascending, presumably somatic and special sensory, systems reaching the same area through the spinal cord and brain stem. One may assume that the brain of these ancestral primordial land vertebrates in its organization and structure resembled that of today's tailed amphibians and thus must have been similar to that of a mudpuppy or salamander. In an excellent paper published in 1921 Herrick [14] has shown how in the amphibian brain, probably in response to new evolutionary challenges presented by life on land, the olfactory apparatus and its central connections and representations were gradually modified leading to increasing differentiation of neuronal cell groups and their specific connections within the ventrolateral forebrain. In the course of this process of differentiation an identifiable primordial amygdala with its well-defined afferent and efferent projection systems seems to have made its first appearance in evolutionary history. The evolutionary innovation, which according to Herrick probably initiated this important reorganization of the brain, was the development of an open passage between the nasal pit containing the olfactory placode and the oropharyngeal cavity. *Pari passu* with this opening of the choanae, a new sensory apparatus, the vomeronasal organ of Jacobson, developed and this led to the differentiation of an accessory olfactory bulb and of its projection system, the ventrolateral olfactory tract ending in a newly differentiated area of grey matter, the primordial amygdala. Little is known about the functional significance of the vomeronasal organ; it seems to have lost much of its importance beyond the reptilian stage of vertebrate evolution. Yet apparently it must have conveyed to the brain of the ancestral land vertebrates, the type of information which necessitated for the first time a clear-cut differentiation of central "rhinencephalic" from "nonrhinencephalic" structures. The former included the important vomeronasal inflow; the latter, further in the course of evolution, gave origin to the striatum and neocortex.

Among amphibian forms still living today, this first step in the development of a clearly identifiable amygdaloid system is found in the brain of tailless amphibians (anura), such as in that of frogs and toads. Herrick's paper of 1921 gives a good account not only of the relevant evolutionary history but also very clearly describes the pattern of connections of the anuran primordial amygdala and its projections to the septal region and the hypothalamus. The most interesting point which emerges from his work, is that the amygdala at the very onset of its evolutionary history laid down a pattern of descending connections to which it has remained faithfully committed throughout the whole span of phylogeny up to and including man. Throughout this time span of millions of years, this pattern suffered only some distortion caused by the enormous development of the mammalian neocortex and the thalamocortical connection systems incorporated in the internal capsule. The fundamental arrangement of the descending connections of the amygdala, however, remained essentially unaffected by this tremendous reorganization of the anatomy of the cerebral hemispheres. In contrast to this conservatism with regard to the descending pathways, the irony of evolutionary history has been that the phylogenetic innovation which provided the initial impetus for the development of the amygdaloid system—namely, the ingrowth of connections from the vomeronasal organ—virtually disappeared again in the more highly developed mammalian brain. Indeed it seems that the most fundamental information we are lacking concerning the mammalian amygdala is that concerning the origins and the organization of its afferent input.

Since very little is known about these afferent connections and because our own work has not been concerned with their study, this review will deal with the organization of the descending amygdaloid projection system and especially with those connections directed towards the ventromedial region of the hypothalamus.

Figure 4–1, taken from Herrick's 1921 paper, demonstrates the fundamental arrangement of amygdaloid connections found in the brains of tailless amphibians. In these forms the amygdala occupies the ventrolateral area of the primitive hemisphere. It gives rise to two descending projection systems, a dorsal and a ventral one, each subdivided into an anterior and posterior portion. The dorsal system is separated from the ventral system by a well-defined fiber tract, the lateral forebrain bundle, which contains mainly ascending fibers of the somatic nervous system which originate at lower brain stem levels and end in the primitive striatum with some fibers also contributing to the primordial neopallium. The anterior portion of the dorsal amygdaloid projection system is called the stria terminalis. It runs forward and medialward to connect with the septum and the preoptic nucleus. The posterior portion of the dorsal system is called the dorsal olfactory projection tract. It is directed backward and medialward to connect with the hypothalamus, more specifically with a well-defined cell mass, the nucleus of the dorsal olfactory tract. Both systems seem to be the homologues of the mammalian stria terminalis. The ventral amygdaloid projection system again is divided into an anterior and posterior portion, the anterior one being the diagonal band of Broca which, after passing ventrally to the lateral forebrain bundle, reaches the septum. The posterior one is the ventral olfactory projection tract directed backward and medialward passing below the lateral forebrain bundle and establishing connections with the preoptic nucleus and the hypothalamus.

This basic pattern of connections, with

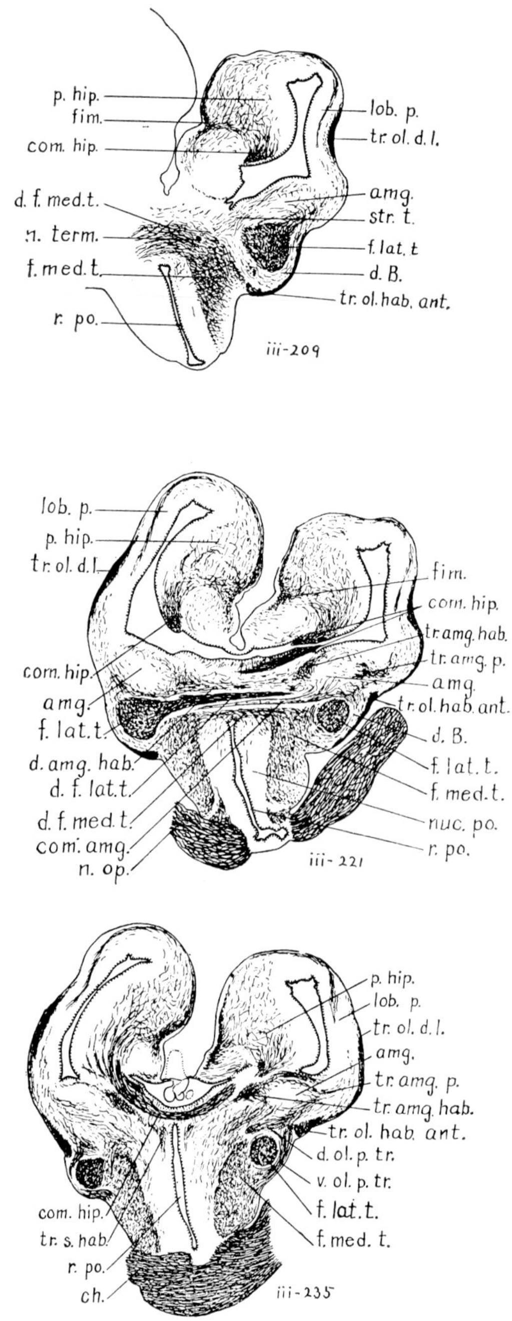

Figure 4–1. Transverse sections through the brain of a frog (*Rana pipiens*) prepared by the silver method of Cajal. The uppermost section is taken immediately rostral to the intraventricular foramen, the middle section is taken through the intraventricular foramen and the anterior commissure, and the lowermost section is taken immediately caudad to the intraventricular foramen. The figures show how the dorsal (str.t., d. ol. p.tr.) and the ventral (d.B., v.ol. p.tr.) amygdaloid projection systems after originating from the amygdala (amg.) are separated from each other in their downward course by the lateral forebrain bundle (f.lat.t.). *Abbreviations:* amg. (nucleus amygdalae), ch. (chiasma opticum), com.amg. (commissure amygdalarum), com.hip. (commissure hippocampi), d.amg.hab. (decussation of tractus amygdalohabenularis), d.B. (diagonal band of Broca), d.f.lat.t. (decussation of lateral forebrain bundles), d.med.t. (decussation of medial forebrain bundles), d.ol.p.tr. (dorsal olfactory projection tract), fim. (fimbria), f.lat.t. (fasciculus lateralis telencephali [lateral forebrain bundle]), f.med.t. (fasciculus medialis telencephali [medial forebrain bundle]), lob.p (lobus piriform), n.op. (nervus opticus), n.term. (nervus terminalis), nuc.po. (nucleus preopticus), p.hip. (primordium hippocampi), r.po. (recessus preopticus), str.t. (stria terminalis), tr.amg.hab. (tractus amygdalohabenularis), tr.amg.p. (tractus amygdalopiriformis), tr.ol.d.t. (tractus olfactorius dorsolateralis), tr.ol.hab.ant. (tractus olfactohabenularis anterior), tr.s.hab. (tractus septohabenularis), v.ol.p.tr. (ventral olfactory projection tract). (From Herrick, J.: *J. Comp. Neurol., 33*:213, 1921.)

a dorsal and a ventral system (the former passing in a dorsal and the latter passing in a ventral position to the lateral forebrain bundle), remained unchanged in the course of further phylogenetic evolution. In mammals, the lateral forebrain bundle undergoes a very great expansion, for its dorsal peduncle evolves into the enormous fiber system of the internal capsule which establishes the main connections between the thalamus and the neocortex. Its great increase in size is linked with the tremendous expansion of the cerebral neocortex. This forces the stria terminalis (together with the tail of the caudate nucleus) to take a long semicircular, looping course around the bulky mass of the internal capsule. In this process the dorsal amygdaloid projection system becomes widely separated from the ventral one, the latter retaining its primitive position at the base of the hemisphere. This is the anatomical arrangement which is found in all mammalian brains including that of man (Figs. 4–2 and 4–3).[16] It is evident, however, that throughout the long scale of evolution each of the two systems has retained to a remarkable degree both its anatomical identity and the general layout of its descending connections.

It seems probable that this conservatism responds to a basic biological need and that the two systems, besides their anatomical individuality, possess and retain a very distinct physiological identity.

In studies carried out in our laboratory

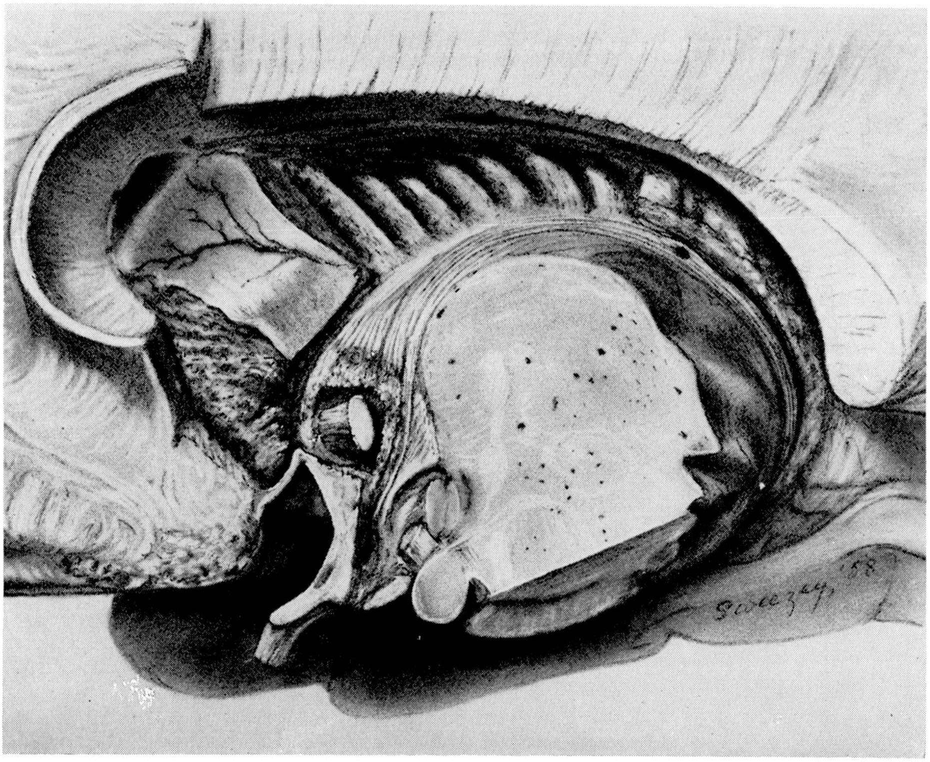

Figure 4–2. Course of the stria terminalis in the adult human brain. Fiber dissection preparation of a right cerebral hemisphere seen from its medial aspect. The stria terminalis can be seen to sweep around the mass of the thalamus and internal capsule, emerging into view where the temporal lobe of the lateral ventricle turns upward. The bundle then fans out anteriorly with some fibers entering the bed nucleus of the stria terminalis surrounding the anterior commissure. The posterior bundle can be seen to descend into the hypothalamus toward the infundibular region. The anterior portion of the tail of the caudate nucleus has been removed to expose the internal capsule behind it as its bundles begin to enter the corona radiata. Also resected were the fornix (except for its last portion entering the mammillary body), the septum pellucidum and the subcallosal area. The medial part of the thalamus was sliced away. (From Klingler, J., and Gloor, P.: *J. Comp. Neurol., 115*:333, 1960).

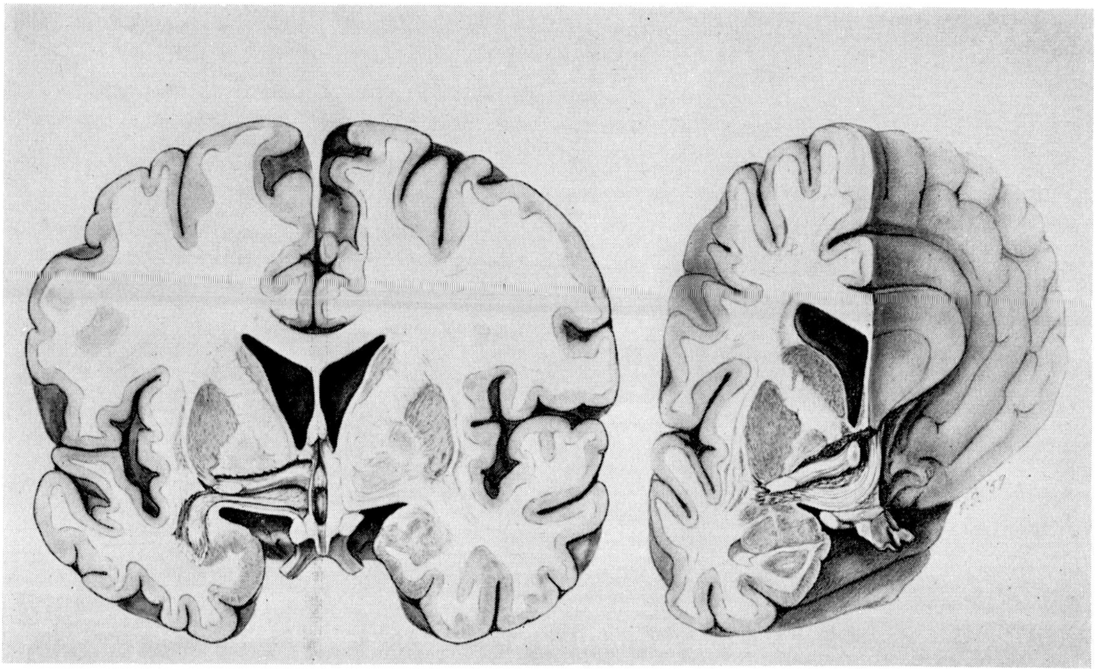

Figure 4–3. The ventral amygdalofugal system in the human brain. Fiber dissection preparations. The specimen on the left side shows a frontal brain slice through the anterior part of the amygdala just behind the anterior commissure. The slice is viewed from its posterior aspect. It shows fibers originating in the lateral part of the amygdala streaming upward and then turning medially beneath the anterior commissure in the sublenticular passage and heading towards the hypothalamus. The specimen on the right is an oblique posteromedial view of the anterior part of the left cerebral hemisphere cut in a frontal plane at a slightly oblique angle from lateral and posterior to medial and anterior. (The amygdala is cut through more posteriorly and the septal region is sliced through more anteriorly than in the specimen on the left.) Part of the ventral amygdalofugal system directed towards the septal region (subcallosal gyrus and paraolfactory area) is shown to emerge from the superior aspect of the amygdada and to curve toward the septal area below the anterior commissure. (From Klingler, J., and Gloor, P.: *J. Comp. Neurol., 115*:333, 1960.)

in the 1950's and again a few years ago, we have tried to explore with electrophysiological means the organization of the descending amygdaloid projection systems and the neurophysiological mechanisms of their actions upon recipient ventromedial hypothalamic neurons.

In the early work done in the 1950's [10,11] single shock and repetitive stimulation of the amygdala was performed in the cat, and the evoked responses were mapped throughout the forebrain and midbrain.

These experiments showed that the amygdaloid projects to a large area of the basal forebrain which extend from the septum through the preoptic area, the hypothalamus and part of the midline thalamus to the upper brain stem tegmentum. Evoked responses could be elicited in all these regions, although in some areas repetitive stimulation was necessary to bring the responses to light.

Within this large projection field, short latency responses, presumably mediated over direct pathways or through connections involving at least only one synapse, were concentrated in the region of the base of the septum, the preoptic area and the anterior hypothalamus. A further analysis of these results indicated that it was impossible that the responses in this primary projection field elicited by stimulation of the basolateral amygdala could have been relayed by the stria terminalis. Indeed as Figure 4–4 shows, basolateral amygdaloid stimulation induced only long latency responses of the order of 15 msec in the stria terminalis, while eliciting responses with latencies of less than 7 msec in the primary projection field in the preoptic region. Obviously this excluded the dorsal amygdaloid projection system of the stria terminalis as being the pathway mediating these responses. Conversely, stimulation of the corticomedial amygdala elicited short latency responses of the order of 6 to 7 msec in the stria terminalis which indicated that the dorsal amygdaloid projection system of the stria terminalis originated within the corticomedial subdivision. It therefore seemed likely that the short latency responses to basolateral amygdaloid stimulation recorded in the preoptic region were mediated by the more direct ventral amygdalofugal fiber system.

In the course of this earlier work, it also became apparent that the ventromedial nucleus of the hypothalamus represented a particularly important focal point of projection of both the dorsal and ventral amygdaloid projection systems, since particularly large evoked responses could be recorded in this nucleus in response to both basolateral and corticomedial amygdaloid stimulation. We have recently reinvestigated the descending amygdaloid projections, particularly those to the ventromedial region of the hypothalamus, by using more modern techniques which included the recording of extracellular action potentials with tungsten microelectrodes, the plotting of poststimulus time histograms of unitary spike discharges with a CAT computer and comparing of the latter with computer-averaged evoked responses.[4,19]

Both the analysis of single-cell discharges and of evoked slow wave responses confirmed the previous supposition that the ventromedial nucleus received a relatively direct and powerful input from both the dorsal and the ventral amygdaloid projection system. Thus, contrary to what one might have expected from previously published anatomical data, the latencies of action potentials recorded in the ventromedial nucleus in response to basal amygdaloid stimulation were shorter than those of action potentials recorded in the dorsal or lateral hypothalamus in the same frontal stereotaxic plane (Fig. 4–5).

Furthermore, the evoked slow wave responses in the ventromedial nucleus of the hypothalamus were much larger in amplitude than in surrounding areas. Two distinctly different responses were found, depending upon whether the corticomedial or the basolateral amygdaloid subdivision were stimulated. Each response differed from the other in both waveform and latency, and each remained essentially unchanged in its morphology throughout the entire extent of the ventromedial hypothalamic nucleus. Figure 4–6 shows that stimulation within the corticomedial amygdala produced a long latency response consisting essentially of a large, positive slow wave which occasionally was preceded by a small negative deflection. The onset latency of this response was of the order of 11 msec. If the stimulating electrode in the corticomedial amygdala which had been used to elicit this response

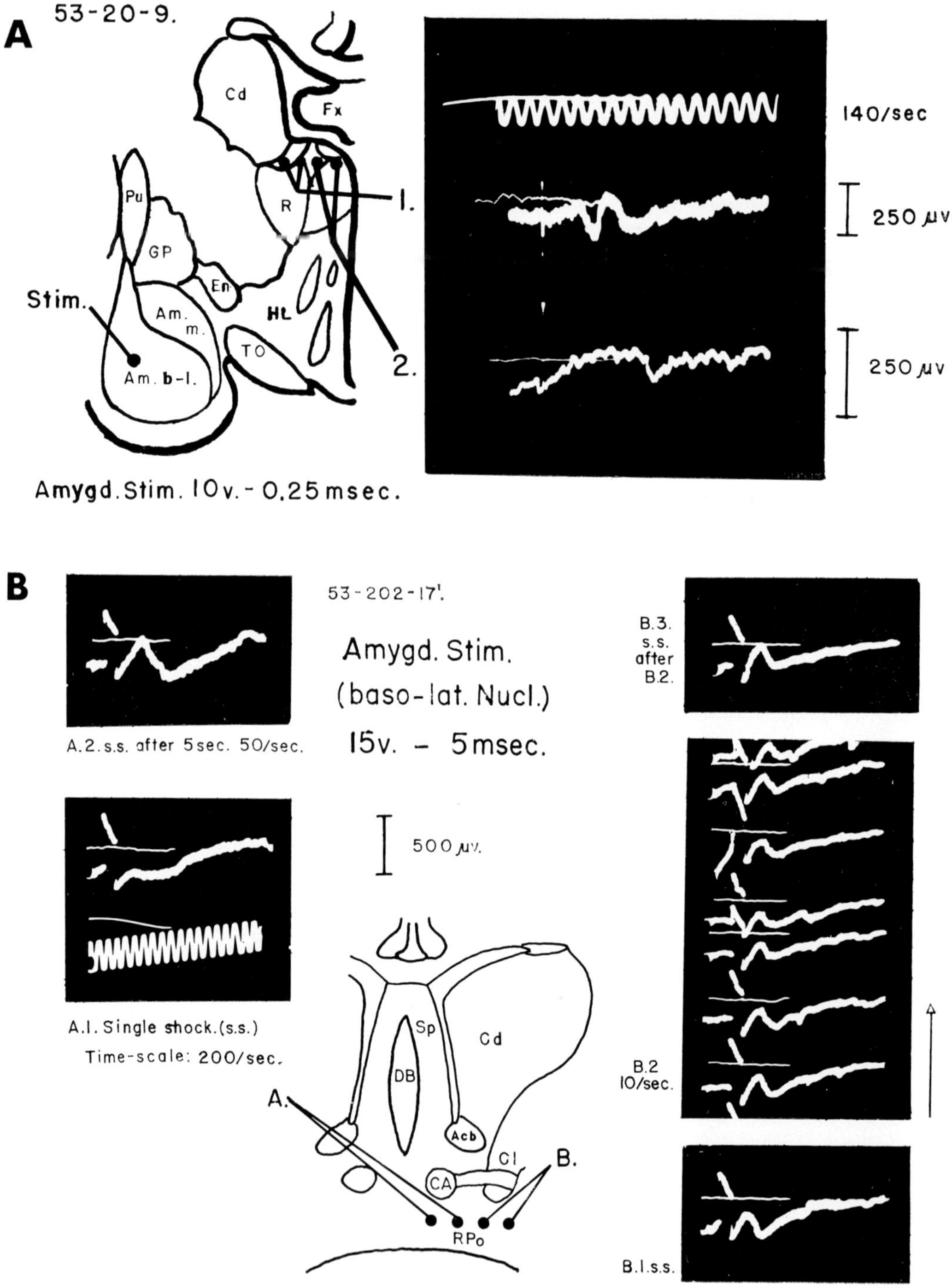
A
53-20-9.
Cd
Fx
Pu
R
GP
En
Stim.
Am. m.
HL
TO
Am. b-l.
1.
2.
140/sec
250 µv
250 µv
Amygd. Stim. 10v. - 0.25 msec.
B
53-202-17'.
Amygd. Stim.
(baso-lat. Nucl.)
15v. - 5 msec.
A.2. s.s. after 5 sec. 50/sec.
500 µv.
A.1. Single shock. (s.s.)
Time-scale: 200/sec.
Sp
Cd
DB
Acb
Cl
CA
A.
B.
RPo
B.3. s.s. after B.2.
B.2 10/sec.
B.1. s.s.

Figure 4–4.

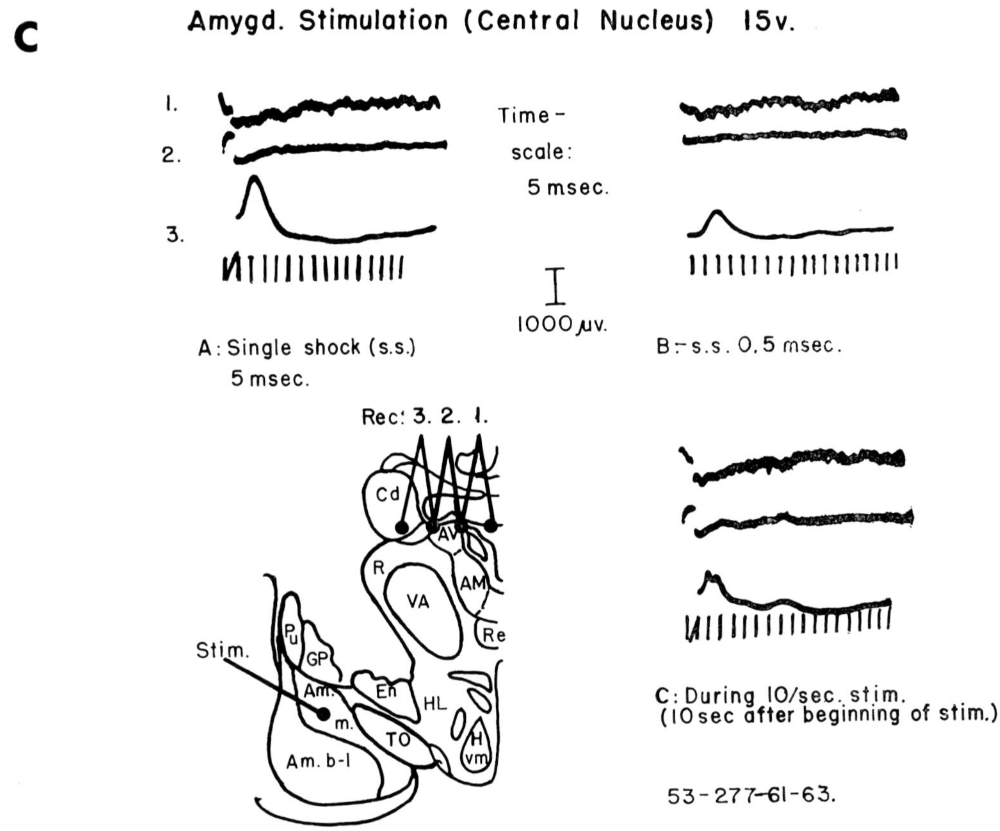

Figure 4–4. (*A*) Long latency (14 msec) response in the stria terminalis (record 1) elicited by stimulation in the basolateral amygdala. (*B*) Short latency responses (5 to 6 msec) elicited in the preoptic region by stimulation in the basolateral amygdala. (*C*) Short latency (6 msec) responses in the stria terminalis (record 3) elicited by stimulation in the corticomedial amygdala (central nucleus). (From Gloor, P.: *Electroenceph. Clin. Neurophysiol.*, *7*:223, 243, 1955.)

was lowered by only a fraction of a millimeter, such that it penetrated the basolateral amygdala, there was a sudden dramatic change of the evoked response in the ventromedial hypothalamic nucleus which now assumed the form of a diphasic, short latency (7 msec), initially negative wave. With further penetration of the stimulating electrode through the basolateral amygdala, this response did not show any further significant change. Figure 4–7 clearly demonstrates that both responses were virtually confined to the ventromedial nucleus of the hypothalamus, and they quickly faded away and lost their specific morphology as soon as the recording electrode was placed outside the region of this nucleus.

These results suggested that the large predominantly positive response elicited with corticomedial stimulation was mediated over the dorsal projection system of the stria terminalis, whereas the shorter latency, diphasic response was mediated over the ventral projection system consisting of the ventral amygdalofugal fibers coursing towards the hypothalamus through the sublenticular passage. The

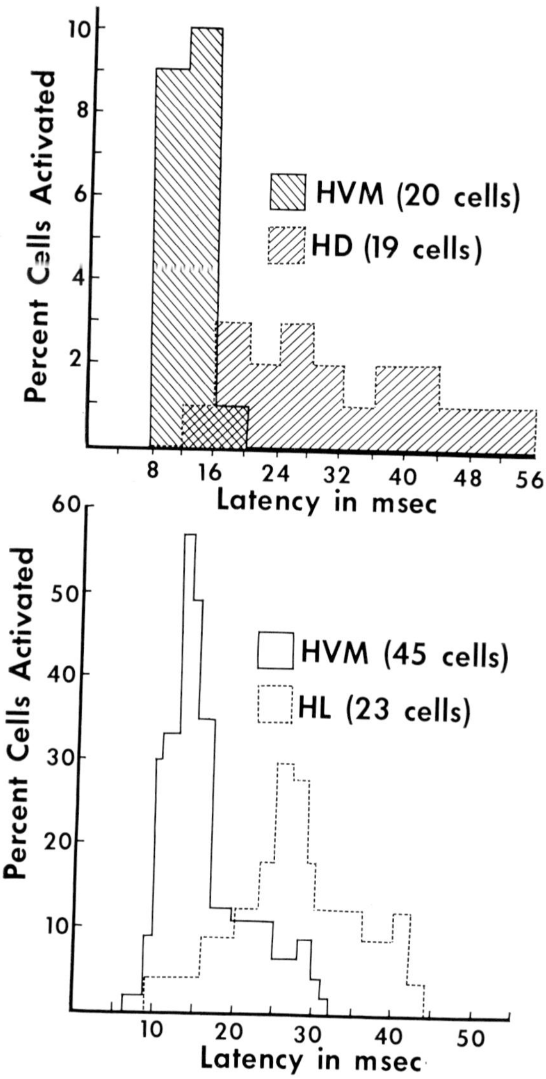

Figure 4–5. Latency distribution of single unit responses to basolateral amygdaloid stimulation in the region of the ventromedial nucleus of the hypothalamus (HVM), the dorsal hypothalamus (HD) and the lateral hypothalamus (HL).

former will therefore henceforth be called the ST response and the latter the VAF response.

Evidence that this conclusion was correct was obtained by the following two sets of experiments:

1. Direct stimulation of the stria terminalis in the floor of the lateral ventricle where it runs in the groove between the tail of the caudate nucleus and the thalamus elicited the ST response in the ventromedial nucleus of the hypothalamus. In contrast, stimulation in the sublenticular passage where the ventral amygdaloid projection system runs elicited the VAF response in the same nucleus.

2. The ST response could be selectively abolished by sectioning the stria terminalis in the floor of the body of the lateral

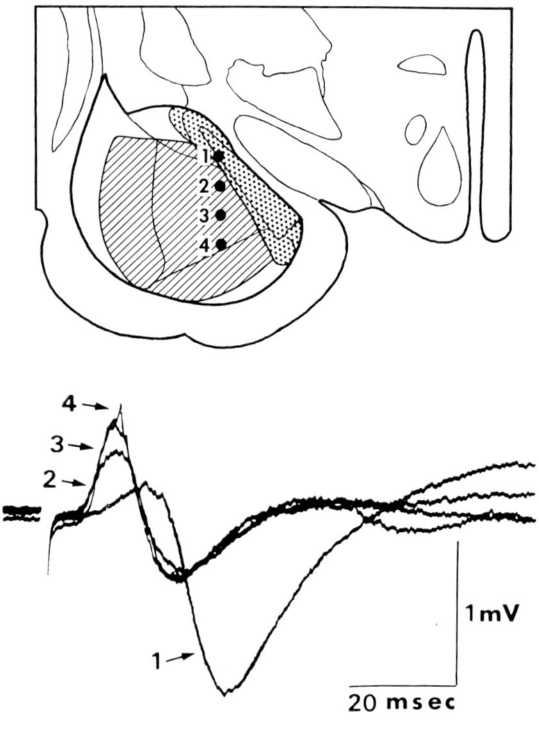

Figure 4–6. (*Top*) Map of the amygdala with reference to the two types of slow potentials recorded in the ventromedial hypothalamic nucleus. Two types are recorded: one from the corticomedial amygdala (stippled area), the other from the basolateral complex (hatched area). (*Bottom*) Representative examples of the two types of slow potentials recorded in the ventromedial nucleus during vertical displacement of a stimulating electrode from points 1 to 4. In this and subsequent figures upward deflection represents negative polarity. (From Dreifuss, J. J., Murphy, J. T., and Gloor, P.: *J. Neurophysiol.*, *31*:237, 1968.)

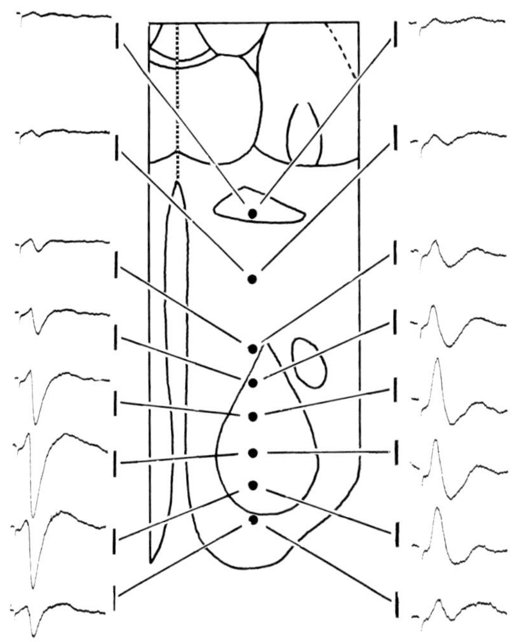

Figure 4–7. The responses evoked by corticomedial amygdaloid stimulation and mediated by the stria terminalis (*left column*) as well as the responses evoked by basolateral amygdaloid stimulation and mediated by the VAF system (*right column*) are virtually confined to the ventromedial hypothalamic nucleus. Calibration 1 mv (vertical) and 50 msec (horizontal). (From Dreifuss, J. J., Murphy, J. T., and Gloor, P.: *J. Neurophysiol., 31*:237, 1968.)

ventricle, at a site far remote from the amygdala. Such a section left the VAF response intact (Fig. 4–8). Conversely section of the ventral amygdaloid projection system along a sagittal plane by means of a stereotactically introduced iridectomy knife completely eliminated the VAF response, while leaving the ST response intact. If, subsequent to this procedure, the stria terminalis was also cut, no responses could be elicited any longer in the ventromedial nucleus of the hypothalamus by stimulation of the amygdala (Fig. 4–9). It should be noted that the VAF response could only be eliminated when the sagittal cut was extended from a position lateral to the septum back to one lateral to the infundibular region of the hypothalamus. This indicates that the VAF system is a loose, fan-shaped, fiber system extending over a long anteroposterior distance within the sublenticular passage in contrast to the stria terminalis which is a very compact fiber bundle (Fig. 4–10).

Having established the fact that the dorsal and the ventral amygdaloid projection systems each have a definite electrophysiological identity in terms of evoked potential morphology, the question arose whether this difference between the two systems could be interpreted in terms of different synaptic mechanisms activated by the two pathways at their sites of termination in the ventromedial hypothalamic nucleus. We therefore tried to establish whether the various phases of the ST and VAF response were related in time to a significant increase or decrease of firing probability of single ventromedial

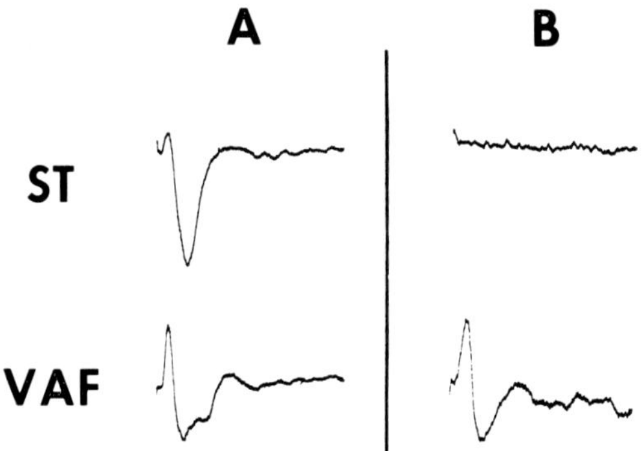

Figure 4–8. (*A*) Evoked potentials in the ventromedial nucleus to corticomedial (ST) and basolateral (VAF) amygdaloid stimulation. (*B*) Response to identical stimulations, but after section of the stria terminalis in the groove between the thalamus and the tail of the caudate nucleus. Note that the ST response has disappeared. *Calibration:* 500μv (vertical); 100 msec (horizontal). (From Dreifuss, J. J., Murphy, J. T., and Gloor, P.: *J. Neurophysiol., 31*:237, 1968.)

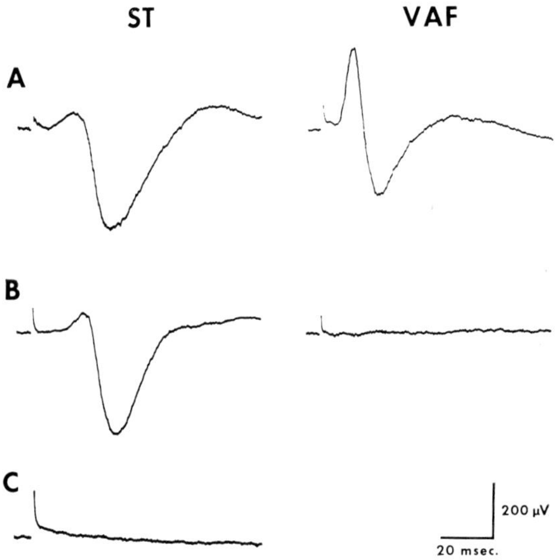

Figure 4–9 (*A*) Evoked potentials recorded in the ventromedial hypothalamic nucleus upon stimulation of the corticomedial (ST) and basolateral (VAF) amygdala. (*B*) Responses recorded in the same animal with identical stimulation but after longitudinal section of the VAF pathway in the sublenticular passage. The VAF response is abolished, the ST response persists. (*C*) Disappearance of all evoked responses in the ventromedial hypothalamic nucleus after additional section of the stria terminalis. (Modified from Dreifuss, J. J., Murphy, J. T., and Gloor, P.: *J. Neurophysiol., 31:*237, 1968.)

hypothalamic neurons. The analysis of raw data (Fig. 4–11) indicated that single unitary action potentials in response to basolateral amygdaloid stimulation tended to occur in conjunction with the negative initial phase of the evoked unitary response. Because these unitary discharges did not in every case occur with the negative deflections of the VAF response, averaging techniques were necessary to confirm the statistical validity of these direct observations. This was even more urgently required for documenting the presence of inhibitory pauses in the ongoing unitary activity, since hypothalamic neurons often fire only at an extremely slow frequency, and it is thus very difficult to detect evidence for inhibition as long as one is restricted to extracellular recording techniques. Two averaging methods were used —namely, simple photographic superimposition of responses on the storage cathode ray tube or computer summation of the slow wave response and comparison of the latter with the poststimulus time histogram of the action potential record from which the slow waves had been eliminated by appropriate filtering. These methods clearly showed that the probability for impulse firing was maximal during the negative deflection of the VAF response and was reduced during the positive phase (Fig. 4–12), whereas for the ST response the probability of firing was drastically reduced during the duration of

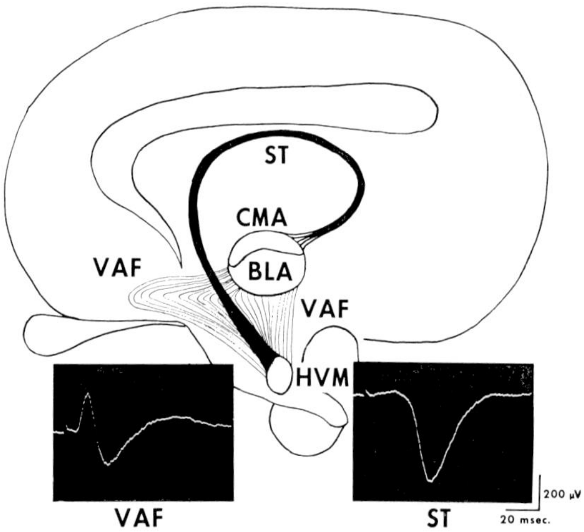

Figure 4–10. The anatomical organization of the two amygdaloid projection systems to the ventromedial nucleus of the hypothalamus. *Abbreviations:* BLA (basolateral amygdala), CMA (corticomedial amygdala), HVM (ventromedial nucleus of the hypothalamus), ST (stria terminalis and stria terminalis-mediated response in the ventromedial nucleus to corticomedial amygdaloid stimulation), VAF (ventral amygdalofugal fiber system and evoked response in the ventromedial nucleus of the hypothalamus mediated by this system upon stimulation of the basolateral amygdala).

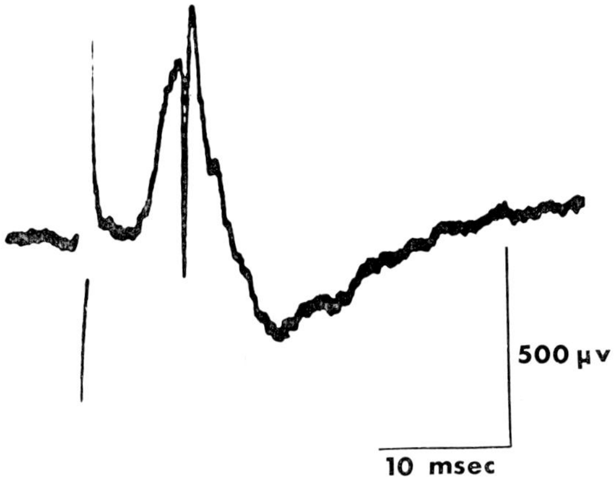

Figure 4–11. Single shock response recorded in the ventromedial nucleus of the hypothalamus to stimulation of the basolateral amygdala. A positive unit spike discharge arises on the crest of the negative phase of the VAF mediated response. *Calibration:* 1 mv and 10 msec.

the main positive deflection (Fig. 4–13). We concluded from this that the basolateral amygdala via its VAF output primarily activates the neurons of the ventromedial hypothalamus and that the negative deflection of the evoked response represents summated EPSPs within this nucleus. This initial activation seems to be followed by a period of secondary inhibition. Conversely the corticomedial amygdala through the stria terminalis seems to provide an inhibitory input to the neurons of the ventromedial nucleus of the hypothalamus.

Although both systems appeared to be functionally antagonistic and to overlap topographically within the neuron population of the ventromedial nucleus, it still remained to be shown whether this convergence of the two pathways extended down to the single cell level. To establish this, it was necessary to demonstrate that one and the same ventromedial neuron was activated by VAF fibers and inhibited by ST fibers. Figure 4–14 demonstrates that this is indeed the case. This illustration shows poststimulus time histograms and averaged slow wave evoked potentials occurring in response to VAF and ST stimulation. These records demonstrate that one and the same ventromedial neuron may be inhibited by ST volleys and excited by VAF volleys. Figure 4–15 shows further evidence for the presence of this convergence and demonstrates how

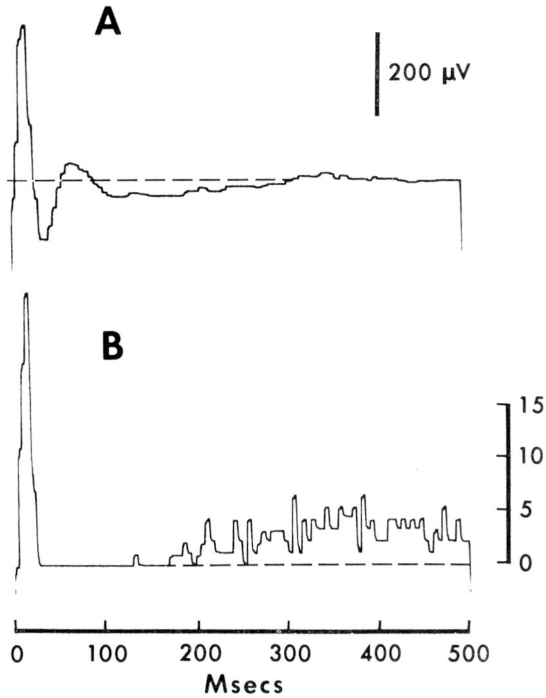

Figure 4–12. Basolateral amygdaloid stimulation. Slow evoked potential (*A*) and poststimulus time histogram of unit firing (*B*) recorded simultaneously through the same microelectrode in the ventromedial nucleus. The time base applies to both records. The evoked slow wave response in A was summated by the CAT computer and in B the poststimulus time histogram was obtained with the same computer, the vertical axis representing the number of action potentials per address summated in 50 consecutive responses. The control firing level was 3 action potentials per address; 400 addresses were used in computing the slow wave; 100 addresses were used in computing the histogram. (From Dreifuss, J. J., Murphy, J. T., and Gloor, P.: *J. Neurophysiol., 31:*237, 1968.)

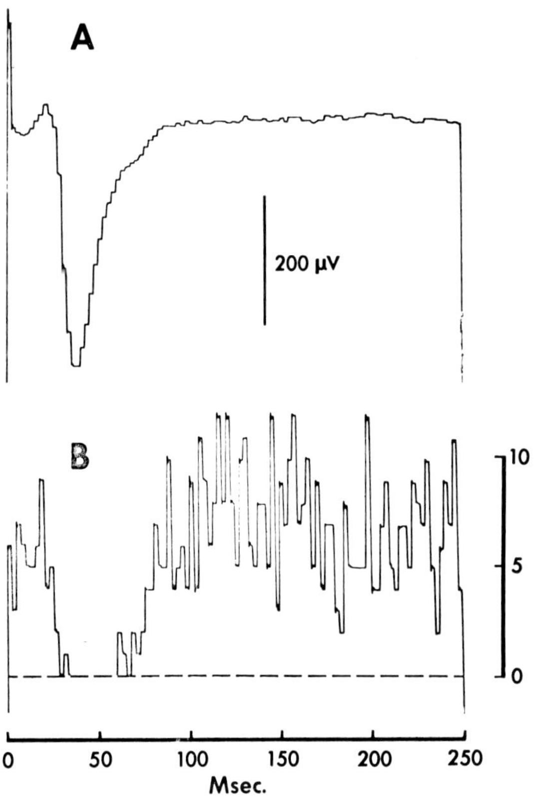

Figure 4–13. Corticomedial amygdaloid stimulation: Slow evoked potential (*A*) and poststimulus time histogram of unit firing (*B*) recorded simultaneously through the same microelectrode in the ventromedial nucleus. Technique as in Figure 4–12; 100 consecutive responses were summated. The control firing level was 6 action potentials per address.

the two synaptic mechanisms interact on an individual ventromedial hypothalamic neuron. The neuron shown in this figure fired off an action potential quite consistently in response to VAF stimulation. These action potentials were closely clustered near the peak of the negative VAF response, as shown in *A*. The same neuron was arrested in its firing during the positive ST slow wave response. The two responses were made to interact in a classical conditioning testing paradigm by applying corticomedial and basolateral stimulation at successively greater intervals. It could thus be demonstrated that the firing probability of the ventromedial neuron was drastically reduced when the latter was under the influence of the ST-evoked inhibition. The curve shown in Figure 4–15, *C*, plotting the time course of reduced firing probability closely espouses the form of the ST-evoked slow wave response. If allowance is made for different latencies in the two pathways, the time functions described by the two curves actually almost match perfectly.

These electrophysiological studies therefore clearly demonstrate that the amygdala projects through two powerful, relatively direct pathways to the ventromedial nucleus of the hypothalamus, establishing positive control of the firing of ventromedial neurons via the VAF system originating in the basolateral amygdala and negative control via the ST system, originating in the corticomedial amygdala. In terms of classical neuroanatomy these rather direct inputs into the ventromedial nucleus are somewhat surprising. Among the older neuroanatomical literature only the work of Adey and Meyer [1] showed some direct connections from the amygdala to the ventromedial hypothalamic nucleus. The traditional descriptions of the connections of the hypothalamus have always emphasized that both the stria terminalis and the ventral amygdaloid projection system are feeding into the medial forebrain bundle and that hence any further connections to other hypothalamic areas would secondarily branch off from presumed relays in the lateral hypothalamus. Clearly both our latency measurements in the lateral hypothalamus and the absence of any very striking evoked potentials in other regions than the ventromedial nucleus suggest that this anatomical concept has to be revised. Fortunately, recent work by Heimer and Nauta [13] has

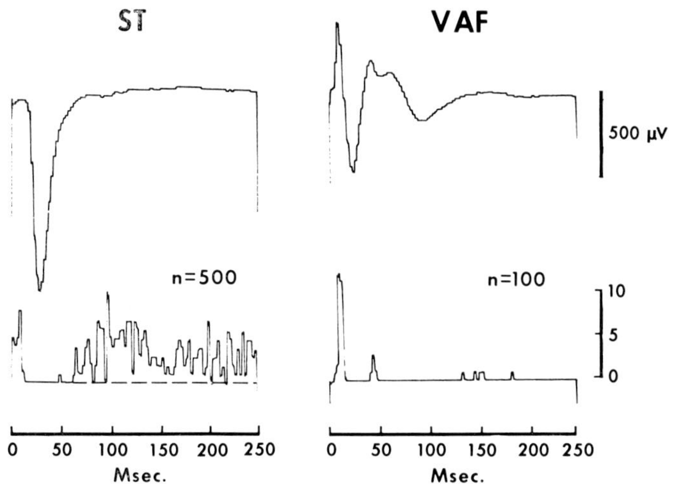

Figure 4–14. (*ST*) Evoked slow potential and poststimulus time histogram of a ventromedial hypothalamic neuron with stimulation of corticomedial amygdala. There is decrease in cell firing during the positive slow potential. (*VAF*) Recording from the same ventromedial hypothalamic neuron, but with stimulation of the basolateral amygdala. There is increased cell firing during negative transients of the slow evoked potential. The letter *n* represents the number of CAT sweeps in the poststimulus time histograms. The vertical axis represents the number of action potentials per CAT address; the control firing level was 3 (*lower left*) and 0.6 (*lower right*) action potentials per address. Four hundred addresses were used to compute the slow potentials, 100 for the histograms. (From Dreifuss, J. J., Murphy, J. T., and Gloor, P.: *J. Neurophysiol.*, *31*:237, 1968.)

demonstrated a direct projection of the stria terminalis to the ventromedial nucleus. The terminal degeneration of this pathway is concentrated in the perinuclear zone probably occupied by the radiating dendrites of ventromedial neurons. Anatomical evidence for a direct or at least oligosynaptic connection from the basolateral amygdala through the ventral amygdaloid projection system to the ventromedial nucleus is however still lacking.

It has thus clearly been established that as far as the ventromedial nucleus is concerned, the dorsal amygdaloid projection system through the stria terminalis is an inhibitory system, whereas the VAF pathway is essentially an excitatory one, even though the excitatory effects are followed by inhibition. Whether this functional dichotomy of the two descending amygdaloid projection systems also applies to other amygdaloid projection areas in the basal forebrain remains unknown. The question evidently arises, however, whether or not the definite functional identity which each of these two amygdaloid projection systems to the ventromedial hypothalamus discloses in electrophysical studies can be translated into specific differences of their biological significance for the organism. Although it is certainly premature to make any definite statements with regard to such a possibility, there are a number of observations, summarized in Table 4–1, which suggest that the corticomedial amygdala with its stria terminalis outflow and the basolateral amygdala with its ventral amygdalofugal outflow subserve biologically distinct functions. What we do not know, however, is to what extent these differences which have been obtained mainly in behavioral

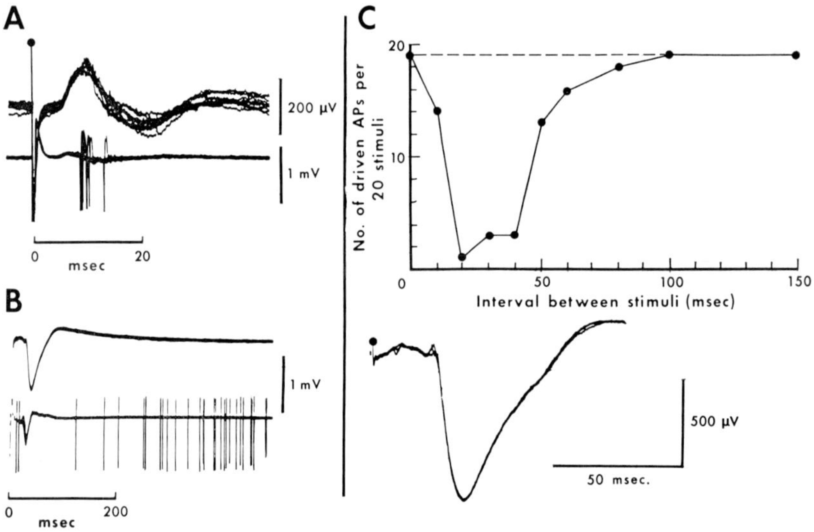

Figure 4–15. (*A*) Photographic superimposition (10 sweeps) of the unfiltered (*upper trace*) and filtered (*lower trace*) records obtained from a ventromedial hypothalamic neuron during stimulation of the basolateral amygdala. The action potentials occur regularly at a short latency after stimulation. (*B*) Inhibition of firing at the same ventromedial hypothalamic neuron during corticomedial stimulation (25 superimposed sweeps). (*C*) (*Top*) Reduction of number of action potentials driven by basolateral amygdaloid stimulation when a shock was applied to the corticomedial amygdala at various intervals before the test stimulus was delivered to the basolateral amygdala. The dotted line represents the control level, obtained with basolateral stimulation alone. (*Bottom*) The corticomedial-induced slow potential shifted to the left by 15 msec with respect to the above graph, in order to take into account the difference in conduction time of the two amygdaloid efferent pathways, mirrors the time function of the basal amygdaloid drive of this ventromedial hypothalamic neuron during the double shock study. (From Dreifuss, J. J., Murphy, J. T., and Gloor, P.: *J. Neurophysiol., 31*:237, 1968.)

studies reflect activities mediated over those portions of the dorsal and ventral amygdalofugal systems which make synaptic contacts with the neurons of the ventromedial hypothalamic nucleus.

Among the behavioral studies which indicate that a dichotomy of the amygdala along the lines of its two main nuclear subdivisions and respective projection systems exists are those concerned with attack and defense, or approach-and-avoidance behavior and their endocrine corollary of ACTH discharge by the anterior pituitary. Hilton and Zbrozyna [15] have shown that stimulation of the basolateral amygdala produces a typical defense reaction and that the integrity of the stria terminalis for the reaction is not required. However, section of the ventral amygdalofugal system abolishes this response. The fact that Fernandez de Molina and Hunsperger [9] have been able to elicit a defense reaction by stimulation of the stria terminalis does not appear to be in conflict with this view, since Hilton and Zbrozyna have demonstrated that after section of the stria terminalis, the aggressive response to stimulation of the stria can only be elicited if electrical stimulation is applied above the cut in the part of the

TABLE 4–1
FUNCTIONAL LOCALIZATION IN AMYGDALA

	Attack & Defense	Approach & Avoidance	ACTH Secretion	Food Intake	Sexual Maturation	Sexual Behavior
Cortico-Medial Group of Nuclei (Stria Terminalis)	–	Approach, Self-Stimulation	–	+	–	+?
Baso-Lateral Group of Nuclei (VAF)	+	Avoidance, Escape	+	–	?	–?

stria still connected to the amygdala, but not when it is applied below the cut. This suggests that the defense response elicited by stria terminalis stimulation is caused by afferent inflow into the amygdala and that the stria terminalis does not serve as the efferent pathway for this particular response.

Closely related to these findings are those of Wurtz and Olds,[26] who studied rats with chronically implanted electrodes and found that self-stimulation could only be elicited with electrodes implanted in the corticomedial division of the amygdala, whereas placements in the basolateral amygdala resulted in escape behavior.

The role of the amygdaloid nucleus in modifying the output of ACTH from the anterior pituitary is probably closely related to these behavioral studies. Our own investigations with Bovard,[3] as well as those reported by Eleftheriou and his coworkers,[5,6] indicate that the corticomedial area of the amygdala inhibits ACTH secretion and that probably the release of ACTH which occurs in response to stimulation of the amygdala is mediated by neurons of the basolateral system discharging over the ventral amygdalofugal pathway.

In view of the fact that the ventromedial nucleus of the hypothalamus is implicated in the control of food intake, studies on modification of food intake in response to amygdaloid stimulation and lesions are of interest with respect to our topic. Again these studies have suggested that the corticomedial and basolateral amygdala may act in an antagonistic fashion in this regard. Lewinska[17] has shown that lesions of the basal nucleus produced an increase in intake of solid and liquid food, whereas lesions involving the corticomedial group of the amygdala render the animals at first totally aphagic. This aphagia is followed by only partial recovery of eating and drinking behavior. She concludes that the corticomedial part of the amygdala is largely concerned with positive control of food intake, whereas the basal nucleus is involved in the inhibitory control of feeding. Since the basal nucleus discharges to the ventromedial nucleus over the VAF system, one may be tempted to speculate that this inhibition of feeding mechanisms elicited from the basal amygdaloid nucleus may be caused by an activation of ventromedial hypothalamic neurons through the VAF input since the ventromedial nucleus of the hypothalamus is thought to represent the neural substrate of the "satiety center."

Finally there are some studies on sexual function which may have some bearing upon the functional and anatomical duality of the two amygdaloid projection systems. Thus Elwers and Critchlow[7,8] and Bar-

Sela and Critchlow[2] have shown that the corticomedial group of nuclei and the stria terminalis are probably involved in delaying sexual maturation in young rats. Section of the stria terminalis produces precocious puberty in these animals; conversely, daily stimulation of the corticomedial nuclei delays sexual maturation. However, whether the basolateral group exerts an antagonistic effect in this respect is unknown. There is also some evidence to suggest that the corticomedial group may be involved in facilitating sexual behavior and in inducing ovulation.[5,6,24,25] Whether the basolateral group exerts the opposite effect is unclear.

In the light of these findings, one may well wonder what relationship, if any, may exist between these mechanisms of attack, defense, approach-and-avoidance, food intake and sexual functions which the amygdala subserves in the mammal and the evolutionary pressures which, once in the distant past, led to the development of that obscure vomeronasal organ which seems to have induced the development of an individualized amygdala and its dual projection system. Herrick,[14] in his classical paper of 1921, speculates that in early land vertebrates this organ subserved what the Germans call *Spürsinn,* a term difficult to translate into English. It denotes a drive mechanism involving exploratory behavior concerned with the analysis of sensory cues related to food intake, tracking of a prey, avoidance of an enemy and the search for a sexual mate. Herrick points out that in the snake the opening of the paired vomeronasal organ is so fashioned as to neatly admit the pointed tips of the serpent's forked tongue which, in this group of reptiles, is an organ which very effectively subserves the *Spürsinn.* It is therefore conceivable that the vomeronasal organ, in spite of its virtual disappearance in higher mammals, nevertheless, left an enduring legacy in the organization of the brain of higher vertebrates in the form of a neural substrate, which now, in higher forms, in addition to olfactory and oral tactile and gustatory cues, has to process data derived from all other sense organs as well as from the mnemonic depositories of the individual's past. These, at least in the human brain, as Penfield's studies on the temporal lobe of man have shown can most easily be accessed from the temporal neocortex which is closely related to the amygdala.[12,18,20-23] For a primitive vertebrate such as an amphibian, the ancestral memories encoded in the genes and expressed in fixed neural mechanisms are probably largely sufficient to subserve the biological needs of survival; in the mammal, and especially in man, the individual life history—that is, learned behavioral patterns—have been evolved as a behavioral superstructure built upon genetically determined ancestral drive mechanisms. This new evolutionary step requires a closer association of limbic structures, such as the amygdala, with the neocortex, and this is reflected in the peculiar mammalian and especially in human anatomy and physiology of this region.[12,16] The place where this fascinating interaction between our individual past and our ancestral heritage occurs is the temporal lobe. This explains why this structure holds so much interest for the physiologist, the psychologist and the clinical neurologist alike.

REFERENCES

1. Adey, W. R., and Meyer, M.: Hippocampal and hypothalamic connections of the temporal lobe in monkey. *Brain, 75:*358, 1952.

2. Bar-Sela, E. M., and Critchlow, V.: Delayed puberty following electrical stimulation of amygdala in female rats. *Amer. J. Physiol., 211*:1103, 1966.
3. Bovard, E. W., and Gloor, P.: Effect of amygdaloid lesions on plasma corticosterone response of the albino rat to emotional stress. *Experientia, 17*:521, 1961.
4. Dreifuss, J. J., Murphy, J. T., and Gloor, P.: Contrasting effects of two identified amygdaloid efferent pathways on single hypothalamic neurons. *J. Neurophysiol., 31*:237, 1968.
5. Eleftheriou, B. E., and Zolovick, A. J.: Effect of amygdaloid lesions on oestrous behavior in the deermouse. *J. Reprod. Fert., 11*:451, 1966.
6. Eleftheriou, B. E., Zolovick, A. J., and Pearse, R.: Effect of amygdaloid lesions on putuitary-adrenal axis in the deermouse. *Proc. Soc. Exp. Biol. Med., 122*:1259, 1966.
7. Elwars, M., and Critchlow, V.: Precocious ovarian stimulation following hypothalamic and amygdaloid lesions in rats. *Amer. J. Physiol., 198*:381, 1960.
8. Elwers, M., and Critchlow, V.: Precocious ovarian stimulation following interruption of stria terminalis. *Amer. J. Physiol., 201*:281, 1961.
9. Fernandez de Molina, A., and Hunsperger, R. W.: Central representation of affective reactions in forebrain and brainstem: Electrical stimulation of amygdala, stria terminalis, and adjacent structures. *J. Physiol.* (London), *145*:251, 1959.
10. Gloor, P.: Electrophysiological studies on the connections of the amygdaloid nucleus in the cat. Part I: The neuronal organization of the amygdaloid projection system. *Electroenceph. Clin. Neurophysiol., 7*:223, 1955a.
11. Gloor, P.: Electrophysiological studies on the connections of the amygdaloid nucleus in the cat. Part II: The electrophysiological properties of the amygdaloid projection system. *Electroenceph. Clin. Neurophysiol., 7*:243, 1955b.
12. Gloor, P., and Feindel, W.: Temporal lobe and affective behaviour. In Monnier, M: *Physiologie des vegetativen Nervensystems.* Stuttgart, Hippokniates Verlag, 1963, Vol. II.
13. Heimer, L., and Nauta, W. J. H.: The hypothalamic distribution of the stria terminalis in the rat. *Brain Res., 13*:284, 1969.
14. Herrick, C. J.: The connections of the vomeronasal nerve, accessory olfactory bulb and amygdala in amphibia. *J. Comp. Neurol., 33*:213, 1921.
15. Hilton, S. M., and Zbrozyna, A. W.: Amygdaloid region for defense reactions and its efferent pathways to the brainstem. *J. Physiol. (London), 165*:160, 1963.
16. Klingler, J., and Gloor, P.: The connections of the amygdala and of the anterior temporal cortex in the human brain. *J. Comp. Neurol., 115*:333, 1960.
17. Lewinska, M. K.: Changes in eating and drinking produced by partial amygdala lesions in cat. *Bull. Acad. Pol. Sci. (Ser. Sci. Biol.), 15*:301, 1967.
18. Mullan, S., and Penfield, W.: Illusions of comparative interpretation and emotion. *Arch. Neurol. Psychiat., 81*:269, 1959.
19. Murphy, J. T., Dreifuss, J. J., and Gloor, P.: Topographical differences in the responses of single hypothalamic neurons to limbic stimulation. *Amer. J. Physiol., 214*:1443, 1968.
20. Penfield, W.: Memory mechanisms. *Arch. Neurol. Psychiat., 67*:178, 1952.
21. Penfield, W.: The interpretive cortex. *Science, 129*:1719, 1959.
22. Penfield, W.: The permanent record of the stream of consciousness. *Proc. 14 Int. Congress Psychol. (Montreal)*, 1954, pp. 47.
23. Penfield, W.: The twenty-ninth Maudsley lecture: The role of the temporal cortex in certain psychical phenomena. *J. Ment. Sci., 101*:451, 1955.
24. Shealy, C. N., and Peele, T. L.: Studies on amygdaloid nucleus of cat. *J. Neurophysiol., 20*:125, 1957.
25. Wood, C. D.: Behavioral changes following discrete lesions of temporal lobe seizures. *Neurology (Minneap), 8*:215, 1958.
26. Wurtz, R. H., and Olds, J.: Amygdaloid stimulation and operant reinforcement in the rat. *J. Comp. Psychol., 56*:941, 1963.

Chapter 5

Synaptic Events Produced by Activation of the Two Amygdalofugal Pathways to the Hypothalamic Ventromedial Nucleus

John T. Murphy and Leo P. Renaud

The discussion in the preceding chapter emphasizes that there are two distinct pathways from the amygdala to the ventromedial nucleus of the hypothalamus, each of which can inhibit ventromedial cell firing. In recent investigations,[6,7] we have extended our study of these two pathways with special emphasis on the implication of inhibitory interneurons. In decerebrate or lightly anaesthetized cats, the experimental procedure consisted of stereotaxically lowering concentric steel electrodes into the ventromedial hypothalamus to apply graded stimuli to various perinuclear regions. This allowed a comparison of the effects of these stimulations with those produced by selective activation of either the ventral amygdalofugal or the stria terminalis pathways. Both field potentials and single neuron spike trains could be recorded extracellularly with high-resistance tungsten microelectrodes inserted into the ventromedial nucleus.

A typical field potential recorded in the ventromedial nucleus of the hypothalamus in response to this local stimulation consisted of an initial negativity lasting only a few milliseconds followed by a larger amplitude positive wave lasting about 20 to 45 msec as shown in Figure 5–1. These potentials were of the same form everywhere within the nucleus, differing only in amplitude, with maximums being recorded in the center of the nucleus. No field potentials were recorded outside the nucleus in response to local stimulation, which indicates that the generators are uniform within the nucleus, thus conforming to Lorente de No's "closed field" formulation.[5] The lowest thresholds for producing these field potentials by local stimulation were found at the lateral edge of the nucleus.

It was determined, by interacting local stimulation with ventral amygdalofugal and stria terminalis pathway stimulation respectively, that the positive field produced by local stimulation reflected inhibitory events within the ventromedial nucleus. Moreover, these effects induced by local stimulation facilitated the stria terminalis evoked positivities, when interacted at suitable intervals, showing that each stimulus activated the same fiber or neuronal elements.

It was observed repeatedly that two functionally distinct types of neurons could be detected within the ventromedial nucleus. One type was of relatively large amplitude in extracellular recordings, usually ranging from 0.5 to 4.0 mV. These cells were most commonly found in the central portion of the nucleus: they fired spontaneously at rates of about 1/sec and were characteristically inhibited by both

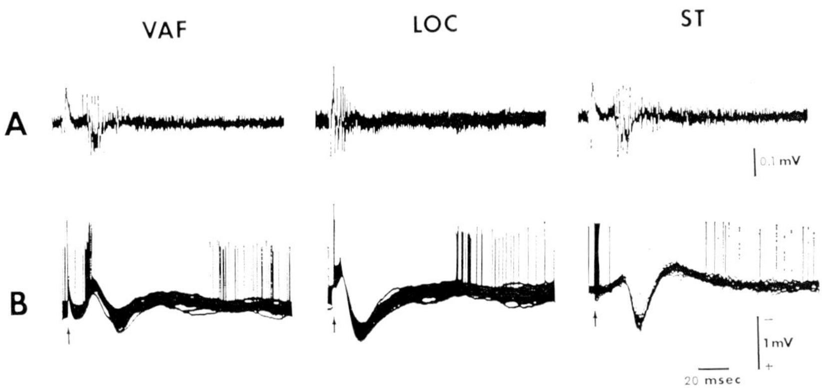

Figure 5–1. (*A*) Convergence of fiber systems activated by ventral amygdalofugal, local and stria terminalis stimulation on the same interneuron. Each tracing represents a single response photographed at high gain after passage through a high-pass filter. Barrage responses produced at a different latency by each pathway are associated in each case with a negative wave B. (*B*) A second unit of larger amplitude recorded at same time as the interneuron in A and photographed at low gain. In addition to being inhibited for about the same duration by all three pathways, this unit was also activated in association with the initial negative wave by ventral amygdalofugal stimulation. The unit channel (high-pass filter) was added to the slow-potential channel (low-pass filter) by the oscilloscope for photography to show the relationship between the unit and slow-wave responses. Each example shows 100 superimposed responses. Arrows refer to onset of stimulation artifact. (From Murphy, J. T., and Renaud, L. P.: *J. Neurophysiol.*, *32*:85, 1969.)

stria terminalis and local stimulation. They responded with activation-depression seqences to stimulation of the ventral amygdalofugal pathway and thus corresponded to those cells examined in previous investigations of the dual amygdaloid pathways.[2,3] These cells are presumably effectors, having long axons. The second type was of small amplitude, usually less than 200μV and rarely fired spontaneously. These cells fired in a rapid burst in response to local stimulation or to stimulation of the ventral amygdalofugal or stria terminalis pathways, the burst usually being about 20 msec in duration and containing 5 to 8 spikes. The duration of the action potential recorded from this latter type of neuron was significantly shorter than that recorded during the brief negativity elicited by any of the stimulations and coincided with the onset of the inhibition of the cells generating the larger amplitude spikes by these stimulations.

We have designated this burst-response cell an inhibitory interneuron. These could most readily be found at the lateral edge of the nucleus but occasionally were recorded within the nucleus. Rarely could activity from both types of neurons be recorded simultaneously by the same microelectrode. An example of such a case is illustrated in Figure 5–1. Two separate channels with different gains and filters were used for this recording. It may be noted that with each stimulation, the interneuron fired with a similar pattern except for the latency (*A*) and that this interneuron was apparently contributing to the inhibition of the neuron producing the larger spike (*B*). It is of interest in this regard that the duration of inhibition, presumably produced in part by this interneuron, was apparently the same in each instance.

An attempt was made to correlate these functional data with the anatomy of this region. Transverse sections through the ventromedial nucleus were stained using the Nissl method. Figure 5–2 shows typical neuronal configurations at high and low magnifications. Our findings confirmed previous Golgi observations that there are primarily two cell types in the ventromedial nucleus of the hypothalamus.[1,8] We found cells of about 7μ in widest diameter with radially bipolar dendritic processes to be concentrated at the perimeter of the nucleus, especially at the lateral edge (Fig. 5–2, upper left). These small cells were usually darkly stained. Larger, paler-staining cells, about 12μ in diameter and having multiple dendritic processes reaching out in various directions, were found in greatest abundance in the central and ventral portions of the nucleus. At times, each of the two different kinds of cell could be found in close proximity. (Fig. 5–2, lower left).

The anatomical and electrophysiological evidence, we believe, best fits the hypothesis that the small bipolar cells at the periphery of the nucleus are inhibitory interneurons which are excited by each af-

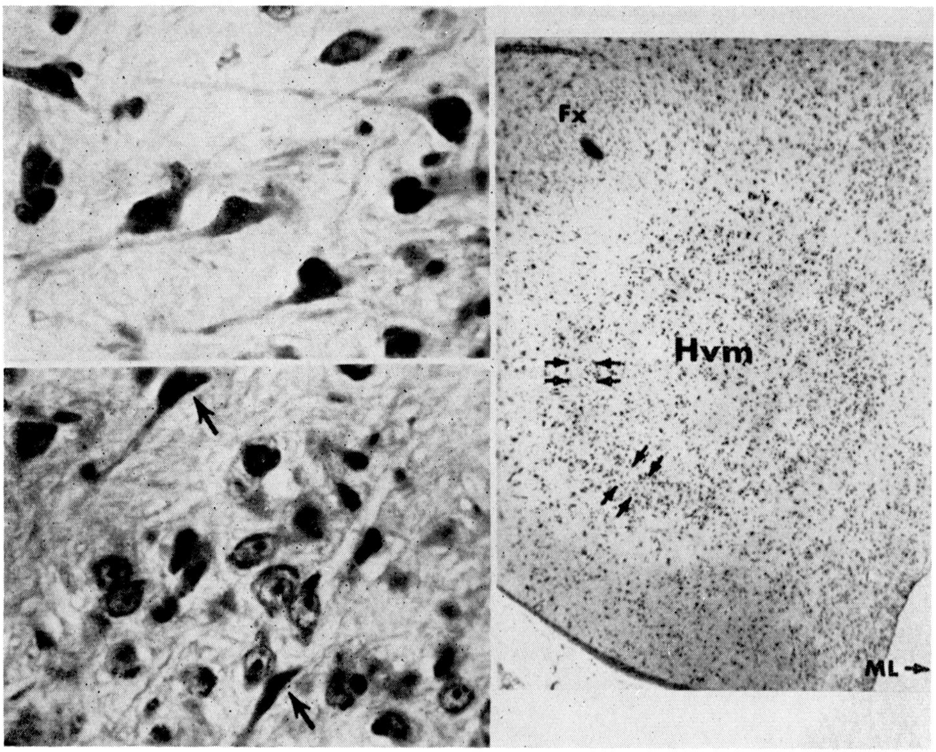

Figure 5–2. Two types of neurons in the ventromedial nucleus of the hypothalamus, thionin-stained sections. (*Right side*) Circular appearance of nucleus as seen under low-power (×50) magnification. Fx, fornix; ML, midline. Photomicrographs at left (×690) were taken from the same section in the areas bounded by the sets of four arrows at right. (*Upper left*) Bipolar neurons at lateral edge of nucleus. Note orientation of dendritic processes. (*Lower left*) Multipolar neurons with round nuclei in ventral portion of nucleus. Arrows indicate nearby bipolar neurons. (From Murphy, J. T., and Renaud, L. P.: *J. Neurophysiol.*, 32:85, 1969.)

ferent amygdaloid pathway, the ventral amydalofugal and the stria terminalis. As a corollary, the larger cells, which presumably are the major effector cells in the nucleus, are the recipients of this inhibition. Supportive evidence for this hypothesis has been obtained, in the case of the stria terminalis in the rat, by the use of the Fink-Heimer method where it was shown that fine terminal endings of the stria terminalis are clustered about the perimeter of the ventromedial nucleus of the hypothalamus (Fig. 5–3).[4] On the basis of latencies, it would appear that the ventral amygdalofugal pathway, which also excites the large cells, exerts its inhibitory influence by a feed-forward mechanism in the same fashion as does the stria terminalis. This hypothesis is schematized in Figure 5–3.

This hypothesis draws attention to some rather interesting points. Firstly, widely divergent effects could be expected as a result of lesioning or stimulating this nucleus, depending upon whether a preponderance of inhibitory interneurons or "effector" cells were involved. Secondly, the hypothesis suggests that the use of terms which imply a singular direction of function for this nucleus, as for example

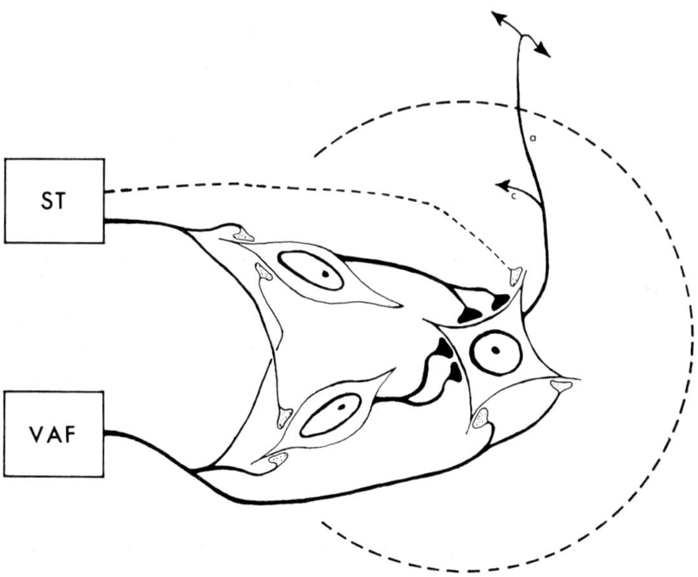

Figure 5–3. Schematic interpretation of experimental results. Light-colored knobs represent excitatory, dark-colored inhibitory presynaptic endings. Cells with bipolar dendritic processes are inhibitory interneurons. Those with multipolar processes are the recipients of this inhibition and are presumably the major effector cells in the ventromedial nucleus. Note manner in which the ventral amygdalofugal pathway might produce excitation-inhibition sequences. The rather ill-defined excitatory effects of the stria terminalis pathway are represented by the dotted line. The major axonal outflow (*a*) from the multipolar neurons courses in a primarily dorsal direction. Axon collaterals within the nucleus exist (*c*), but their termination on inhibitory interneurons is not yet certain. The apparent concentration of inhibitory interneurons at the lateral edge of the nucleus places these neurons in an excellent position to act as transmission cells for the amygdala's inhibitory efferent pathways. (From Murphy, J. T., and Renaud, L. P.: *J. Neurophysiol.*, *32*:85, 1969.)

"satiety center," may be misleading. In certain input situations, for instance, the discharge of one of the two types of neuron might be expected to produce a "feeding center" type of effect. Moreover, this reasoning could also be extended to other functions in which the ventromedial nucleus has been shown to be implicated, and it reinforces the concept that this neuronal network must be plastic in its functional role. Finally, it is of general interest that this phylogenetically older neuronal network has a control system which, in respect to the presence of local inhibitory neurons, may be considered at least superficially similar in design to those found in more recently developed regions, such as the cerebral and cerebellar cortices. This design may thus be considered an effective one in the context of evolutionary requirements. This effectiveness may be due in large part to the fact that such a network would be more accurate in its response to the input and as well would reduce the distorting effects of any nonlinearities contained in the input.

REFERENCES

1. Cajal, Ramon Y. S.: *Histologie due Système Nerveux de l'Homme et des Vertèbres.* Paris, Maloine, 1911, Vol. 2.
2. Dreifuss, J. J., Murphy, J. T., and Gloor P.: Contrasting effects of two identified amygdaloid efferent pathways. *J. Neurophysiol., 31:*237, 1968.
3. Gloor, P., Murphy, J. T., and Dreifuss, J. J.: Anatomical and physiological characteristics of the two amygdaloid projection systems to the ventromedial hypothalamus. In Hockman, C. H. (Ed.): *Limbic System Mechanisms and Autonomic Function.* Springfield, Charles C Thomas, 1972.
4. Heimer, L., and Nauta, W. J. H.: The hypothalamic distribution of the stria terminalis in the rat. *Brain Res., 13:*284, 1969.
5. Lorente de No. R.: Analysis of the distribution of the action currents of nerve in volume conductors. *Studies Rockefeller Inst. Med. Res., 132:*384, 1947.
6. Murphy, J. T., and Renaud, L. P.: Inhibitory interneurons in the ventromedial nucleus of the hypothalamus. *Brain Res., 9:*385, 1968.
7. Murphy, J. T., and Renaud, L. P.: Mechanisms of inhibition in the ventromedial nucleus of the hypothalamus. *J. Neurophysiol., 32:*85, 1969.
8. Szentagothai, J., Flerko, B., Mess, B., and Malasz, B.: *Hypothalamic Control of the Anterior Pituitary.* Budapest, Akademizi Kiado, 1968.

DISCUSSION

Dr. Hall: I was wondering if you could tell us whether the electrode was placed only in the large-celled part of the basal nucleus or did it traverse both parts? I ask because I found that following lesions in the most medial part of the basal nucleus, degenerated fibers were present not only in the longitudinal association bundle but also in the stria terminalis.

Dr. Gloor: Dr. Murphy may want to comment on this, too, if I don't cover all the relevant aspects. We looked into this matter. We put electrodes in various positions in a number of areas in the medial and lateral portions of the nucleus. We didn't explore the medial part of the basal nucleus too much, at least not in a very systematic fashion. Since we were interested mostly in distinguishing the two efferent projection systems of the amygdala, we usually used the vertical electrode track type of exploration (as shown in Fig. 4–6). The chances are that with this approach one may leave unexplored the most lateral and the most medial parts of the amygdala. Thus, if you do find fibers that go from the most medial part of the basal nucleus to the stria terminalis, we do not have any data which would contradict these findings.

Dr. Hall: I would like to mention that anatomical studies have not shown as clear cut a separation of the basolateral and corticomedial divisions as your observations would suggest, nor do the individual nuclei appear to be homogeneous structures. For example, the small-celled part of the basal nucleus cannot be separated sharply from the cortical nucleus in Golgi preparations. There is an overlapping of their dendritic trees that prevents a definition of their adjacent borders. Acetylcholinesterase studies of the amygdala have demonstrated that only the large-celled part of the basal nucleus gives a strong, positive reaction. In our department, Dr. Lescault has evidence that certain neocortical afferents to the lateral nucleus are not diffusely distributed throughout the nucleus but are concentrated in the dorsolateral region. These differences may eventually prove significant as anatomical and physiological data are brought together to explain how the amygdala functions.

Dr. Gloor: I would certainly agree that the organization is much more complex than the simple dorsal-ventral division we have been speaking about. I would also be willing to accept the fact that the lines of division, if one takes into account the more detailed organization of the amygdala, do not necessarily coincide everywhere with those of the classical subdivisions visible in Nissl-stained preparations. The boundaries may well have to be redrawn to some extent, according to the Golgi technique or others. The two systems are separate in that they have their physiological identity, but exactly where the boundary line between the two systems lies is not clearly established throughout the whole extent of the amygdala, except that in the intermediate region along a vertical track of the stimulating electrode, the boundary seems to be quite sharp and appears to coincide with the boundary between the corticomedial and basolateral subdivision of the amygdala.

Dr. Mogenson: I was just trying to relate your Table 4–1, Dr. Gloor, with Figure 5–3 shown by Dr. Murphy. I was wondering, in view of the reciprocal effects you were talking about, especially in the lesioning and stimulation of the amygdala, if it is your proposal that the outflow of these large cells of the VMH, the axons of which go into the lateral hypothalamus feeding systems, and that with the stria terminalis you are inhibiting this outflow to the lateral hypothalamus which, in itself, is inhibitory. The ventral amygdalofugal pathway, on the other hand, activates the outflow to the VMH. Is this how you reconcile the two diagrams?

Dr. Gloor: Maybe I can answer this question first, and then Dr. Murphy may express his views on this. I would partially agree with what you said. The VAF certainly activates the outflow of the large VMH cells, but this is followed by inhibition of these cells. It is a two-phased response, really, activation followed by inhibition. In contrast, the stria terminalis seems to be almost a purely inhibitory pathway for the large VMH cells. There are a few exceptions, as Dr. Murphy pointed out, but they are so few that I would not have any qualms about describing the stria terminalis as a purely inhibitory system with regard to VMH. On the other hand, I am not so sure that I can agree with you regarding your statements on the "outflow of VMH to the lateral hypothalamus," because I just don't know where the axons of the large VMH neurons go. We could not find anything in the anatomical literature which would give us precise information on this, nor do we have any information from our own studies.

Dr. Mogenson: Evidence for connections from the VMH to the lateral hypothalamus is quite inconclusive with lesions produced by gold thioglucose. We don't know quite where the lesion is, although degeneration is observed in the lateral hypothalamus associated with the system we are talking about.

Dr. Murphy: The degeneration shown in Arees and Mayer's illustration appeared to be quite sparse. It is certain that more anatomical data is needed. I don't believe that there is sufficient physiological evidence at present to indicate that the ventromedial nucleus cells inhibit lateral hypothalamic neurons. The only evidence I know of in this regard is Oomura's cross-correlation studies. Some of his results may be due to postactivation depression rather than inhibition.

Dr. French: I am quite confused about the relationship between what you said, Dr. Gloor, and what Dr. Murphy's diagram showed. Let me give you an example. Out our way, Dr. Crandall is implanting electrodes in the amygdala and hippocampus of patients with temporal lobe seizures. Dr. Mandell is working with these patients and has found that stimulation of the amygdala (and I agree it is very difficult to say exactly in which part of the amygdala the stimulating electrode is located) produces an increase in ACTH output as in your diagram, while stimulation of the hippocampus produces inhibition of ACTH secretion which seemed to conform with your diagram. Now I have difficulty in distinguishing between the inhibiting influence of the amygdala on the medial hypothalamus, on the one hand, and the excitatory phenomena described, on the other. Would you respond simply by saying whether you think Doctors Crandall and Mandell were stimulating the corticomedial or the ventrobasal part of the amygdala to produce these effects.

Dr. Gloor: Well, there are far more good endocrine studies on the effects of amygdaloid stimulation on ACTH discharge with respect to the *activation* of ACTH discharge than on any other neuroendocrine aspect of amygdaloid physiology. Take for instance, McHugh's work that showed that amygdaloid stimulation facilitates ACTH discharge. Unfortunately, he doesn't exactly say what part of the amygdala he is stimulating. He just says that he is stimulating the amygdala. Now, if you just aim at the amygdala in a monkey or any primate, the chances are that about nine times out of ten you will be somewhere in the basolateral group, because the corticomedial area is so much smaller. This would fit quite well with what I wish to propose, although we are dealing here with a reasonable assumption and not with proven facts. But at least this assumption allows one to conceptualize this system in a way that agrees with our data. We may hypothesize that the VAF pathway is the activatory pathway of the discharge, although no one has shown this conclusively. But this would fit with the fact that Hilton and Zbrozyna find that the defense reaction is mediated by this pathway. Now, one would expect that if an animal gets angry or is frightened, its ACTH secretion would increase. McHugh's animals with the implanted electrodes looked frightened, and when he measured the ACTH output, it was elevated. Also, Wurtz, in his studies on rats, found that the animal does not want to self-stimulate and escapes from self-stimulation when the electrodes are placed in the lateral part of the amygdala, but if they do self-stimulate, the electrodes are located in the corticomedial zone. The work we have done with Bovard, in which we made small lesions bilaterally in the corticomedial region, showed that the ACTH output after these lesions is raised. This was not a stimulation but a lesion experiment. It showed that there is apparently more ACTH output when a presumably inhibitory system with regard to ACTH secretion is destroyed. These experiments, therefore, again suggest that the much smaller corticomedial group is probably an area that inhibits ACTH discharge, whereas the lateral area promotes discharge of this pituitary hormone. In man, I think that it would be extremely difficult to find a good electrode placement that would stimulate just the corticomedial group, because in man the corticomedial group is very small in comparison with the basolateral—even more so, relatively speaking, than in other animals. The basolateral nuclei form almost the whole bulk of the human amygdala.

Dr. French: Then, do you think our people are stimulating the stria terminalis?

Dr. Gloor: No, the VAF system.

Dr. French: It seemed to me your chart showed that if you make a lesion in the VAF system you get an increase in the ACTH production.

Dr. Gloor: No, the other way around.

Dr. French: Then I have noted your description of the diagram incorrectly.

Dr. Gloor: Let's look at Table 4–1 again. This table summarizes the work of a number of investigators, obtained in a variety of stimulation and lesion experiments. The third column lists the effects on ACTH secretion. ACTH discharge presumably is inhibited by the corticomedial group of nuclei. So far, no evidence for this has been obtained from stimulation experiments, but localized lesions in this area produce an increase in circulating corticoids. Other experiments show that amygdaloid stimulation may increase the output of ACTH, with stimulation being presumably applied to the basolateral area in these instances. There is one interesting aspect to this: McHugh's work has shown that if you implant electrodes into the amygdala and the hypothalamus of a monkey and stimulate in the amygdala, you increase the plasma corticosteroid level from a resting value to a new higher level. If you give the animal plasma corticoids beforehand and this artificially increase its plasma corticosteroid level to the same value as that achieved by amygdaloid stimulation, no further increase can be obtained by electrical stimulation of the amygdala. If you raise the level only half the way, amygdaloid stimulation increases the corticosteroid level only by an additional equal amount, but if you stimulate the hypothis artificially increases its plasma corticosteroid level is from which you start, you get an increase. I think that this means that the feedback control is in the hypothalamus. What the amygdala does is to reset the "set-point." McHugh didn't state his conclusions exactly in these terms, but his experimental results suggest to me that this is the proper explanation for his findings. What is happening, I believe, is that when one stimulates the hypothalamus, one directly activates the machinery that puts out the substances from the anterior pituitary. One overwhelms the feedback control system by an artificial and overpowering stimulus, but if one stimulates the amygdala, the hypothalamic feedback control is maintained, and amygdaloid stimulation merely resets the gain of the loop.

Dr. Reis: I just wondered if Dr. Gloor and Dr. Murphy think that these studies throw any light on the conflicting data from experiments in which both a lesion or electrical stimulation of the ventromedial nucleus of the hypothalamus can produce sham rage behavior in cats? In other words, the same behavior can be produced by lesion or stimulation. It would seem that now you have made clear by your experiments that perhaps a paradox can be resolved by assuming that there are regional differences of organization within the nucleus. Thus a lesion might release inhibition, while stimulation would excite within the nucleus.

Dr. Murphy: Yes, that is the way I interpret it.

Chapter 6

Some Cerebellar Influences on Autonomic Function

Ray S. Snider

This short chapter lists certain experiments which contribute data to the field of visceral motor control by the cerebellum, and illustrates relationships which one observes from electrical stimulation of the cerebellum. It is not possible within the space alloted me to evaluate data collected from experiments with lesions of the cerebellum.

GALVANIC SKIN RESPONSES

In my opinion, the best paper published on this topic is the one by Wang and Borrison [14] in 1956. They showed that inhibition of the galvanic skin reflex in the cat under chloralose anesthesia could be inhibited by high-frequency stimulation of a medial zone of the anterior cerebellum. This is rather significant, since we ordinarily think of sweat glands as being innervated only by the sympathetic division of the autonomic nervous system. These investigators believed that the cerebellum was acting through the ventral medial bulbar reticular formation to produce the effect.

URINARY BLADDER

There are numerous observations scattered through the literature on the effects of changes in urinary bladder pressure and induction of urination by cerebellar stimulation. I shall refer only to the study by Bruhn, Foley, Emerson and Emerson,[3] since some of these experiments were started in our laboratory and were continued after Dr. Emerson moved to another site. In cats without cerebral cortex and the basal telencephalic nuclei, the cerebellum was stimulated (control for spread of current to the brain stem was done). Either an elevation or depression of the bladder pressure was observed depending upon the initial bladder pressure. The best responses were obtained when the medial zone of the cerebellum was stimulated, particularly that portion of the median zone that projects through the nuclei fastigii.

DIGESTIVE SYSTEM

I am not going to present data on the digestive system since this is one weak point in cerebellar physiology. If you wish, however, this can be handled during the discussion period.

MOTION SICKNESS

The experiments on motion sickness were carried out while I was in the Department of Physiology at Johns Hopkins. Bard, Woolsey, Snider, Mountcastle and Bromiley [1] showed that removal of the floccular-nodular lobe prevented motion sickness. The experiments were well controlled histologically. After removal of the floccular-nodular lobe, the animals showed some signs of discomfort when tested in a swing, but they never vomited. If given apomorphine, however, vomiting was induced quickly.

CHANGES IN THE EYE

There are numerous experiments reporting autonomic changes in the eye. David Ferrier,[6] for example, in 1876 saw constriction of the pupils, and Mussen [11] observed it in his studies on the monkey in 1927. Orbelli [12] reported it in 1932, and Hampson, Harrison and Woolsey [7] also reported it in 1952. A significant aspect of some reports is that dilatation of the pupil by sciatic nerve stimulation can be changed to constriction by stimulation of midline cerebellar structures.

This point comes out repeatedly in experiments on the visceral motor structures. In order to observe cerebellar effects, one must enhance basic physiological mechanisms. For example, produce a good pupillary dilatation then stimulate or induce an increase in blood pressure and then stimulate.

SHAM RAGE

The most interesting experiments were done by Moruzzi [9] in 1947 and 1948.[10] He was able, at the height of sham rage, to stimulate midline structures of the cerebellum and quiet the animal down. Not only that, but some animals with thalamic lesions that did not show rage (unanesthetized animals), did show a parasympathetic effect during stimulation and a rebound sympathetic effect when the electrical stimulus was terminated.

RESPIRATION

Stimulation of the cerebellum does not appear to alter normal respiration in any way. Wiggers,[16] in 1943, was able to induce a fast respiratory movement by the injection of potassium cyanide, and stimulation of the cerebellum quietened this down. On the other hand, he saw no effect on the spontaneous breathing of the dog.

METABOLISM

I include one reference on metabolism for historical reasons. In 1858, Claude Bernard [2] noticed that a puncture in the posterior cerebellum of the rabbit produced a glycosuria. This work has been criticized by those who claimed that the brain stem was damaged; however, Claude Bernard controlled this part of the experiment. It is true that glycosuria can be produced by puncturing the posterior medulla, but it can also be produced by puncturing the cerebellum alone. Eckhard,[5] in 1871, observed both glycosuria and polyuria following stimulation of the posterior cerebellum, particularly the uvula. He controlled for spread of current by stimulating other cerebellar structures. He also noted that sectioning of the splanchnic nerves abolished this effect. It was not until 1935 that it was shown that the blood sugar rise caused by cerebellar puncture was due to adrenaline release.

In 1943, Wiggers[16] showed that there was a difference in the sugar tolerance level of dogs following lesions of the posterior cerebellum. He could not obtain these results in cats or monkeys. Apparently no one else has tried to elucidate these effects, and this is an oversight that should be corrected.

Believe it or not, a first report on possible cerebellar influences on visceral structures was made in 1664 by Willis.[17] He reported that such involuntary activities as heartbeat, respiration, intestinal contractions and so forth, which occur constantly and independently of our knowledge, are due to cerebellar control. This speculation was not supported by experimentation.

Camis[4] considered the cerebellum as the leading autonomic center and believed that it regulated sympathetic tonus on muscle, whatever that is. Orbelli[12] was the leader of a Russian School which considered the cerebellum as a "higher autonomic center." Orbelli obtained his data via conditional reflex experiments.

In 1954, Zanchetti and Zoccolini[18] studied thalamic cats and demonstrated a pressor response associated with sham rage which was altered both at the onset and termination of cerebellar stimulation. Koizumi and Suda[8] recorded discharges in single sympathetic postganglionic fibers and parasympathetic preganglionic fibers following microinjections of sodium glutamate into the cerebellar cortex and observed reciprocal activities in the sympathetic and parasympathetic fibers as well as alterations in blood pressure.

The question arises as to how these complex effects can be produced by cerebellar stimulation. The ascending tracts are difficult to trace. Whiteside and Snider[15] were the first investigators to trace widespread electrical effects to the midbrain tegmentum, including areas adjacent to the periaqueductal gray which Dr. Nauta referred to in Chapter 2. We were not able to trace short latency responses into the hypothalamus, nor can we explain the ascending influences to the limbic system.

REFERENCES

1. Bard, P., Woolsey, C. N., Snider, R. S., Mountcastle, V. B., and Bromily, R. B.: Delimitation of central nervous mechanisms involved in motion sickness. *Fed. Proc., 6:*72, 1947.
2. Bernard, C.: *Lecons sur la Physiologie et la Pathologie du Systeme Nerveux.* Paris, J. B. Balliere, 1858, Vols. 1, 2.
3. Bruhn, J. M., Foley, O. J., Emerson, G. M., and Emerson, J. D.: Autonomic response to cerebellar stimulation in the decorticate cat. *Amer. J. Physiol., 201:*700, 1961.
4. Camis, M.: Das Kleinhirn als Regulationszentrum des sympatischen Muskeltonus. *Arch. Ges. Physiol., 197:*441, 1922.
5. Eckhard, C.: Untersuchungen uber hydrurie (Forsetzung). *Beitr. Anat. Physiol. (Giessen), 6:*51, 1871.
6. Ferrier, D.: *The Functions of the Brain.* London, Smith-Elder, 1876.
7. Hampson, J. L., Harrison, C. R., and Woolsey, C. N.: *Res. Publ. Ass. Res. Nerv. Ment. Dis., 30:*299, 1952.
8. Koizumi, K., and Suda, I.: Induced modulations in autonomic efferent neuron activity. *Amer. J. Physiol., 205:*738, 1963.
9. Moruzzi, G.: Sham rage and localized autonomic responses elicited by cerebellar stimulation in the acute thalamic cat. *Proc. XVII Int. Congr. Physiol. (Oxford)*, 114, 1947.
10. Moruzzi, G.: Ricerche sperimentali e una nu-

ova ipotesia sulla natura del rimbalzo cerebellare. *Boll. Soc. Ital. Biol. Sper., 24*:397, 1948.
11. Mussen, A. T.: Experimental investigations on the cerebellum. *Brain, 50*:313, 1927.
12. Orbelli, L. A.: New conceptions on the functions of the cerebellum (In Russian). *Usp. Sovr. Biol., 13*:207, 1940.
13. Simkina, A. M., and Orbelli, L. A.: Effects of the stimulation of the cerebellum (In Russian, with German summary). *Fiziol. Zh. (Kiev), 15*:557, 1932.
14. Wang, G. H., and Borrison, V. W.: Suprasegmental inhibition of an autonomic reflex. *J. Neurophysiol., 19*:564, 1956.
15. Whiteside, J. A., and Snider, R. S.: Relation of cerebellum to upper brain stem. *J. Neurophysiol., 16*:397, 1953.
16. Wiggers, K.: The influence of the cerebellum on vegetative functions. I. A Review. *Arch. Physiol., 27*:286, 1943.
17. Willis, T.: *Cerebri Anatome cui Nervorum Descriptio et usus.* London, Flesher, 1664.
18. Zanchetti, A., and Zoccolini, A.: Autonomic hypothalamic outbursts elicited by cerebellar stimulation. *J. Neurophysiol., 17*:475, 1954.

Chapter 7

Cerebellar Influences on the Cardiovascular System

Barry J. Hoffer, J. Mitra and Raymond S. Snider

The physiological role for cerebellar control of some functional aspects of the autonomic nervous system has been debated for centuries.[34] But it was Eckhard in 1872 who first showed that electrical stimulation of the cerebellum could produce unequivocal changes in the circulatory system. Only a few investigators have studied this problem since that time, and there is much controversy as to the duration and magnitude of these changes. However, changes in heart rate and usually both pressor and depressor responses are consistently observed.[9,19,23,36] Some of the observed variability of these circulatory responses relates to the type and depth of anesthesia, stimulation parameters and the presence or absence of diencephalic centers.

The classical circulatory response parameters themselves represent another important source of variability. Blood pressure is, at best, a secondary variable representing the summation of resistance changes in the various organs and/or alterations in cardiac output. During the past fifteen years, it has been apparent that the intra-organ and inter-organ distribution of cardiac output may be the most critical parameter in the CNS regulation of circulatory dynamics and that major redistributions may occur both experimentally[31] and physiologically[3,28] with negligible changes in blood pressure. Vasodilation in some organs is often precisely balanced by vasoconstriction in others and/or alterations in cardiac output.

Blood flow studies have also indicated greater heterogeneity in the classical central nervous pressor and depressor pathways. Feigl,[12] for example, has shown that stimulation of some midbrain tegmental points elicits pressor reactions associated with a marked renal vasoconstriction and little change in skeletal muscle resistance. Similar pressor responses from other tegmental loci were accompanied by large skeletal muscle vasoconstrictions and a negligible change in renal flow. Such functional heterogeneity is masked by the study of blood pressure alone.

The present investigation was undertaken to reexamine the blood pressure responses to cerebellar stimulation and to analyze the effects of cerebellar stimulation upon blood flow in skin, skeletal muscle and kidney as well. These three organs were chosen for a variety of reasons. Firstly, each organ possesses different proportions of extrinsic neural activity and intrinsic myogenic activity in its "resting vascular tone." Cutaneous vascular resistance is almost wholly determined by efferent sympathetic activity,[14] whereas the kidney shows little or no vasoconstrictor fiber activity at rest.[24] Skeletal muscle vasomotor tone occupies a middle position between these two extremes.[18] Secondly, these three organs actively participate in many "physiological" flow redistributions, such as those occurring with exercise and temperature regulation. Finally, the arterial inflow and venous outflow from these organs can be isolated and quantitatively studied.

METHODS

A total of seventy-seven cats was used. After induction with ether, surgical anesthesia was maintained by the intravenous injection of 40 to 45 mg/kg of chloralose. In an earlier study, Nembutal ® (30 mg/kg), Dial ® (0.6 cc/kg) and urethane (1.5 mg/kg) were tried. The circulatory responses to cerebellar stimulation with these anesthetics were much smaller than those in chloralose-anesthetized preparations.

The cerebellar cortex was stimulated with bipolar nichrome electrodes, approximately 0.3 mm in diameter, with tips separated 1 to 1.5 mm. The electrodes were lowered into the cortex until the tip of the more superficial member just disappeared beneath the surface. Local procainization of many of the active loci was used to control for possible current spread. All stimuli were trains of monophasic rectangular pulses of 0.1 msec duration and of 0.5 to 15 v intensity. Stimulation frequency was 300 sec unless otherwise noted. Stimulated cortical areas are abbreviated as follows: ant. vermis, vermal anterior lobe; ant. lob. simplex, anterior lobulus simplex; post. lob. simplex, posterior lobulus simplex; int. ctx., intermediate cerebellar cortex. Brain stem areas were stimulated through similar bipolar electrodes implanted stereotaxically.

Arterial blood pressure (BP) was measured by cannulation of the femoral or carotid artery. Renal (RAF) and skeletal muscle (SMAF) arterial flow was measured with an electromagnetic flow meter. Skeletal muscle flow was measured in the hindleg after skinning the leg and tying off the paw. Renal (RVF) and cutaneous (SVF) venous flow was measured by a drop counter similar to that described by Lindgren,[16] with the exception that an electrical, rather than mechanical, readout was used. Silicone oil was used in the counting chamber to minimize variations in drop size with flow rate. Drop size was 0.12 cc at 1 cc/min and 0.1 cc at 35 cc/min. Preliminary *in vitro* experiments were performed to insure that the resistance of the drop counter circuit did not materially reduce the rate of blood flow. Renal outflow was measured by cannulation of the renal vein. Cutaneous outflow was measured by cannulation of the venae saphena magna of one of the hindpaws. Heparin (5 mg/kg) was employed to prevent clotting in those experiments dealing with venous outflow. Flaxedil (3 to 4 mg/kg) was used periodically to insure that the circulatory responses to cerebellar stimulation were not secondary to somatomotor activity.

Central nervous lesions were produced either by suction (decerebration, five animals; bilateral thalamectomy, eleven animals) or electrolytically (posterior hypothalamic lesion, nine animals). All lesioned animals were perfused at the termination of the experiments, and the extent of the lesion was verified histologically. In order to denervate the kidney, all nerves to it were sectioned under a dissecting microscope. Following this, the adventia was completely stripped away from a portion of the renal artery and the media was painted with phenol.

RESULTS

Blood Pressure Changes

Three different types of blood pressure changes are elicited by stimulation of the cerebellum: (a) pressor (Figs. 7–1,B and C), (b) depressor (Figs. 7–1,A and E) responses to the onset of stimulation and (c) rebound[1] pressor reactions (Figs. 7–1,A, B, C, and E) at the termination of the stimulation. Responsive cortex is limited to the vermal zone[15]; however, there is no localization of the above-mentioned types of responses within this zone. The persistence of the responses after systemic injection of Flaxedil (Fig. 7–1,C) and their disappearance after local application of procaine (Figs. 7–1,D and F) around the site of stimulation indicates that neither current spread nor somatic movement is involved in the pressure changes.

It is difficult to generalize concerning the magnitude of the blood pressure changes from experiment to experiment, since there was considerable variability. Most responses ranged from 20 to 100 mm Hg; rarely were changes seen of greater magnitude than 100 mm. Much of this variability probably derives from the cerebellum itself. Cardiovascular reactions in approximately 35 percent of the experiments could no longer be elicited after several hours of stimulation. In an additional 30 percent of the animals, no circulatory changes were ever obtained to cerebellar stimulation. In both groups, there was no visible damage to the cerebellum

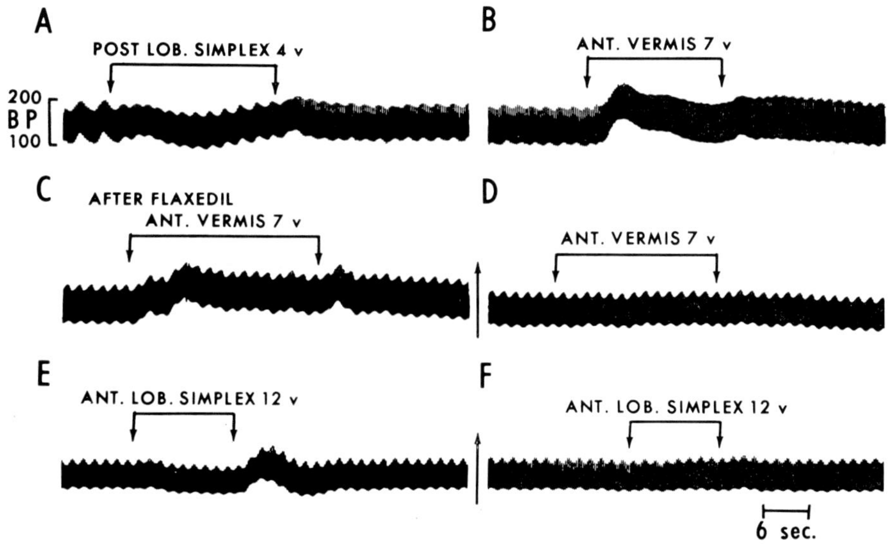

Figure 7–1. Effects of cerebellar stimulation on systemic blood pressure (BP). (All blood pressure calibrations are in millimeters of mercury. The onset and termination of electrical stimulation is indicated by the arrows, the duration of stimulation by the length of the bracket. All stimulated cerebellar loci are within the vermal zone unless otherwise noted.) Combinations of the three response types shown in *A* and *B*. After administration of Flaxedil, the responses persist as shown in *C* and *E*. Subsequent procainization of the cerebellar loci activated in *C* and *E*, as indicated by the arrows, abolishes the pressure changes. This is shown in *D* and *F* respectively.

and circulatory responses to stimulation of central nervous structures in the brain stem were present. One might assume that the activity of the cerebellar cortex is particularly capricious, a finding often reported in electrophysiological studies.[8] Such a propensity might easily account for much of the variability observed in blood pressure studies.

Variation of stimulus frequency had a marked effect upon the blood pressure responses produced by cerebellar stimulation, even if pulse width was simultaneously changed to provide an equal duty cycle at all frequencies. Responses were maximal at stimulation frequencies of 200 to 300/sec and decreased below 150/sec (Fig. 7–2). Little or no response was seen at stimulation frequencies below 50/sec. This appeared to be true for all three response types studied.

Brain stem pathways mediating these effects have been a subject of considerable controversy. Precollicular decerebration has been reported to abolish circulatory responses to cerebellar stimulation,[22,36] although these negative data must be interpreted with caution. After precollicular decerebration (Fig. 7–3) in the present experiments, the direct pressor responses to cerebellar stimulation disappeared whereas depressor and rebound responses usually remained intact. Loci which when stimulated evoked direct pressor patterns prior to the lesion often subsequently produced depressor responses at different stimulus strengths after the lesion was made. This lends support to the belief that there is an absence of topographical localization of pressor and depressor areas in the vermal cortex. A prolonged recovery time of 90 to 120 minutes was usually necessary for the return of any autonomic responses to cerebellar stimulation following brain stem transection. Electrolytic lesions of the posterior hypothalamus produced a differential abolition of responses induced by electrical stimulation, similar to that seen following brain stem transection (Fig. 7–4). Bilateral ablation of the entire diencephalon by suction, sparing the hypothalamus, yielded no decrement in the direct pressor response (Fig. 7–5). Thus, the hypothalamus appears to be the essential diencephalic structure for this response.

Renal Blood Flow

Stimulation of the vermal cerebellar cortex often induced pronounced vasoconstriction[2] in the kidney. The increased renal resistance was seen regardless of

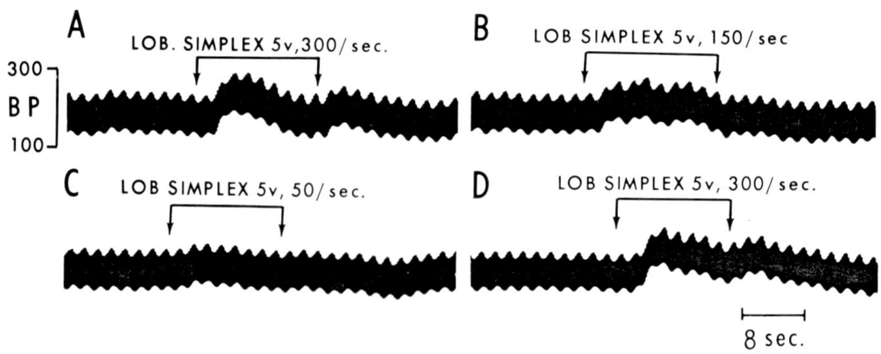

Figure 7–2. Effects of variation of stimulation frequency on the blood pressure changes produced by cerebellar stimulation. (*A*) Stimulation at 300/sec. (*B*) Stimulation at 150/sec. (*C*) Stimulation at 50/sec. (*D*) Stimulation at 300/sec.

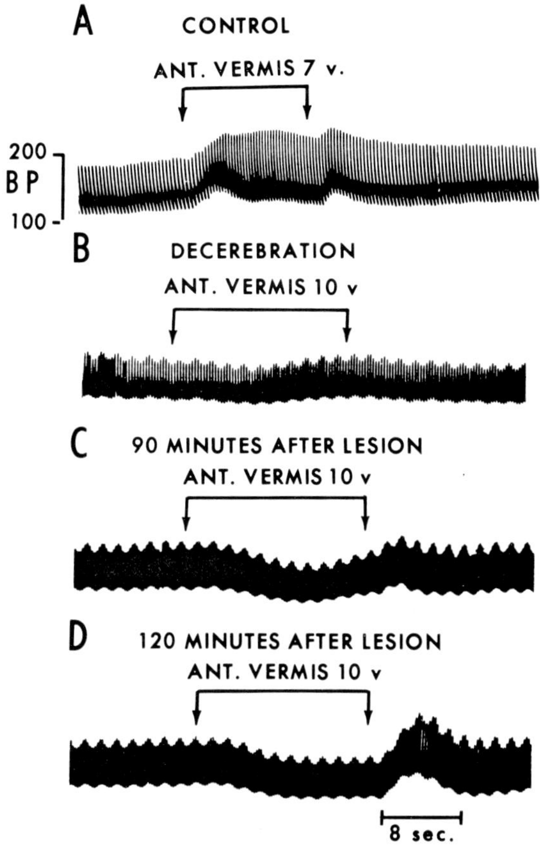

Figure 7–3. Effects of precollicular decerebration on the blood pressure responses to cerebellar stimulation. (*A*) Control. (*B*) Five minutes after decerebration. (*C*) Ninety minutes after the lesion. The "off" pressor response remains intact whereas the "on" pressor response is replaced by a depressor response. Note the prolonged recovery time needed for the depressor response to develop D.

which of the three types of blood pressure changes was observed and often occurred without any sign of systemic pressure response.

Surgical denervation of the kidney abolished the effects of cerebellar stimulation on renal resistance (Fig. 7–6). Intra-arterial injection of phentolamine, a powerful and relatively short-acting alpha sympatholytic agent, also abolished the effect (Fig. 7–7). These data indicate that the renal responses are mediated solely by adrenergic vasoconstrictor neurons. This finding is consistent with conclusions of Celander [4] on the predominant role of sympathetic neurons in the nervous control of blood flow. The renal resistance changes showed the same stimulation frequency optima, 200 to 300/sec, noted for blood pressure.

The absence of renal vasodilation in response to cerebellar stimulation is not surprising in view of the minor neural contribution to resting vasomotor tone in this organ.[24] To ascertain whether cerebellar stimulation can inhibit renal vasoconstrictor discharge, such discharge was induced artificially by stimulation of the brain stem. When sympathetic tone was increased in this fashion, simultaneous activation of cerebellar cortex produced a marked inhibition of both the systemic pressor response and the increased renal resistance (Fig. 7–8). These same cerebellar areas usually inhibit sympathetic responses produced by not just one but several brain stem areas successively stimulated. Thus, they appear to produce generalized inhibition of sympathetic centers rather than specific inhibition of any one brain stem locus. Inhibition of brain stem cardiovascular changes by concurrent cerebellar activation also manifests specificity for stimulus frequency (Fig. 7–9). The inhibitory effect was most marked at frequencies of 200 to 300/sec, less marked at frequencies below 150/sec; little effect was induced when stimulation frequencies below 50/sec were used. Figure 7–9 illustrates that some response specificity can exist, since excitatory responses evoked by brain stem stimulation (pressor reaction, renal vasoconstriction) were effectively suppressed by simultaneous cerebellar stimulation, while inhibitory responses (bradycardia) often were not.

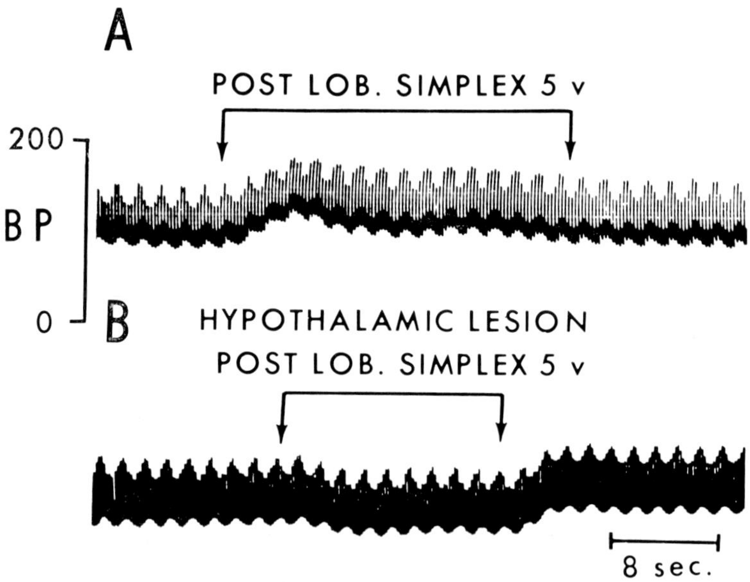

Figure 7–4a. Effects of bilateral hypothalamic electrolytic coagulation on blood pressure changes produced by cerebellar stimulation. (*A*) Control. (*B*) Thirty minutes after the lesion.

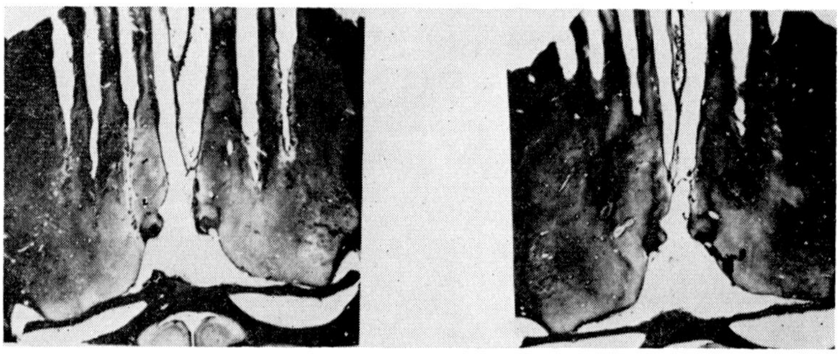

Figure 7–4b. Cross-sction of brain-stem showing extent of lesion in hypothalamus (Weil stain).

Skeletal Muscle Blood Flow

Vermal stimulation usually elicited decreased resistance of the skeletal muscle blood vessels (Fig. 7–10a). These responses were usually independent of blood pressure changes. Increased resistance was seldom seen. The changes were rarely more than twofold and were abolished by intra-arterial injection of phentolamine. The responses were also markedly reduced by division of the lumbosacral plexus. Systemic injections of Flaxedil or intra-arterial methylatropine, on the other hand, had little or no effect on the reduction of skeletal muscle vascular resistance. These findings are interpreted to indicate that the decreased resistance is due to inhibition of tonic vasoconstrictor discharge and that cholinergic vasodilation or somatic movement play little role in the response.

Stimulation of the fastigial nucleus produced considerable vascular change in skeletal muscle (Fig. 7–10b). In this prep-

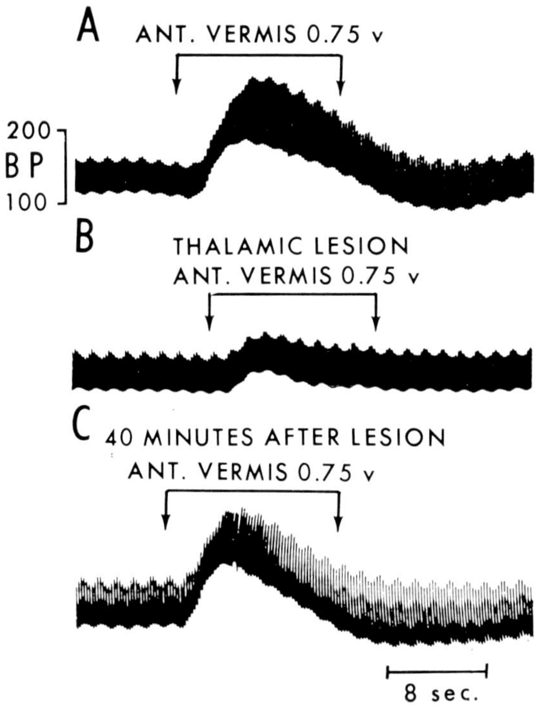

Figure 7–5a. Effects of bilateral thalamic ablation on the direct pressor response evoked by cerebellar stimulation. (*A*) Control. (*B*) Five minutes after the lesion. (*C*) Forty minutes after the lesion.

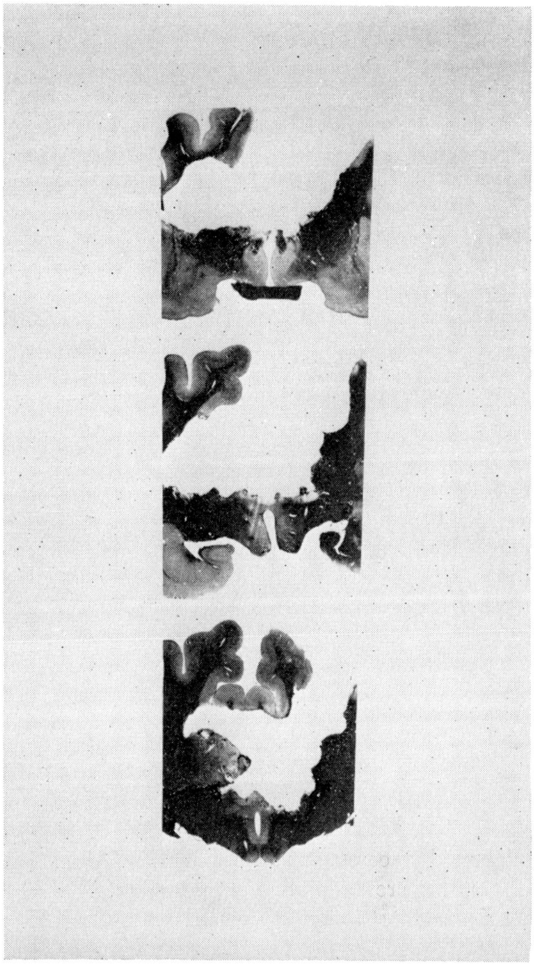

Figure 7–5b. Cross-sections of diencephalon showing extent of thalamic lesions (Weil stain). Frontal sections at anterior 13.5, 9.5, and 7.5 respectively (Horsley-Clarke planes).

aration treated with 4 mg/kg of Flaxedil there was an initial decrease of blood flow during stimulation which was followed after "OFF" by a rebound increased blood flow lasting for more than a minute. Since there were no discernible changes in heart rate and blood pressure and since the limb was free of skin (the hindpaw was ligated and blood flow measured from femoral artery), these data are interpreted to indicate decreased blood flow to the musculature. Placement of the stimulating electrode into the nucleus interpositus only 2 mm away failed to induce the effect when two times the stimulating current—that is, 1200μA, were used—so current spread to nearby structures cannot explain the data. Some of the effects obtained from stimulating the nucleus fastigii are opposite to those obtained as a result of stimulating the cerebellar cortex. Cortico-nuclear counteraction has been similarly

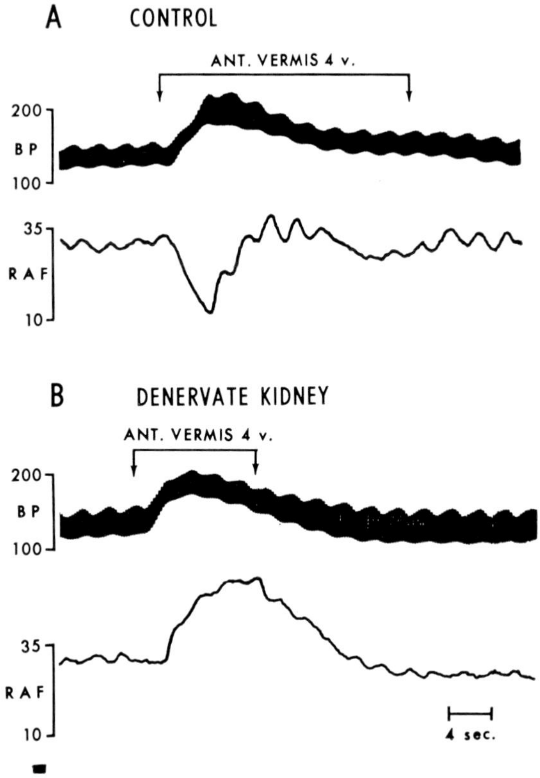

Figure 7–6. Renal arterial flow (RAF) changes induced by cerebellar stimulation. (All flow calibrations are in milliliters per minute.) (*A*) Renal vasoconstriction associated with a pressor response. Renal resistance increases from 5.4 to 60.0. (*B*) After renal denervation, blood flow increases passively.

demonstrated for posture and movement by Chambers and Sprague.[5] Recent work by Eccles and his associates[10] indicates these antipodal corticonuclear responses are probably produced by Purkinje cell inhibition of the deep nuclei.

Skin Blood Flow

Increased cutaneous vascular resistance was also produced by stimulation of the cerebellar cortex. Vasoconstrictor reactions were elicited by both the onset (Fig. 7–11,A) and termination (Fig. 7–11,B) of stimulation.

As with renal and skeletal muscle vascular reactions, the responsive points were limited to the vermal zone (Fig. 7–11,A). Within this area, active and inactive loci were closely intermingled. As opposed to renal and skeletal muscle resistance changes, however, cutaneous vasoconstrictions to the onset of stimulation were always associated with pressor responses. Rebound cutaneous vasoconstriction, on the other hand, need not be so associated.

The abolition of the cutaneous vasoconstriction following local (Fig. 7–12) or combined local and systemic (Fig. 7–13) administration of phentolamine indicated that this reaction was produced by increased sympathetic efferent discharge. The direct pressor response shown in Figure 7–13 was also abolished by systemic injection of phentolamine. The disappearance of circulatory changes after local procaine application to the active locus in both experiments was done to demonstrate that current spread to nearby structures was not involved. The importance of using fast frequencies of stimulation to induce both the cutaneous resistance and blood pressure changes is shown in Figure 7–14.

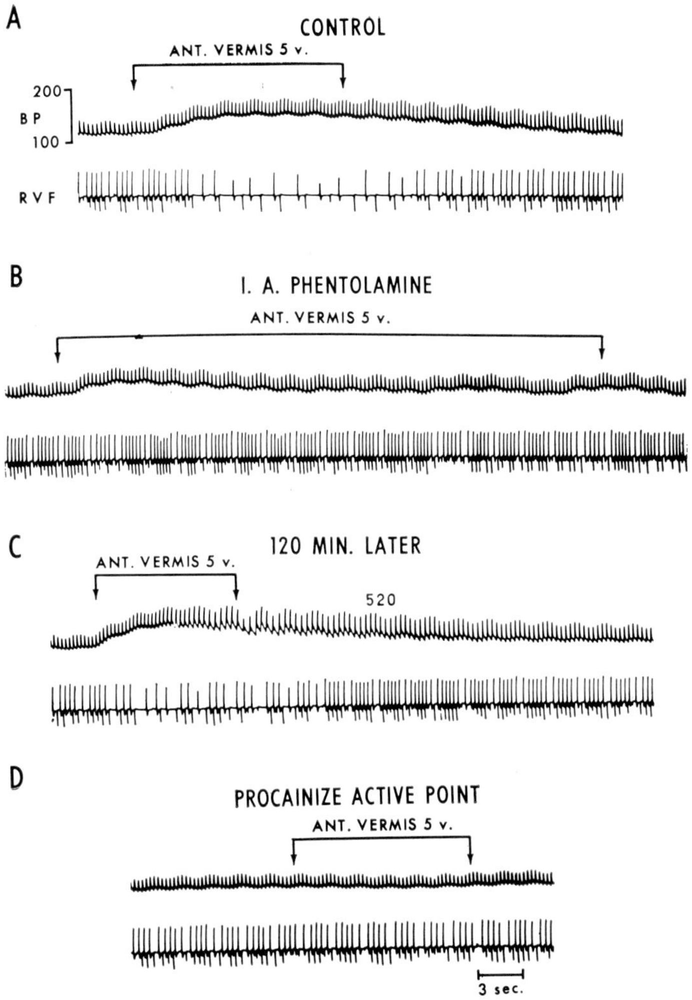

Figure 7–7. Effects of local phenotolamine on the renal vascular resistance changes elicited by cerebellar stimulation. (*A*) Cerebellar stimulation produces a pressor response associated with renal vasoconstriction. (*B*) Five minutes after intra-arterial injection (IA) of phentolamine (renal artery—0.5 mg/kg), the change in renal blood flow is no longer apparent. (*C*) Partial recovery of the flow response occurs 120 minutes later. (*D*) Both the pressure and flow changes are abolished by procainization of the active cerebellar point.

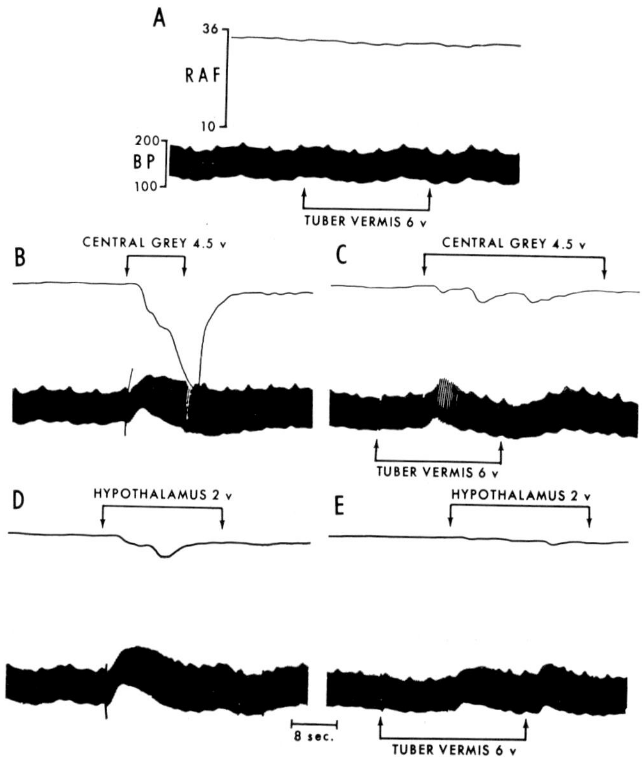

Figure 7–8. Inhibition of brain-stem "pressor" areas by the cerebellum. Stimulation of a cerebellar area, which has no overt effects upon blood pressure and renal arterial flow (*A*), may inhibit circulatory responses elicited by brain stem stimulation. Activation of the central gray (*B*) and posterior hypothalamus (*D*) produces pressor reactions accompanied by renal vasoconstrictions. Resistance changes are 4.5 to 22 and 4.3 to 7.6 respectively. Concurrent stimulation of the "inactive" cerebellar locus (*C* and *E*) inhibits these circulatory responses. Resistance changes in C and E are only 4.3 to 5.6 and 4.3 to 4.6 respectively.

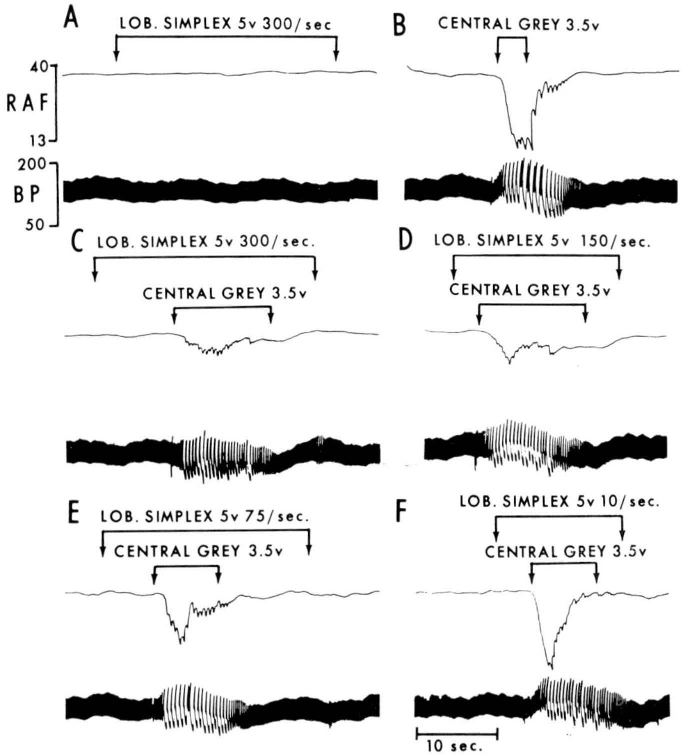

Figure 7–9. Effects of changing stimulation frequency upon the inhibitory interaction between brain stem and cerebellum. The pressor response and renal vasoconstriction (resistance change 3.2 to 9.4) elicited by stimulation of the central gray (*B*) is markedly inhibited by concurrent stimulation (*C*) of the cerebellum at 300/sec (resistance change 3.2 to 3.4). As the stimulation frequency is reduced (*D*, *E*), the inhibition diminishes. At 10/sec (*F*), no inhibition is apparent (resistance change 3.2 to 9.8). Note that stimulation of the cerebellum itself (*A*) has no overt effect upon blood pressure or renal blood flow.

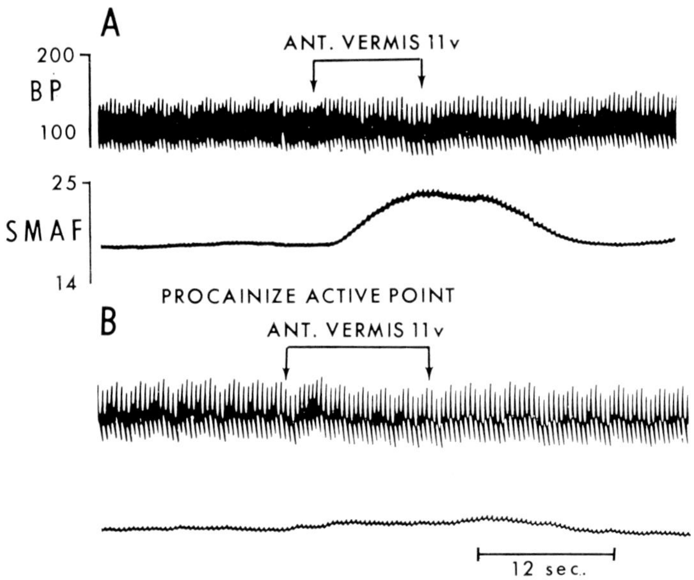

Figure 7–10a. Skeletal muscle vasodilation elicited by cerebellar stimulation. (*A*) Control. The increase in skeletal muscle arterial flow is not accompanied by any blood pressure change. (*B*) After procainization of the active cerebellar point, this flow change is greatly reduced.

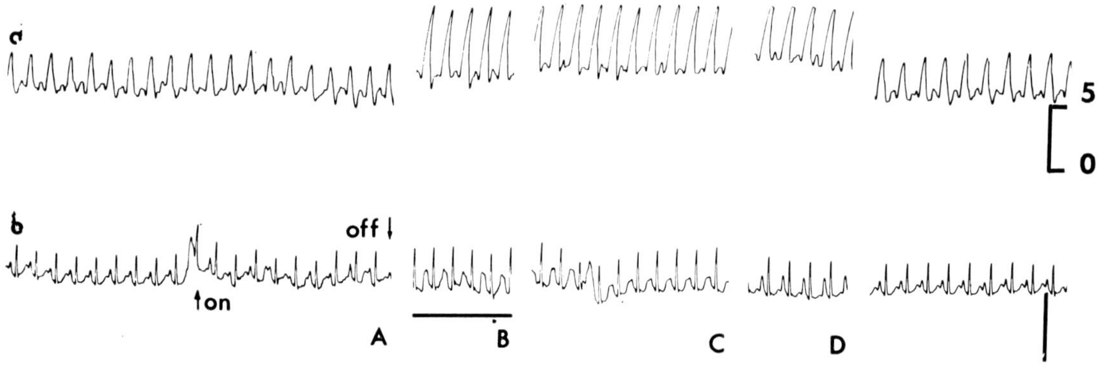

Figure 7–10b. Skeletal muscle vascular resistance changes elicited by stimulation of the fastigial nucleus. Changes produced in (*a*) blood flow records and (*b*) EKG when left nucleus fastigii is stimulated for 15 seconds (ON-OFF) with 600μA (300/sec, 0.1 msec duration). At A, 6 seconds of record were removed; at B, 5 seconds; at C, 8 seconds; and at D, 80 seconds. Horizontal calibration line = 2 sec; vertical line (a) = 5.0 ml/min, vertical line (b) = 0.5 mV/cm. EKG = lead I (arm-to-arm). Electromagnetic blood flow record taken from femoral artery to right leg following skin removal and paw ligation. Note that blood flow changed from 7 to 4 ml/min during stimulation and increased to 15 ml/min after "off." Total time of change equaled 103 seconds. Heart rate and blood pressure (left femoral artery) did not change.

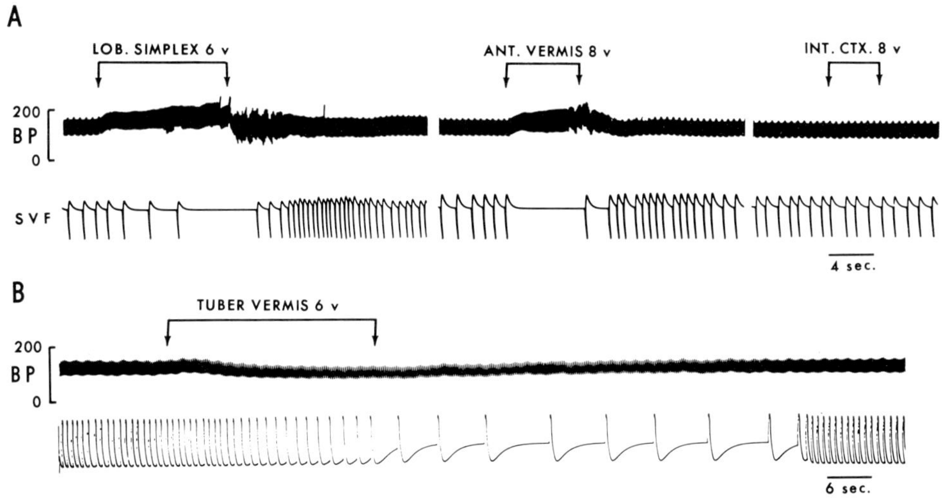

Figure 7–11. Cutaneous vasoconstriction evoked by cerebellar stimulation. (*A*) Stimulation of two areas in the vermal zone (lobulus simplex and anterior lobe) produces a marked diminution in cutaneous venous outflow (SVF) associated with pressor responses. Stimulation of a nearby nonvermal point (intermediate cortex) produces no circulatory changes. (*B*) Rebound cutaneous vasoconstriction observed during a second experiment.

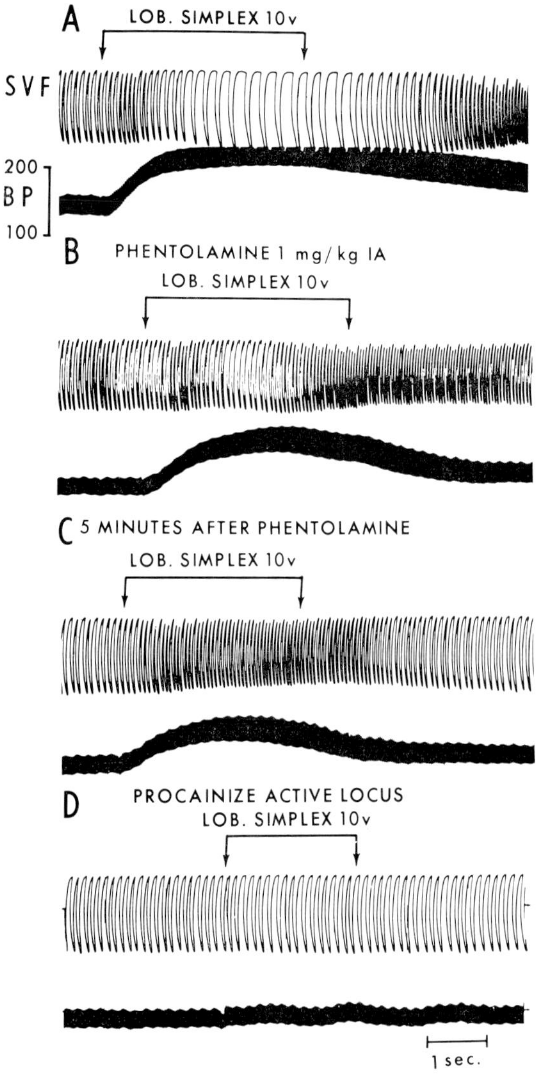

Figure 7–12. Abolition of cutaneous resistance changes by local phentolamine. (*A*) Control. Resistance changes from 19.0 to 72.0 during the cutaneous vasoconstriction. (*B*) Thirty seconds after intra-arterial injection of 1 mg/kg of phentolamine. (*C*) Five minutes later, the effects of the drug are more marked. Blood flow increases passively during the pressor response with no cutaneous resistance change. (*D*) Abolition of the pressor response after procainization of the active cerebellar point.

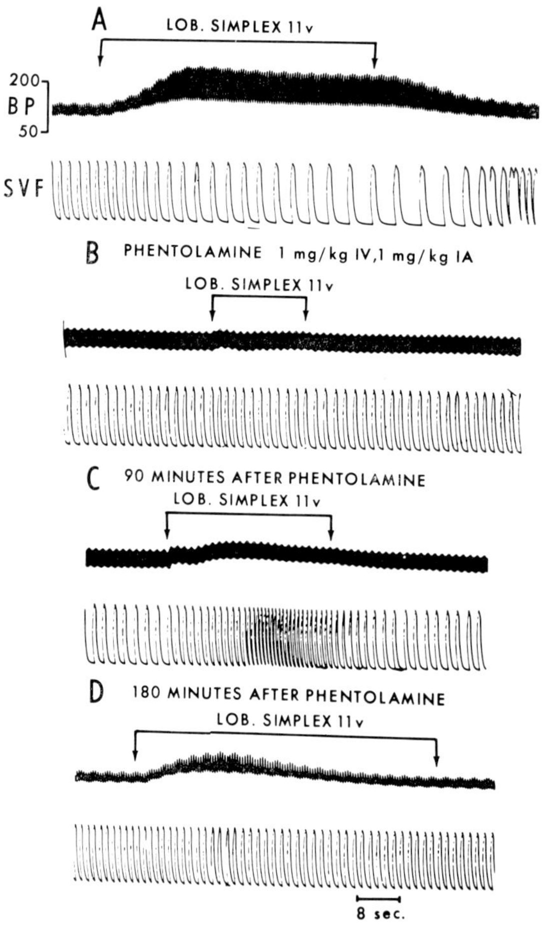

Figure 7–13. Abolition of the circulatory changes induced by cerebellar stimulation after local and systemic phentolamine. (*A*) Control. Cutaneous resistance changes from 17 to 64. (*B*) Five minutes after phentolamine administration 1 mg/kg IA, 1 mg/kg IV. (*C*) Partial recovery of the pressor response 70 minutes after the phentolamine administration. Cutaneous blood flow increases passively. (*D*) After 180 minutes, there is further recovery. Cutaneous resistance changes from 17 to 24 during stimulation.

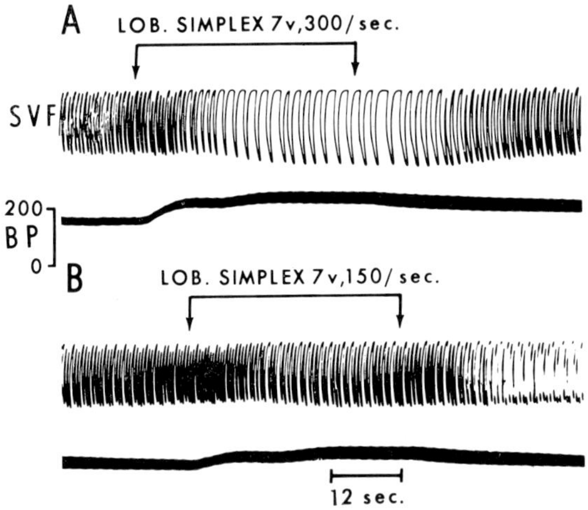

Figure 7–14. Effects of varying cerebellar stimulation frequencies on cutaneous resistance changes. (*A*) Stimulation at 300/sec. Cutaneous changes from 19 to 156. (*B*) Stimulation at 150/sec. Cutaneous resistance changes from 16.2 to 30.5.

DISCUSSION

Blood Pressure

Blood pressure responses previously reported to be elicited by electrical stimulation of the cerebellum were all observed in this study: pressor,[2,23,36] depressor[2,9,23] and rebound.[9,23,36] Active loci, at reasonable stimulus strengths, were restricted to vermal cortex. However, there was no clear anatomical separation of the loci within this medial zone; all three reactions could be induced from neighboring points during some experiments. Similar conclusions about the anatomical and physiological homogeneity of vermal cortex were made by Chambers and Sprague,[5] while studying the effects of cerebellar lesions on posture and motoricity. On the other hand, Ban[2] and Zanchetti and Zoccolini[36] report some anteroposterior localization of areas related to blood pressure responses. Some of these differences can be explained by the different anesthetic agents used. Evoked potential studies by Combs[7] indicate that localization of responses within the cerebellum can be markedly altered by an anesthetic agent.

The anatomical substratum related to these responses can be speculated on. In mammals, the majority of vermal Purkinje cell axons terminate in the fastigial nuclei. Efferent projections from the fastigial nuclei to the medullary, pontine and mesencephalic reticular formation, periaqueductal gray substance, and the posterolateral and dorsolateral hypothalamus have been demonstrated.[6,30] The fastigioreticular pathways show a diffuse projection.[32] Evoked potential studies[1,2,33] also show widespread fastigiobulbar connections.

The present studies suggest that depressor and rebound responses are probably mediated by fastigiofugal pathways to the pontine and medullary reticular formation, whereas the direct pressor response pathway involves hypothalamic areas. A major problem in evaluating deficits following brain stem lesions is the length of the recovery time. Often cardiovascular reactions did not return for several hours which is far longer than the time necessary for restoration of resting blood pressure levels, brain stem circulatory reflexes and postural responses following cerebellar stimulation. If ample time for recovery were not allowed after decerebration, it might be concluded that all pressure responses were mediated through a diencephalic locus. Such an effect may explain our failure to confirm the disappearance of circulatory responses after surgical decerebration, reported by Moruzzi,[9] Zanchetti and Zoccolini,[36] and Ban.[2]

Blood Flow

Cerebellar stimulation, in this study, produced a redistribution of cardiac output from kidney and skin to skeletal muscle, independent of muscular movement or current spread to nearby brain stem structures. The resistance changes in all three organs appear to be mediated by modulation of adrenergic-sympathetic neuronal discharge, with increased firing in the constrictor innervation of the kidney and cutaneous vascular beds and decreased firing in that of skeletal muscle. Renal and skeletal muscle flow changes were not associated with any one particular class of blood pressure response and often occurred independently of any pressure change whatsoever. A similar dissociation of pressure and flow changes has been reported following diencephalic,[13] mesencephalic [12] and rhombencephalic [29,35] stimulation.

At no time was active renal vasodilation produced by cerebellar stimulation, confirming the widely accepted opinion concerning the absence of renal vasodilator fibers or resting vasoconstrictor tone. Takeuchi and his associates [29] reached similar conclusions following studies involving diencephalic and medullary stimulation. The determination of cerebellar inhibitory influences upon the renal vasoconstrictor fiber pool, consequently, depends upon the artificial production of vasoconstrictor tone. Suppression of brain stem induced pressor reactions and renal vasoconstriction by concurrent cerebellar stimulation furnishes evidence that such inhibitory influences do exist. The fact that many brain stem sites, serially activated, can be inhibited from a given cerebellar locus suggests widespread inhibitory influences within central areas of the autonomic nervous system.

The frequency of electrical pulses used for stimulation was critical for the production of circulatory responses. The specificity of stimulation frequencies has been demonstrated for cerebellar inhibition and facilitation of movements induced by stimulation of the cerebral cortex.[25,26] Moruzzi [9,20] has reported reversal of somatomotor responses to cerebellar stimulation when various stimulation frequencies are used. However, reversal of autonomic responses was never found in the present study. Recent studies on cerebellar synaptology by Eccles and his associates [10] have revealed possible intracortical mechanisms whereby the frequency of stimulation may alter both the magnitude and direction of the fastigiobulbar discharge.

Significance of the Flow Redistribution

Speculation on possible roles played by the cerebellum in physiological cardiovascular responses may be hazardous since macroelectrode stimulation of the cerebellar cortex can never reproduce exactly the natural temporal and spatial discharges of populations of Purkinje cells. It is also probable that such stimulation simultaneously influences more than one autonomic response pattern.

Despite these reservations, there were circulatory changes which occurred with such sufficient reliability that additional comments appear worthwhile and may be worth relating to natural physiological adjustments. A redistribution of blood flow from skin and kidney to skeletal muscle is seen in the early stages of exercise.[21] Perhaps the cerebellum, with its well-known functional role in regulating posture and somatic movements, is concerned with the integration of circulatory patterns providing the nutrient supply for the muscles subserving these movements. Further experiments are needed to ascertain whether the cerebellum can differentially alter the blood supply to flexors and extensors concurrently with differential facilitation and inhibition of these muscles.

The cerebellar "suppressor" areas, which inhibit vasoconstrictor fiber discharge, may participate in regulation of brain stem circulatory adjustment patterns. The cerebellum is known to have a similar influence in the sphere of somatomotor responses.[25,26]

Cerebellar stimulation is also known to produce emotional changes.[17,27] Furthermore, sham rage, in thalamic preparations, may be induced or inhibited by excitation of the cerebellum.[36] Suppression of effects is often followed by rage "rebounds." As major redistributions of cardiac output are known to accompany many affective states, these findings on cerebellar stimulation indicate that this organ may play a role in the integration of affective behavior and the autonomic reactions accompanying such behavior. The inhibitory interaction with brain stem areas, stimulation of which in intact animals often produces rage, is especially interesting in this respect.

In conclusion, despite the absence of overt cardiovascular deficits after cerebellar lesions, electrical stimulation of this structure produces many profound circulatory reactions. Many of these reactions resemble those seen during exercise, affective behavior, temperature regulation and other natural circulatory responses. Analyses of the actual role of the cerebellum in these physiological response patterns must await experiments on animals chronically implanted with devices to monitor phasic circulatory changes and to produce reversible cerebellar lesions.

REFERENCES

1. Anand, B. K., Malhotra, C. L., Singh, B., and Dua, S.: Cerebellar projections to limbic system. *J. Neurophysiol., 22*:451, 1959.
2. Ban, T.: Cerebellar autonomic function. *Recent Advances Res. Nerv. Syst. 3*:555, 1959.
3. Brouha, L., and Radford, E. P.: The cardiovascular system in muscular activity. In Johnson, W. R. (Ed.) *Science and Medicine of Exercise and Sports.* New York, Harper & Bros., 1960, pp. 178.
4. Celander, O.: The range of control exercised by the sympathetico-adrenal system. *Acta Physiol. Scand., 32 (Suppl. 116)*, 1954.
5. Chambers, W. W., and Sprague, J. M.: Functional localization in the cerebellum. *Arch. Neurol. Psychiat., 74*:653, 1955.
6. Cohen, D., Chambers, W. W., and Sprague, J. M.: Experimental study of the efferent projections from the cerebellar nuclei to the brain stem of the cat. *J. Comp. Neurol., 109*:233, 1958.
7. Combs, C. M.: Electro-anatomical study of cerebellar localization. *J. Neurophysiol., 17*:123, 1954.
8. Crawford, J. M., Curtis, D. R., Voorhoeve, P. E., and Wilson, V. J.: Acetylcholine sensitivity of cerebellar neurons in the cat. *J. Physiol., 186*:139, 1966.
9. Dow, R. S., and Moruzzi, G.: *The Physiology and Pathology of the Cerebellum.* Minneapolis, University of Minnesota Press, 1958.
10. Eccles, J. C., Ito, M., and Szentagothai, J.: *The Cerebellum As a Neuronal Machine.* New York, Springer-Verlag, 1967.
11. Eckhard, C.: Uber den Einfluss des kleinen Gehirns auf die Herz- und Atembwegungen sowie auf die Urinsekretion nach Versuchen an Hunde. *Beitr. Anat. Physiol., 6*:175, 1872.
12. Feigl, E. O.: Vasoconstriction resulting from diencephalic stimulation. *Acta Physiol. Scand., 60*:372, 1964.
13. Feigl, E. O., Johansson, B., and Lofving, B.: Renal vasoconstriction and the defense re-

action. *Acta Physiol. Scand., 62*:429, 1964.

14. Folkow, B.: Role of the nervous system in the control of vascular tone. *Circulation, 21*:760, 1960.
15. Jansen, J., and Brodal, A.: Experimental studies on the intrinsic fibers of the cerebellum. *J. Comp. Neurol., 73*:267, 1940.
16. Lindgren, P.: An improved method for drop recording of arterial or venous blood flow. *Acta Physiol. Scand., 42*:5, 1958.
17. McDonald, J. V.: Responses following electrical stimulation of the anterior lobe of the cerebellum in cat. *J. Neurophysiol., 16*:69, 1953.
18. Melander, S., and Johansson, B.: Control of resistance, exchange, and capacitance functions in the peripheral circulation. *Pharm. Rev., 20*(3):1, 1968.
19. Moruzzi, G.: Sham rage and localized autonomic responses elicited by cerebellar stimulation in the acute thalamic cat. *Proc. XVII Int. Physiol. Congress Oxford,* 1947, pp. 114.
20. Moruzzi, G.: Effects at different frequencies of cerebellar stimulation upon postural tonus and myotatic reflexes. *Electroenceph. Clin. Neurophysiol., 2*:463, 1950.
21. Robinson, S.: Physiology of muscular exercise. In Bard, P. (Ed.): *Medical Physiology,* 11th ed. St. Louis, C. V. Mosby, 1961, pp. 512.
22. Sawyer, C. H., Hilliard, J., and Ban, T.: Autonomic and EEG responses to cerebellar stimulation in rabbits. *Amer. J. Physiol., 200*:405, 1961.
23. Simkina, A. M.: Present views on the cerebellar influence on the autonomic and sensory functions. *Usp. Sovr. Biol., 25*:345, 1948.
24. Smith, H. W., Rovenstine, E. A., Goldring, W., Chasis, H., and Ranges, H. H.: The effects of spinal anesthesia upon the circulation of normal unoperated man with reference to the autonomy of the arterioles, and especially that of the kidney. *J. Clin. Invest., 18*:319, 1939.
25. Snider, R. S., and Magoun, H. W.: Facilitation produced by cerebellar stimulation. *J. Neurophysiol., 12*:335, 1949.
26. Snider, R. S., McCulloch, W. S., and Magoun, H. W.: A cerebellobulboreticular pathway for suppression. *J. Neurophysiol., 12*:325, 1949.
27. Sprague, J. M., and Chambers, W. W.: Control of posture by reticular formation and cerebellum in the intact, anesthetized and unanesthetized and in the decerebrate cat. *Amer. J. Physiol., 176*:52, 1954.
28. Strom, G.: Central nervous regulation of body temperature. In Field, J., Magoun, H. W., and Hall, V. C. (Eds.): *Handbook of Physiology.* Baltimore, Williams & Wilkins, 1960, Vol. II, Sec. I, pp. 1173.
29. Takeuchi, J., Inoue, J., Tokeda, J., Uchida, E., Yagi, S., Ishii, M., and Ueda, H.: Experimental studies on the nervous control of the renal circulation. *Jap. Heart J., 4*:364, 1963.
30. Thomas, D. M., Kaufman, R. P., Sprague, J. M., and Chambers, W. W.: Experimental studies of the vermal cerebellar projections to the brain stem of the cat *J. Anat., 90*:371, 1956.
31. Uvnas, B.: Sympathetic vasodilator system and blood flow. *Physiol. Rev., 40 (Suppl. 4)*:67, 1960.
32. Wallberg, F., Pompeiano, O., Westrum, L. E., and Hauglie-Hanssen, E.: Fastigii-reticular fibers in the cat. *J. Comp. Neurol., 119*:187, 1962.
33. Whiteside, J. H., and Snider, R. S.: Relations of cerebellum to upper brainstem. *J. Neurophysiol., 16*:397, 1954.
34. Willis, T.: *Cerebrei anatome; cui assessit nervorium descripto et uses,* Amsterdam, Shagen, 1664, pp. 139.
35. Wise, B. L., and Ganong, W. F.: Effect of brainstem stimulation on renal function. *Amer. J. Physiol., 198*:1291, 1960.
36. Zanchetti, A., and Zoccolini, A.: Autonomic hypothalamic outbursts elicited by cerebellar stimulation. *J. Neurophysiol., 17*: 475, 1954.

DISCUSSION

Dr. Murphy: We have recent observations which show how subtle changes in stimulating current applied to the cerebellar cortex may produce either excitation or inhibition of Purkinje cells in the *same* location. Thus one might expect at times to obtain opposite or contrasting autonomic effects by stimulating the same cortical locus with different currents. Did you ever observe such contrasting effects?

Dr. Hoffer: This is really a very difficult problem to analyze. In this context, I was particularly glad to hear Dr. Andy's presentation, again showing different responses, presumably from activation of different pathways, produced by stimulation of the same area. Moruzzi and his co-workers demonstrated a similar phenomenon in the production of somatomotor responses with stimulation of the cerebellar cortex.

Dr. MacLean: Did you control for electrical after-discharges in your stimulation, or don't you see it in the encéphale isolé?

Dr. Hoffer: You mean electrical after-discharges in the cerebellum?

Dr. MacLean: Yes, in the cerebellum itself. Have you done any electrophysiological recordings in the cerebellum while stimulating?

Dr. Hoffer: No, I haven't.

Dr. MacLean: Ray, do you think that this ever enters the picture—that is getting local after-discharges?

Dr. Snider: I very definitely do, and I refer to the work in 1952 by Granit and his associates in which they showed by stimulating midline structures of the cerebellum (the anterior lobe) switching effects in either the gamma efferent system or the alpha efferent system. They speculated at that time that maybe part of the switching device was the interaction between the cortex and the nucleus. Dr. Hoffer is considering another switching effect in which the visceral motor system helps to induce more blood flow to the muscle (skeletal) by diminishing blood flow to the viscera. This may be something peculiar to the cerebellar cortex, but a feedback circuit from the nuclei cannot be ruled out.

Dr. Reis: This is very interesting. Miura and I have recently discovered a powerful pressor response evoked by electrical stimulation highly localized to the rostral pole of the fastigial nucleus and its medial ventral segment. The pressor response is very marked and can be as large as 100 mm Hg. As seen in Figure 7–15, as one lowers an electrode through the cortex, an initial mild depressor response turns pressor as the electrode reaches the localized region in the fastigial nucleus. The threshold stimulation is of the order of 0.15 mA or less, which is very low. The response is definitely not due to spread of the stimulus current to the brain stem. The response is mediated by the fastigial bulbar tract which projects through the restiform body to the paramedian reticular nucleus. It is therefore a cerebellar-medullary reflex arc and does not involve structures lying above the rostral medulla. Bilateral lesions of the paramedian reticular nucleus abolish the response without changing the resting blood pressure. The paramedian nucleus, by the way, is the area to which the carotid sinus nerve projects monosynaptically. It therefore appears to serve as a common site for termination of both baroreceptor fibers and the cerebellar projections affecting blood pressure.

Dr. Snider: Do you see a rebound effect in your experiments?

Dr. Reis: No, very rarely.

Dr. Hockman: I should like to add that we have stimulated in the same region of the fastigial nucleus as just described by Don. We have also observed tremendous increases in blood pressure with and without rebound; furthermore, we have also induced alterations in heart rate and rhythm by stimulating the same region with slightly higher stimulus intensities.

Dr. Snider: Did you use animals treated with Flaxedil?

Dr. Hockman: Yes, we did, and we also used animals immobilized with succinylcholine.

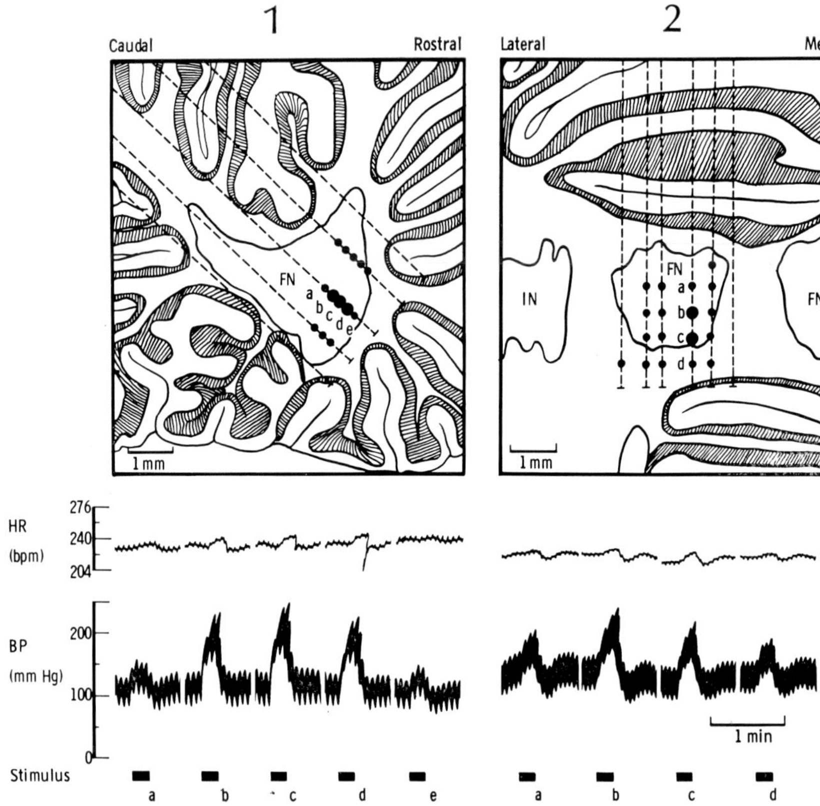

Figure 7–15. Localization for optimal loci for fastigial pressor response in two representative experiments. Column *1* is a sagittal section of cerebellum; column 2 is a coronal section. Electrode tracks penetrating cerebellum are reproduced by dotted lines. Responsive sites are shown by solid circles. Small circles represent weak responses, and large circles represent more powerful pressor responses. Positive points were identified by stimulation 200μ steps (sagittal section) or at 500μ steps (coronal section) with a 12-second stimulus train (0.1 msec duration, 50 cps and constant intensity of 0.2 ma). Points along tracks identified by letters are represented by appropriate polygraph tracings below each cross section showing heart rate (HR) in beats per minute (bpm) and blood pressure (BP). Note that maximal responsive sites are localized to rostral and ventromedial portion of fastigial nucleus. FN (fastigial nucleus), IN (interposed nucleus). (From Miura, M., and Reis, D. J.: *Amer. J. Physiol., 219:*1330, 1970.)

Dr. Hoffer: Is there any problem with current spread in your preparations? As you know, the deep cerebellar nuclei are quite close to the brain stem.

Dr. Hockman: No. Advancing the electrode a millimeter or two was sufficient to lose the response. We also recorded gross electrical activity with the stimulating electrode at stimulus termination, but we never observed any after-discharge.

Dr. Nauta: Dr. Snider, have I correctly understood you to say that the effect which you showed the cerebellum to have on peripheral vasomotor functions is essentially an anticipatory one? If so, the instructions provided by the cerebellum to central vasomotor control mechanisms must be extremely detailed. It must convey, literally, a copy of the somatic motor blue print to these autonomic control mechanisms. I was wondering if one could possibly approach this matter in the classical operant-conditioning situation in which a monkey is withholding a response because the final "now go" signal has not come yet, although the previous signal has told him what response will be required of him. Could one possibly, in this short interval, expect to be able to measure blood flow in muscle groups prominently involved in the anticipated movement?

Dr. Abrahams: An experiment of this type was done by Brod in Czechoslovakia on dogs trained to work in which he conditioned vasomotor changes in a muscle on the basis of the preparation for work, but he didn't do a detailed regional flow, muscle by muscle.

Dr. Snider: That is a very challenging concept. Another challenging one is the well-known observation that the cerebellum is one of the last portions of the brain to mature. Can one equate latency of maturation with acquired motor skills of a special type? Perhaps these anticipatory responses are very real. If so, bear in mind that the proprioceptive response may reach the cerebellum at least 5 msec before it reaches the cerebral cortex. The auditory click response gets to the cerebellum 4 msec before it gets to the auditory cortex. Maybe the training of motor skills in young individuals deals more intimately with cerebellar systems than has been considered.

Dr. Reis: The lag in the loop from the output for motor neurons in contrast to output along fine myelinated fibers and the tremendous latency of transmitter release at an artery would not make this very realistic. I think that your pressure changes and flow changes occur in the order of seconds, whereas motor changes occur in the order of milliseconds. So while your information can get to the cerebellum very rapidly, the effector end is going rather slowly.

Dr. Hoffer: Yes, but we are talking not about the fact that the muscle is moving, engaging in exercise and "telling" the cerebellum to send more blood as a secondary adjustment. We are talking about an organism which knows that it is going to be exercising. There are certain learned patterns, anticipatory responses, if you will, prior to the onset of exercise. This point could only be tested by Dr. Nauta's suggestion—that is, by having a monkey trained so that he could say, I'm going to move my biceps in about five seconds, and then observing what happens with cerebellar stimulation or other techniques of reversibly influencing the cerebellum.

Dr. Abrahams: Hilton and I attributed that to the hypothalamus in 1960, and I think that we called them "preparatory reflexes."

Dr. Hoffer: According to Dr. Nauta, the cerebellum does project there. Furthermore, Ban has shown that cerebellar responses may be influenced by hypothalamic stimulation and vice versa. However, the projection to the hypothalamus cannot be the only one involved since some circulatory responses to cerebellar stimulation remain after interruption of this projection.

Dr. Calaresu: I was very intrigued by your experiments showing a reversal of the effector response before and after decerebration. I wonder what is a possible explanation for that?

Dr. Hoffer: Well, I view the cerebellar cortex as an admixture of areas producing pressor and depressor responses. Any particular response means that you are stimulating more points of one than of the other. After you decerebrate the animal, you presumably block the pathways for the direct pressor responses, and the depressor elements you are stimulating at the same time now come through. Presumably, they were previously masked by the pressor elements.

Dr. Calaresu: I was wondering if the change in arterial pressure may be due to the different vagal level.

Dr. Hoffer: I have found, by and large, with light chloralose, you can have a very reactive autonomic nervous system with an active baroreceptor regulatory system. After you decerebrate and wait a while, the pressure usually comes back up to where it was, maybe 5 to 10 mm lower. Furthermore, responses to baroreceptor stimulation and brain stem stimulation in decerebrate animals usually returned to prelesion levels. Consequently, I do not believe that the absence of some responses to cerebellar stimulation after decerebration is due to differences in "resting" vascular tone. Those animals that showed a marked difference in "resting" vascular tone or baroreceptor responses after decerebration were eliminated from the study.

SESSION III

Chairman: **Paul Dell**

Chapter 8

Implications of Microelectrode Findings on Exteroceptive Inputs to the Limbic Cortex

PAUL D. MACLEAN

THE EXPERIMENTS to be described were partly motivated by the following question: What is it that psychologically distinguishes each one of us as individuals? Introspection suggests that the condition most essential to our feeling of individuality is a twofold source of information from the external public world and the internal private world.[22] Signals to the brain from the world within are entirely private, whereas those from the outside world can be publicly experienced and lend themselves to comparison among individuals. A sense of individuality would therefore seem to depend on mechanisms that conjoin public signals with those that are entirely private.

For many years, I have been interested in the question of how forebrain mechanisms account for the fusion of internal and external experience and the feeling of individuality. In giving a little background for the microelectrode and neuroanatomic studies, I will touch on some evolutionary considerations and then mention some pertinent symptoms of patients suffering from psychomotor epilepsy. Finally, I will point out how the problem under consideration is relevant to mechanisms underlying memory and learning.

In approaching the analysis of cerebral functions I have been guided by the simplification that in its evolution, the brain of man retains the pattern of organization of three basic brain types which for purposes of discussion I refer to as reptilian, old mammalian and new mammalian.[15,16,18,20,21,23] Despite their great differences in structure and chemistry all three types must intermesh and function together as a triune brain.[24,25] The prototype for man's most ancient brain is basically reptilian. As schematized in Figure 8–1, it forms the matrix of the upper brain stem and comprises much of the reticular system, midbrain and basal ganglia. The reptilian brain has only a rudimentary cortex. The evolving old mammalian brain is distinctive because of a marked evagination and differentiation of the primitive cortex, while the outstanding feature of the neomammallian brain is the great development of more highly differentiated type of cortex called neocortex.

In popular terminology, the three subbrains might be imagined as biological *computers*, each with its own peculiar form of subjectivity and intelligence and its own time-measuring, memory, motor and other functions.[21,23]

The detailed behavioral descriptions of ethologists would allow the inference that the reptilian-type brain programs stereotyped behaviors "according to instructions based on ancestral learning and ancestral memories."[20] In other words, it seems to

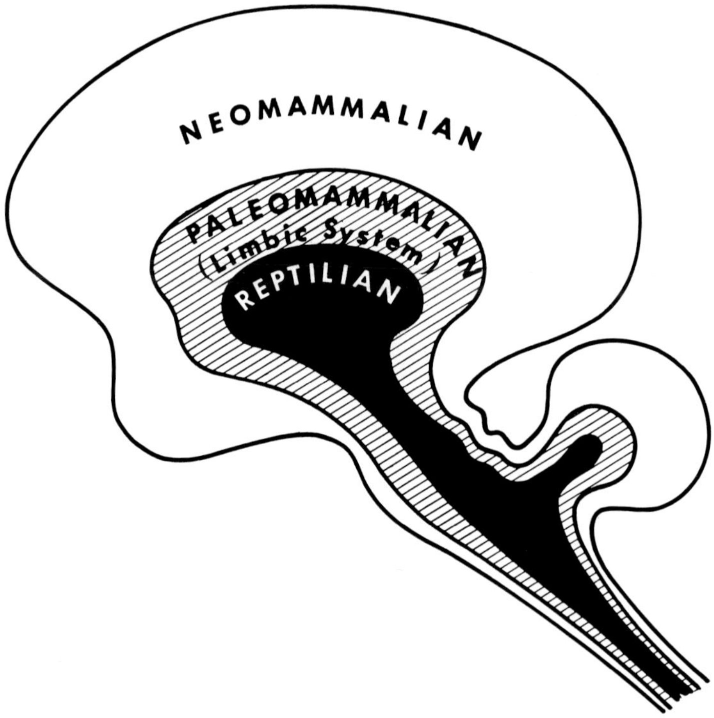

Figure 8–1. Hierarchic organization of three basic brain types which represent major developments in the evolution of man's brain. For purposes of simplification, they are referred to in ascending order as reptilian, paleomammalian and neomammalian. Greatly unlike in structure and chemistry, they are joined together as a *triune* [24,25] brain. Man's counterpart of the paleomammalian brain comprises the so-called limbic system [14] which is primarily discussed in this chapter in connection with affective processes underlying a feeling of individuality and involved in mechanisms of learning and memory. (From MacLean, P. D., *J. Nerv. Ment. Dis.*, *144*:374, 1967.)

play an important role in genetically constituted forms of behavior involved in establishing territory and social hierarchies, finding shelter, foraging, hunting, homing, mating, breeding and the like. At the same time there is evidence that it is not well designed for learning from experience.

The evolutionary development in lower mammals of a respectable cortex appears to represent Nature's attempt to provide the reptilian brain with a "thinking cap." [21] Memories of current experiences, it would seem, begin to take precedence over ancestral memories in guiding behavior.

The primitive cortex is contained in the large convolution which Broca [3] called the great limbic lobe because it surrounds the brain stem. The limbic cortex has similar features in all mammals and is structurally primitive compared with the neocortex. In a review paper in 1952, I used the descriptive term "limbic system" to refer to the limbic cortex and structures of the brain stem with which it has primary connections.[14] Restrictive definitions of this kind are operationally useful in dealing with such a complicated structure as the brain where, so to speak, all roads eventually lead to Rome.

The evolutionary stability of the limbic cortex stands in contrast to the burgeoning neocortex which mushrooms late in evolution and culminates in man "to become the brain of reading, writing, and arithmetic."[20] The evolution of this new brain goes hand-in-hand with the elaboration of visual, auditory and somatic systems, which, more than any of the other "sensory" systems, provide a refined differentiation and discrimination of happenings in the external environment. In this land of Marshall McLuhan, one is reminded that the signals to which these three systems are receptive are the only ones that lend themselves to electronic amplification and radiotransmission. Smells, tastes and interoceptions have no such avenue for communication.

Clinical observations suggest that the limbic system, unlike the neomammalian brain, derives subjective information in the form of emotional feelings which influence behavior required for self-preservation and the preservation of the species.[15] The most cogent evidence for this is provided by clinical cases with epileptogenic foci in or near the limbic cortex. As Penfield and Jasper have demonstrated during surgical intervention in such cases, either with the epileptic discharge itself or with electrical stimulation of the involved cortex, patients may experience a wide variety of vivid emotional and visceral feelings.[31] On the basis of clinical and experimental evidence, it is probable that the hippocampus is nearly always involved in the seizure discharge, with the discharge either arising in it or spreading to it from related structures. It is of fundamental importance in regard to the question of individuality that some patients experience during an aura a heightened sense of conviction of the reality of themselves and their environment. There may also be the reverse situation in which they experience a depersonalization—or what Hughlings Jackson called a "mental diplopia"[9]—characterized by a feeling as though they are looking at themselves from a distance. Finally, of further relevance, there may be distortions of perception involving any one of the sensory systems.

In the "visceral brain" paper[13] of 1949, I showed a diagram illustrating the hypothesis that all the sensory systems feed into the limbic cortex of the parahippocampal gyrus which in turn is an origin of impulses that reach the hippocampus and hypothalamus. It was then known that the olfactory system was connected with the hippocampal gyrus, but there was no experimental evidence of a representation of the other senses.

In 1952 we reported that gustatory and somatic stimulation elicited olfactory like responses in the anterior hippocampal gyrus of the rabbit.[27] Subsequently, Green and Arduini found that all forms of sensory stimulation elicited rhythmic theta activity in the hippocampus.[8]

Since then it has been shown anatomically[6] and physiologically[8] that the septum acts as a connecting link between the hypothalamus and the hippocampal formation. Fibers from the septum to the hippocampus course through the fornix. This would provide a source of interoceptions.

Various authors from time-to-time have reported that visual, auditory and somatic stimulation evokes slow wave potentials in different areas of the limbic cortex, but the authenticity of these responses has remained in doubt because of the possibility of volume conducted responses from neighboring structures.

In order to be certain about the source of the generators we have investigated sensory inputs to the limbic cortex by microelectrode techniques. All experiments have been performed on squirrel monkeys prepared with a chronically fixed stereo-

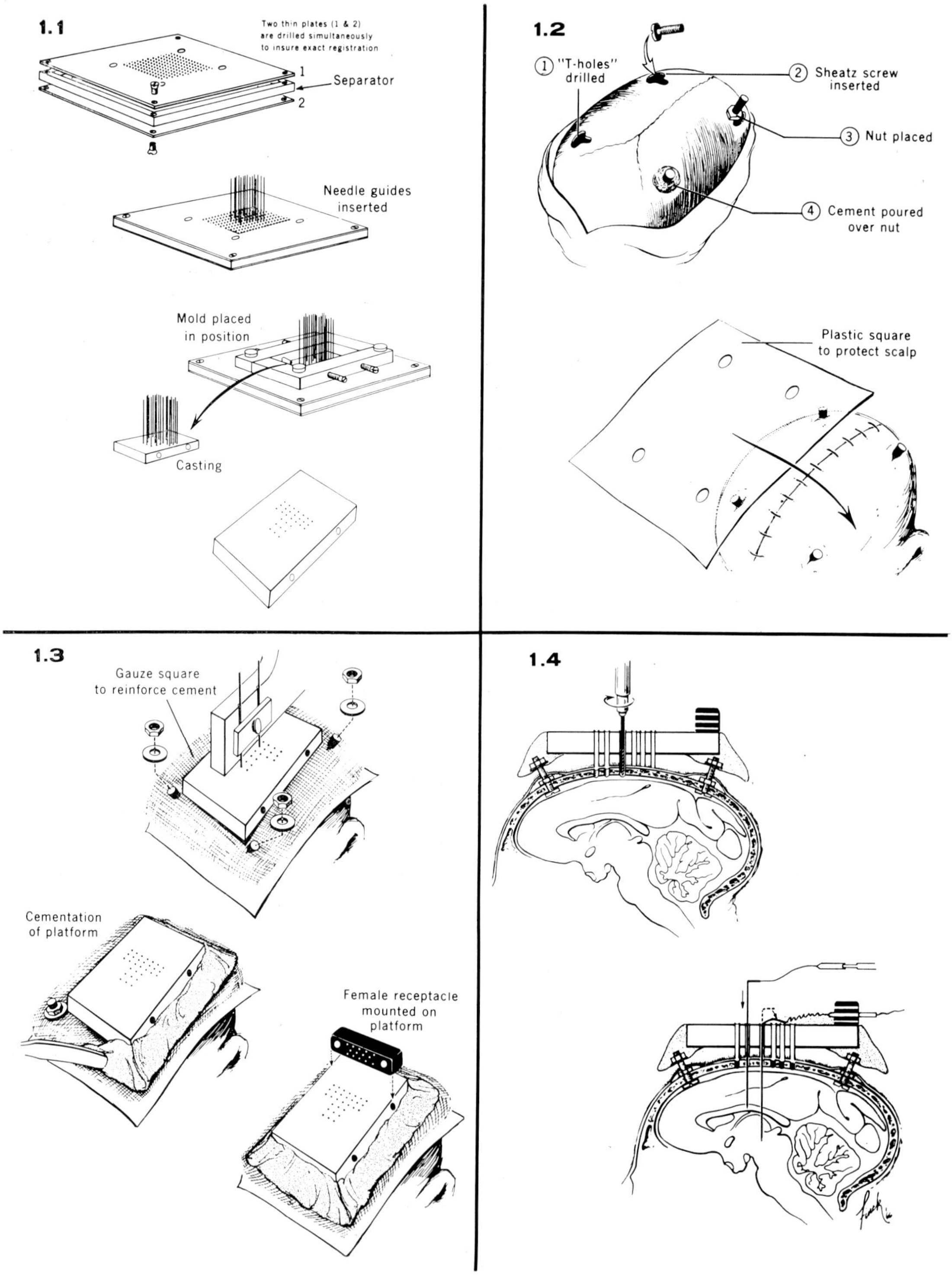

Figure 8–2. Steps in fabrication and attachment of stereotaxic device used for exploration of the brain (in the standard frontal plane) with either metal or glass microelectrodes. It provides, among other advantages, an essentially closed system and makes it possible to obtain histological sections in the same plane as all the electrode tracks. (From MacLean, P. D., *Electroenceph. Clin. Neurophysiol., 22*:180, 1967.)

taxic device that provides a closed system for intracerebral exploration with either metal or glass microelectrodes.[19] Figure 8–2 illustrates the stereotaxic platform with guides for the electrodes and shows how it is fixed above the scalp on four screws cemented into the skull. Among its other advantages, the technique makes it possible to obtain histological sections in the same plane as all of the electrode tracks. During an experiment the monkey sits in a special chair which *prevents flexion of the neck.* At the end of each experiment the electrode is usually fixed at a desired point for histological confirmation of its locus. About eight microelectrode penetrations are made on each animal over a period of six weeks.

Figure 8–3 shows the type of platinum irridium electrode designed for use with the stereotaxic device. It substitutes a tough paint for glass insulation. Figure 8–4 charts data on 5,000 units successively recorded with these electrodes. It indicates that in a typical experiment one may expect about 85 percent of the unit spikes to be negative in sign. The majority have an amplitude of about 300μV. With glass micropipettes we have been successful in obtaining intracellular recordings in awake, sitting monkeys.

Because of the fundamental role of vision in man, attention was focused first on the question of visual connections with the limbic cortex. The traditional emphasis on the close topographical relationship of the hippocampal formation to the rhinal fissure appears to have diverted attention from its interesting relationship to the calcarine fissure.[17] As illustrated by the sagittal section of the brain of man shown in Figure 8–5, there appears to be almost as much of the hippocampal formation tucked up in the region of the calcarine fissure as in the region of the rhinal fissure. In this section the hippocampus reminds one of a double-pointed boat capable of sailing in either direction.

Long ago Elliot Smith emphasized that the calcarine is one of the three oldest furrows of the brain[35] and that its counterpart, the stem of the splenial sulcus, in carnivores and ungulates marks the boundary between the striate and limbic cor-

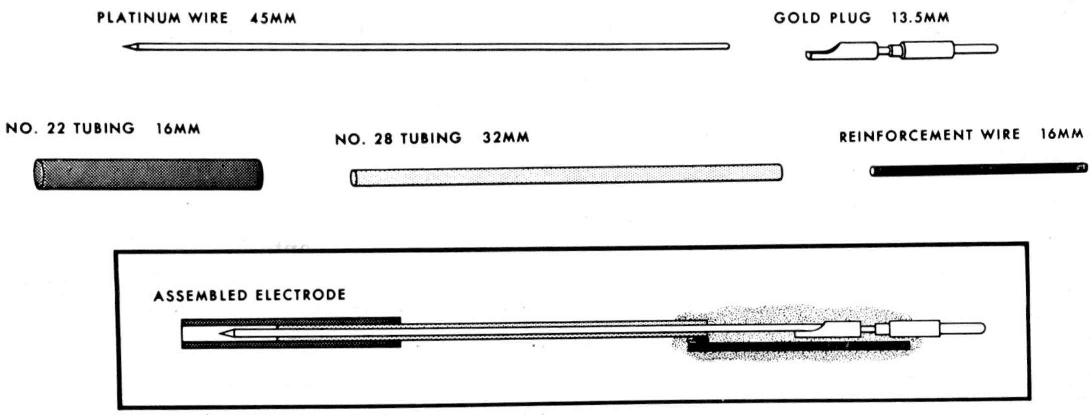

Figure 8–3. Components of platinum microelectrode devised for use with stereotaxic device shown in preceding figure. Electrode is ensheathed in guide which protects tip upon insertion into the brain and thereafter maintains it in desired frontal plane while it is lowered by a micromanipulator. (From Kinnard and MacLean, *Electroenceph. Clin. Neurophysiol.,* 22:183, 1967.)

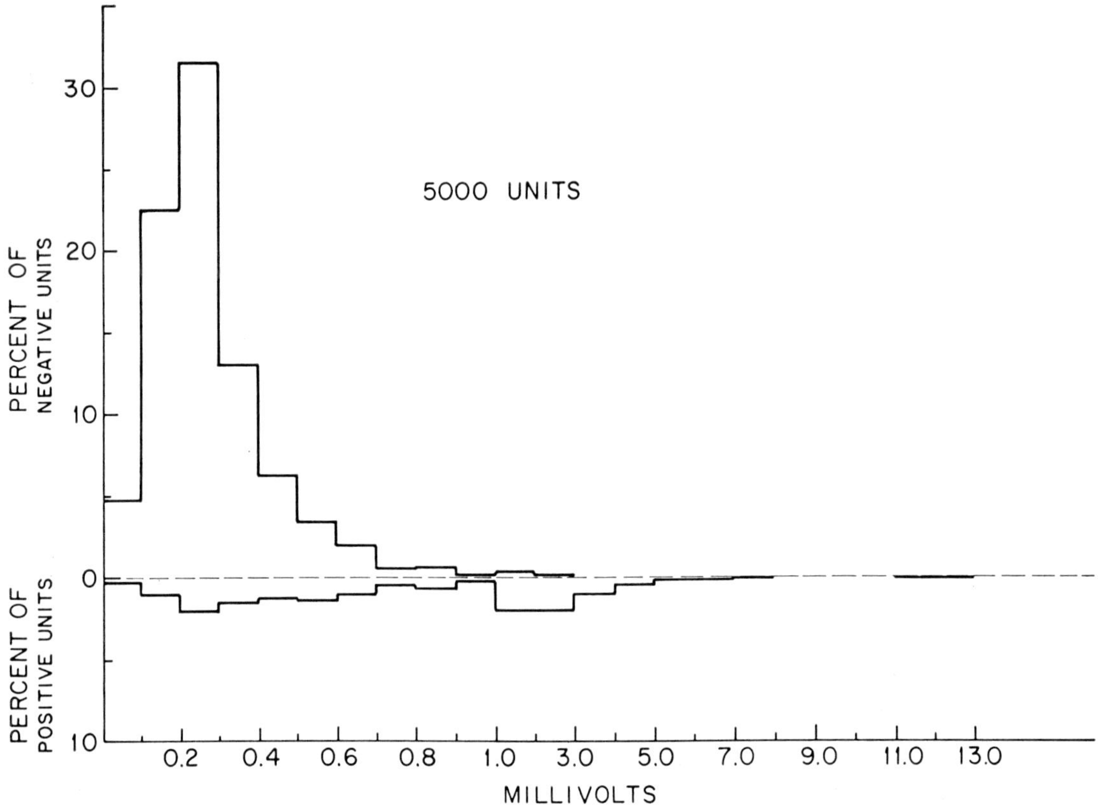

Figure 8–4. Histogram showing sign and amplitude of 5000 successively recorded units in experiments employing type of electrode shown in preceding figure. (From Kinnard and MacLean, *Electroenceph. Clin. Neurophysiol., 22*:183, 1967.)

tex.[36] In primates the abrupt transition occurs near the junction of the anterior and posterior calcarine sulci (cf. Fig. 8–6). In primates generally, and in man in particular, there is a great expansion of the perilimbic and perivisual cortex in the medial parieto-occipitotemporal region. Indeed, the fusiform gyrus, represents a new convolution in the brains of higher primates.[2]

In a recently published study we tested the effects of photic stimulation on more than 4500 units located in the limbic cortex, visual system and elsewhere.[28] As topographically shown in Figure 8–7, in the awake monkey, photic stimulation specifically evoked unit potentials in the posterior hippocampal gyrus (H), the parahippocampal portion of the lingual gyrus (L), and the retrosplenial cortex (R). Units were also activated in the perilimbic cortex of the fusiform gyrus (F). It was found that the responsive area did not extend forward into the entorhinal area (see arrow in Fig. 8–7) in the anterior part of the hippocampal gyrus. This negative finding was of interest in the light of Cajal's observation that in macrosmatic animals the entorhinal cortex has a number of similarities to the visual cortex.[33] As will be commented upon later, none of the 600 units recorded from the hippocampus itself were responsive.

A majority of responsive cells in the pos-

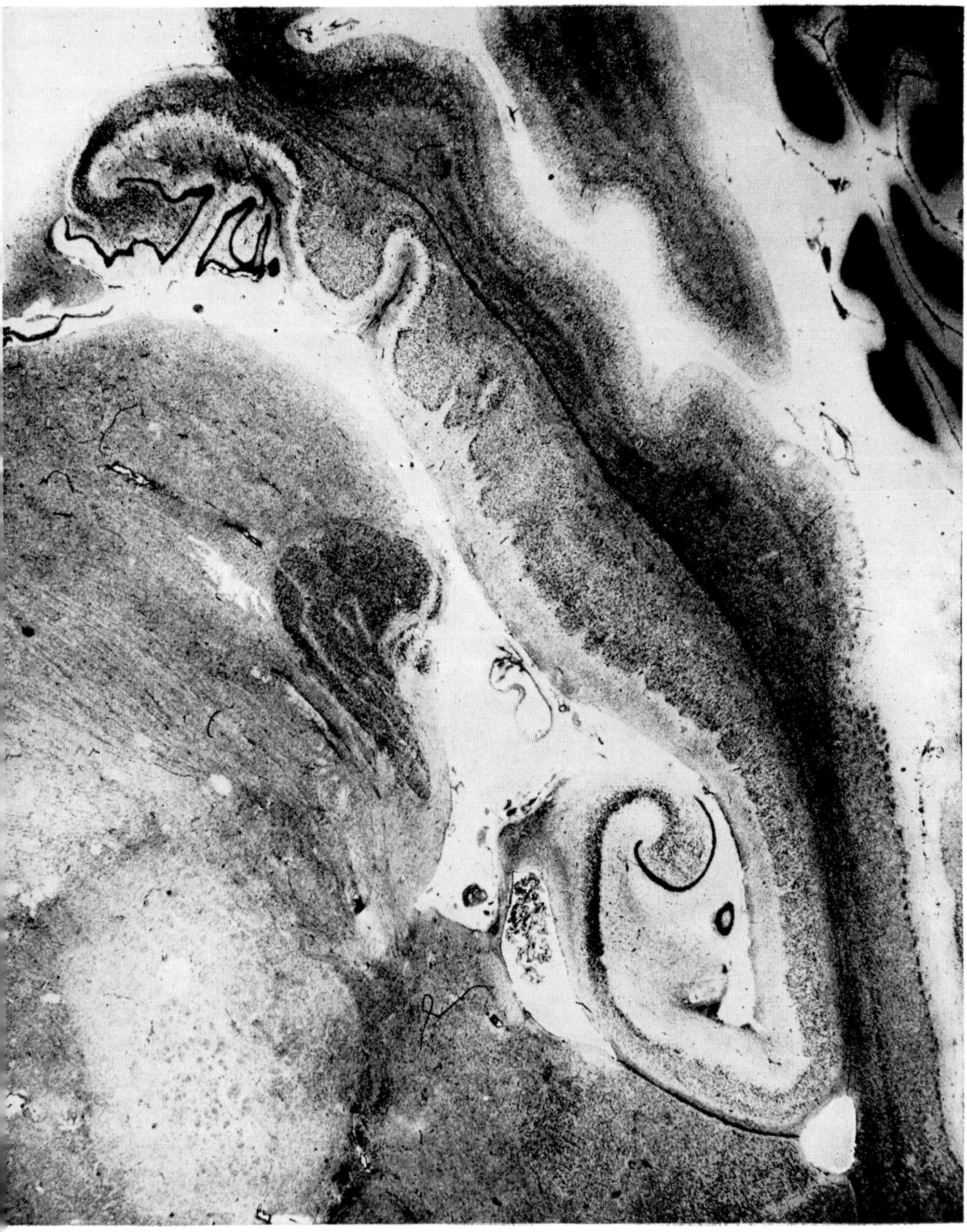

Figure 8–5. Sagittal section of human hippocampus, illustrating the folding that occurs near the rhinal fissure and calcarine sulcus. Note lateral geniculate body just above "belly" of the hippocampus. The transition between the entorhinal area and more posterior cortex of the hippocampal gyrus occurs at the level of the blood vessel in the space above the cerebellum. (From the slide collection of Dr. John M. Van Buren.)

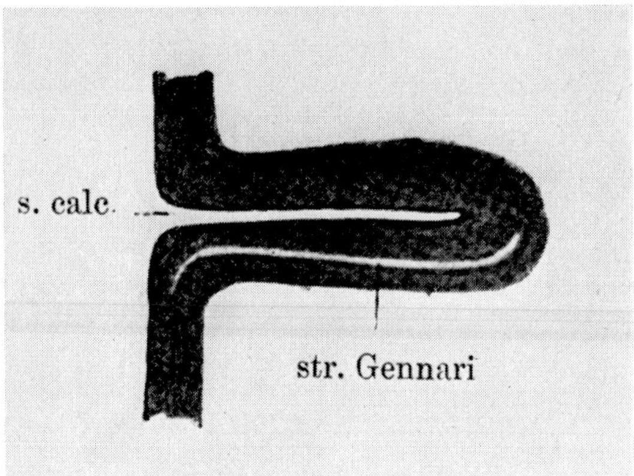

Figure 8–6. Illustration from one of the early papers of Elliot Smith, showing how the anterior calcarine sulcus marks "the boundary between the striate visual cortex and the gyrus fornicatus." (From Smith, G. Elliot, *Anat Anz., 24*:436–451, 1903–1904.)

terior hippocampal gyrus (H) were distinctive from those in other limbic areas and in the visual cortex because they gave a sustained on-response during illumination of the eye. The oscilloscopic tracing below the photograph in Figure 8–7 illustrates a sustained on-response of this type of unit. It is possible that these "tonic" units in the posterior hippocampal gyrus are involved in mechanisms by which light contributes to a state of wakefulness and changes of light induce alerting and attention. It is also possible that they may play some role in neuroendocrine functions affected by diurnal or seasonal changes in light. Elsewhere, we found such sustained responses only in the lateral geniculate body and lateral tegmental process of the pons.[28]

How do visual impulses reach the posterior parahippocampal cortex? In an attempt to answer this question Creswell and I placed lesions in or near the geniculo-pulvinar complex of twenty-three squirrel monkeys.[26] With modifications of the Nauta stain for showing fine cortical fibers, it was found that a lesion in the ventrolateral part of the lateral geniculate body resulted in a continuous band of degenerating fibers extending into the core of the hippocampal gyrus (see Fig. 2 of Ref. 26). Some fibers entered the cortex of this gyrus, as well as the contiguous areas labeled *L* and *F* in Figure 8–7. The inferior temporal part of the band corresponds to Meyer's loop in man. It has never been clear why this part of the optic projections makes a detour through the temporal lobe (cf. Fig. 8–7), but it would now appear on the basis of the new findings that it takes this roundabout course in order to distribute fibers to the posterior parahippocampal cortex and adjoining areas. Of added significance was the finding that the inferior pulvinar, commonly regarded as a visual association nucleus, projects to these same cortical areas by way of a band of fibers just lateral to the optic radiations.[26]

The parahippocampal cortex transmits impulses to the hippocampus which projects to the hypothalamus, midthalamus and other structures of the brain stem involved in emotional, endocrine and somatovisceral functions. Through such connections there exists one possible mechanism by which the melding of visual and visceral experience contributes to a sense of individuality. The sublety of this psychological process is illustrated by the déjà vu experienced by some patients with psychomotor epilepsy. It is characterized by a vivid feeling that one has already seen and experienced what is transpiring at the moment. The feeling has an important affective quality that seems to be indispensable for a sense of familiarity and personal identification with what is visually experienced. This feeling, in turn, appears to be basic to the memory of visual experiences.

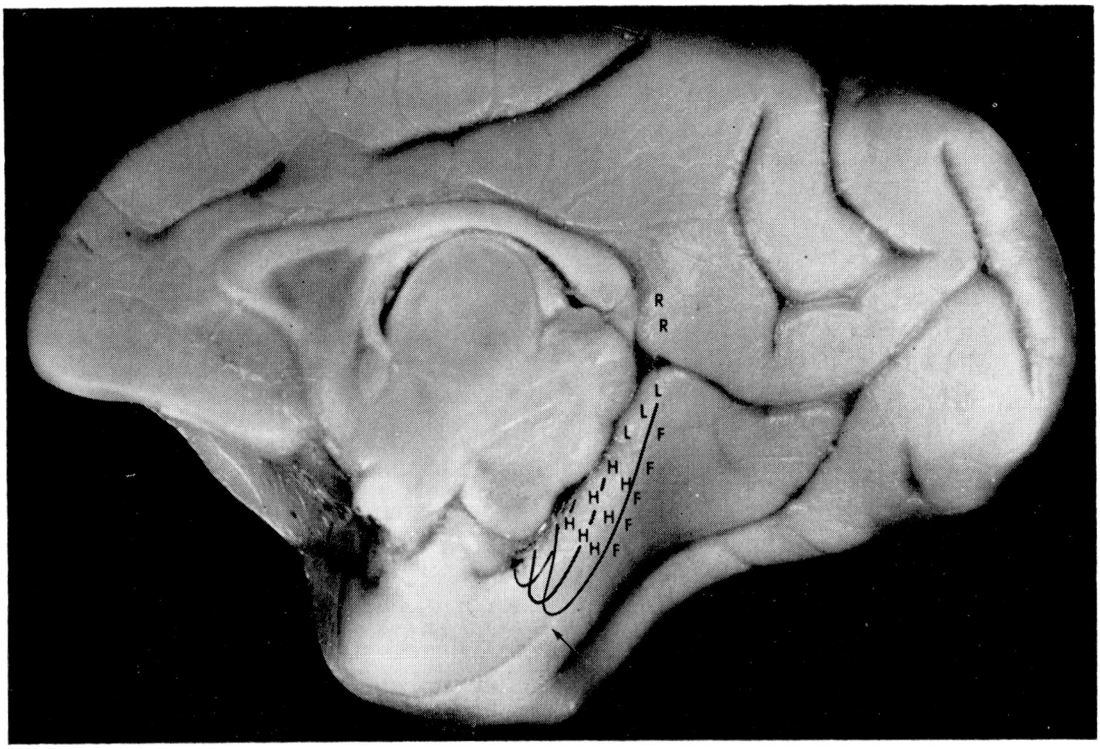

Figure 8–7. Medial view of squirrel monkey's brain showing approximate location of limbic cortical areas in which single nerve cells were activated by photic stimuli [28]—namely, the posterior hippocampal gyrus (H), parahippocampal portion of the lingual gyrus (L) and restrosplenial cortex (R). The responsive area in the fusiform gyrus (F) falls outside the limbic cortex. The curved black lines schematize the circuitous path of the optic fibers that have been traced anatomically to these areas.[26] Arrow marks termination of rhinal fissure and caudal limit of entorhinal cortex. Some nerve cells found only in area H gave sustained responses to ocular illumination. An example is shown below in the oscilloscopic tracing. The response of a photo cell in the record immediately underneath indicates the 2.5-second duration of the stimulus. Negativity up.[22,28]

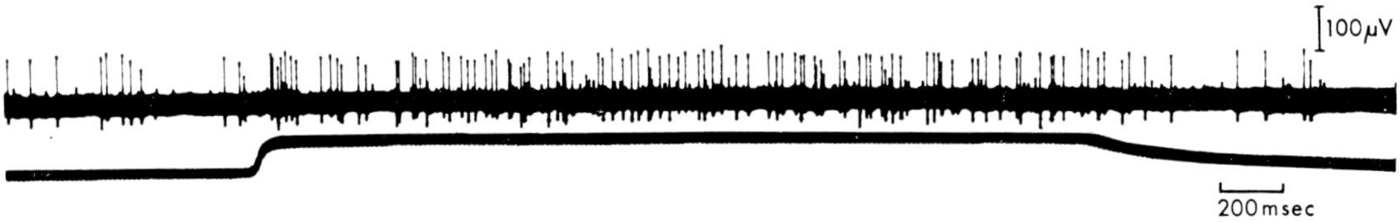

AUDITORY AND SOMATIC INPUTS

There next arises the question about auditory and somatic inputs. In the awake monkey, routine testing with clicks and sample testing with somatic stimuli failed to evoke unit responses in any of the limbic structures that were explored in the visual study. We therefore decided to explore the limbic cortex overlying the claustrum because it lies in close proximity to the auditory and somatic areas. The insular cortex overlying the claustrum (claustrocortex of Brockhaus)[4] is by definition limbic because it forms part of the phylogenetically old cortex surrounding the hilus of the hemisphere. Neuronographic findings indicate that the claustral insula fires into the anterior hippocampal formation.[32]

For auditory stimulation we employed clicks as well as pure tones applied in the form of a 5-msec diamond envelope at frequencies ranging from 500 cycles to 20 kc. In performing somatic stimulation we applied light touch with a camel's hairbrush and sharp and blunt pressure by means of a probe attached to a transducer for signaling the onset, duration and strength of the stimulus.

We tested more than 1800 units, 497 of which were located histologically in the insula overlying the claustrum.[37] Figure 8–8 shows the loci of responsive auditory and somatic units plotted on a lateral-view diagram of the insula.

Fifty-three (10.7 percent) of 497 units responded to auditory stimulation. There were two main types of such units. One type responded at a short latency (7 to 15 msec) with a discharge of 1 to 6 spikes. The other type responded at longer latencies (up to 125 msec) with discharges persisting as long as 250 msec. These two types of units were further distinguished by their response to repetitive stimuli. The first type followed stimuli with a high probability of response at rates up to 10/sec, whereas units with long latency had a low probability of response at repetition

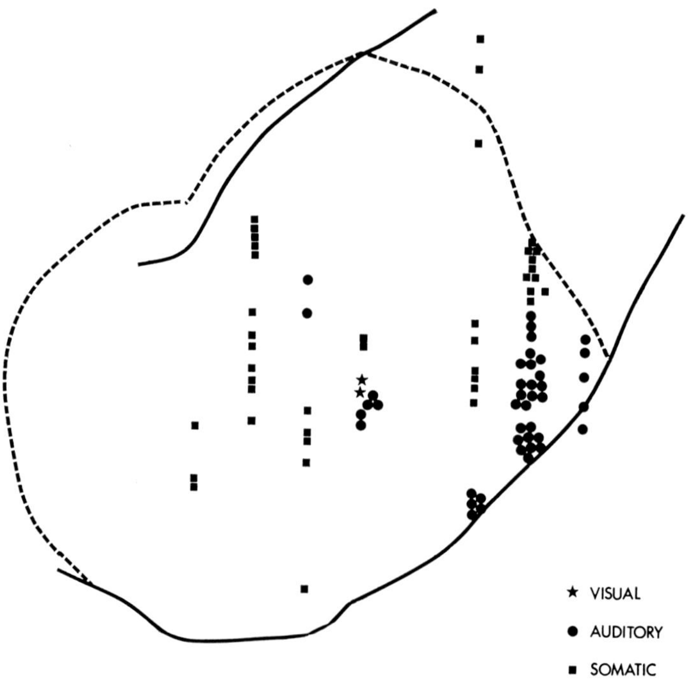

Figure 8–8. Lateral view of the insular cortex overlying the claustrum (bounded by broken line), showing loci of units responding to auditory and somatic stimulation. The claustral cortex is by definition limbic because it comprises part of the phylogenetically old cortex bordering the brain stem. The nonclaustral part of the insula lies caudally to the right of the broken line.

rates faster than one stimulus every 1 to 2/sec. A few units were isolated in the claustral insula which responded to tones only in the range between 500 cps and 1.5 kc. Parenthetically, it is of interest to mention a unit in the frontal operculum, which was found by a chance occurrence to respond only to the vocalization of another monkey.

About 9 percent of the units in the claustrocortex responded to some form of somatic stimulation. The latencies of the responses ranged from 30 to 300 msec. All but three units were activated by light touch, as well as by blunt and sharp pressure. The three exceptions were units that responded only to stimulation of a noxious character. The receptive fields were usually large and bilateral. Some units were activated by stimulation of any part of the body surface. Fields confined to one side of the body were always contralateral to the hemisphere with the recording electrode. The plotting of the results with respect to receptive fields revealed that units responding to stimulation of the head and upper extremities were for the most part located nearer to the frontal operculum than those for the trunk, tail and lower extremities. In the frontal operculum 75 (14.5 percent) of 518 units were activated by somatic stimulation, and most of the receptive fields (70 percent) involved the head and/or upper extremities. It would therefore appear that the insula and the frontal operculum represent a functional continuum.

Only two units in the claustrocortex responded to photic stimulation, indicating that the insula is little affected by changes in luminous flux. A new type of unit was encountered in the claustrocortex and frontal operculum that responded only to approaching objects in the visual fields of the monkey. These units were unresponsive to photic stimulation and side-to-side movements of objects in the visual fields were ineffective. Approach movements made in darkness were likewise ineffective, ruling out the possibility of excitation of tactile receptors by currents of air. Further experiments, including the recording of extraocular movements, must be done in an attempt to learn how these units are activated. Their mode of activation raises the question as to whether they are implicated in the aura of patients who experience macropsia in association with discharges in the circuminsular region. One such patient described by Penfield and Jasper [31] reported that "objects seemed to come quite close to him." His aura was followed by an automatism with mastication.

It deserves emphasis that none of the units recorded from the claustral insula responded to more than one modality. It is also noteworthy that there was a statistically significant difference in the localization of auditory and somatic units; auditory units were predominantly more caudal and somatic units more anterior.

Since the claustrocortex projects to the hippocampal formation,[32] the foregoing findings suggest at least one corticofugal pathway by which auditory and exteroceptive somatic information becomes combined in the hypothalamus with that of internal origin.

RELEVANCE OF CENTRAL THEME TO MEMORY AND LEARNING

As mentioned in the introduction, the union of internally and externally derived experience seems to be an essential condition for a sense of individuality. Kubie [11] would claim that memory depends on a similar duality of experience.[22] If so, the same might be said of learning, because learning depends on memory. There is a growing body of clinical and other evidence that the hippocampal formation is somehow important in laying down memories (see Ref. 21 for some key references).

As conditioning reactions are a first step to memory, the question arises as to how hippocampal cells might become conditioned. Gergen and I reported some microelectrode and neuroanatomic observations on the squirrel monkey that are possibly relevant to this problem.[7] The septal and olfactory pathways to the hippocampus may be considered as representative of internal and external inputs. In animals anesthetized by α-chloralose, it was found that septal stimulation evoked a negative slow wave in *stratum oriens* which was associated with a discharge of cells in the pyramidal layer; whereas stimulation of the olfactory tract elicited a large negative wave in *stratum radiatum* which was poorly correlated with pyramidal cell discharge.

There was previous evidence that olfactory impulses probably follow the perforant pathway from hippocampal gyrus and terminate in the distal portions of the apical dendrites of hippocampal pyramids. As opposed to this situation, our anatomical studies[7] indicated that septal fibers terminate in the *stratum oriens* which contains basal dendrites of the hippocampal pyramids as well as internuncial cells.

The essential anatomical differences are schematized in Figure 8–9. As a working hypothesis, we suggested that impulses of internal origin transmitted by the septum

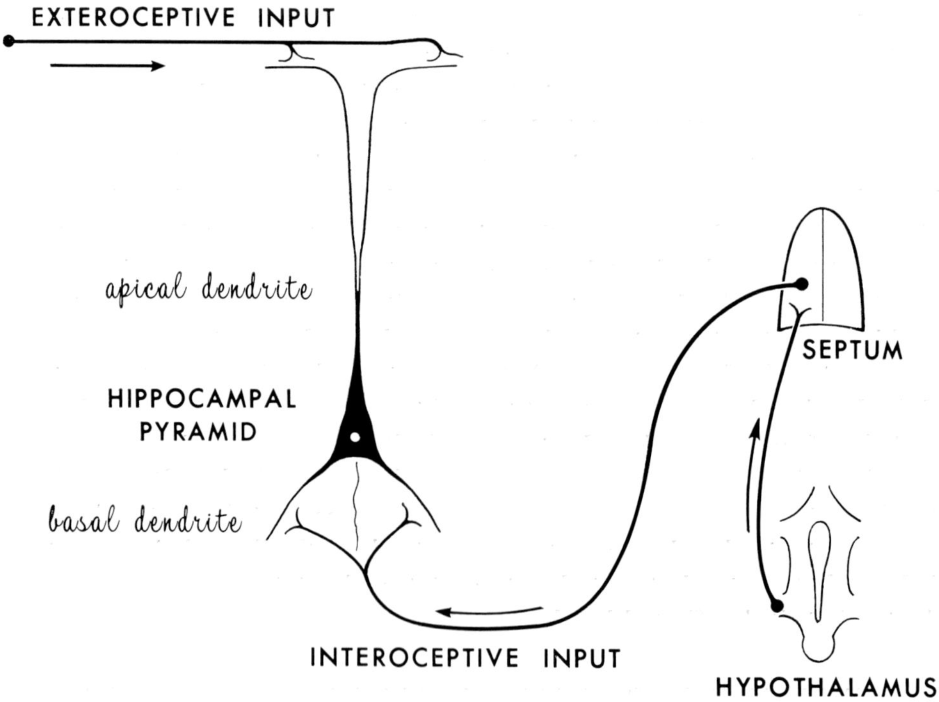

Figure 8–9. Anatomical distinctions that possibly account for differential action of interoceptive and exteroceptive inputs on hippocampal neurons. See text for implications regarding "conditioning." (From MacLean, P. D., *J. Nerv. Ment. Dis.*, *149*:40, 1969.)

act predominantly on the basal dendritic and perisomatic regions of hippocampal cells where they are highly effective in causing neuronal discharge; whereas olfactory and other exteroceptive stimuli are relatively ineffective because they result in excitation of distal portions of the apical dendrites.

Although useful for detecting the discharge of single nerve cells, as well as slow potentials, extracellular recording with microelectrodes is inadequate for revealing changes of excitability within individual cells. In order to obtain more information about the differential action of septal and olfactory inputs on hippocampal neurons, Yokota, Reeves and I performed experiments involving intracellular recording in awake, sitting squirrel monkeys with glass micropipettes.[39] The results were in agreement with the findings of the original study. Stimuli applied to the olfactory bulb elicited excitatory postsynaptic potentials (EPSPs) comparable in size to those induced by septal volleys, but only the septal EPSPs were associated with spike discharges. Examples are illustrated in Figure 8–10. Statistical analysis showed that for the two groups of cells showing EPSPs with septal and olfactory volleys,

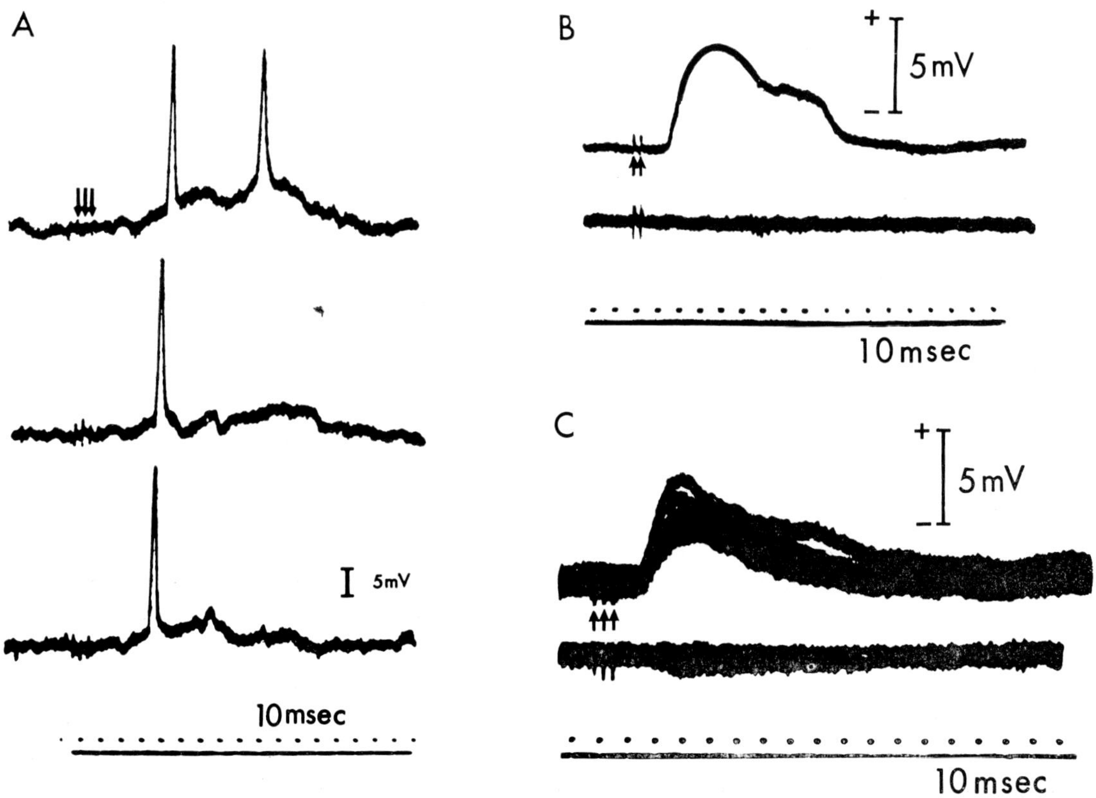

Figure 8–10. Recordings from *inside* hippocampal neurons in awake, sitting squirrel monkeys. The three successive responses shown in (*A*) illustrate that stimulation of the septum was highly effective in eliciting excitatory postsynaptic potentials (EPSPs) and discharge of the cell. On the contrary, as illustrated in (*B*) and (*C*), stimulation of the olfactory bulb induced only EPSPs without cellular discharge. In C several responses are superimposed. Resting potentials of the cells were stable and measured between −40 and −50 mV. See text regarding significance of the findings.

there was no significant differences in regard to resting membrane potentials or peak amplitudes of the EPSPs. There was, however, a highly significant difference with respect to the occurrence of spikes in the one case and their absence in the other ($p = 0.005$). Among the possible explanations was the suggestion that septal volleys might result in the initiation of spikes in the basal dendrites and their propagation to the soma.[39]

How might the electrophysiological findings be construed in terms of classical conditioning? Through the septum, the hippocampus receives impulses from the hypothalamus (see Fig. 8–9) which is involved in aversive, appetitive, visceral and humoral reactions of an *unconditional* nature. The electrophysiological findings would indicate that impulses from the septum are comparable to unconditional stimuli insofar as they are capable by themselves of causing neuronal discharge. On the contrary, olfactory impulses conducted by the perforant pathway appear to be incapable, when acting alone, of inducing a discharge. In this respect they would be comparable to conditional stimuli. It is probable that visual impulses from the posterior hippocampal gyrus, as well as auditory and somatic impulses from the insula, also utilize the perforant pathway. If so, it might explain the failure, as in the case of olfactory excitation, to evoke unit spikes in the hippocampus by visual, auditory and somatic stimulation.[28]

SUMMARY

This chapter deals with the neurophysiological question of mechanisms underlying a feeling of individuality. Introspection suggests that a sense of individuality depends on an integration of internally and externally derived information. An analysis of the problem concerning neural mechanisms begins with a consideration of cerebral evolution. In its evolution, the human brain expands along the lines of three basic patterns which are here referred to as reptilian, old mammalian, and new mammalian. The *limbic system* represents the counterpart of the old mammalian brain. It merits special attention with respect to the present topic because of clinical evidence that it is fundamental for feelings of individuality and reality. How might this system afford an integration of internal and external experience? In this regard there has been a notable lack of information about inputs to the limbic cortex from exteroceptive systems. Microelectrode and neuroanatomic experiments designed to answer this question have provided evidence in the monkey of visual connections with posterior limbic cortex. Recording of unit activity has also revealed inputs from auditory and somatosensory systems to the limbic insular cortex overlying the claustrum. These cortical areas are a source of afferents to the hippocampus which in turn projects to the hypothalamus and other brain stem structures. Intracellular recording in awake, sitting squirrel monkeys have shown a differential effect of interoceptive and exteroceptive inputs on the excitability of hippocampal neurons. As schematized in a neural model, this situation may reflect differences in the sites at which the inputs terminate on the hippocampal pyramids. In addition to the matter of individuality, the electrophysiological findings are relevant to the question of archicortical conditioning and the role of such in memory and learning.

REFERENCES

1. Andersen, P., and Lomo, T.: Mode of activation of hippocampal pyramidal cells by excitatory synapses on dendrites. *Exp. Brain Res., 2:*247, 1966.
2. Ariëns Kappers, C. U., Huber, G. C., and Crosby, E. C.: *The Comparative Anatomy of the Nervous System of Vertebrates, Including Man.* New York, Macmillan Co., 1936, p. 864.
3. Broca, P.: Anatomie comparée des circonvolutions cérébrales. Le grand lobe limbique et la scissure limbique dans la série des mammifères. *Rev. Anthrop., 1:*385, 1878.
4. Brockhaus, H.: Die Cyto und Myeloarchitektonik des Cortex claustralis und des Claustrum beim Menschen. *J. Psychol. Neurol. (Leipzig), 49:*249, 1940.
5. Cuenod, M., Casey, K. L., and MacLean, P. D.; Unit analysis of visual input to posterior limbic cortex. I. Photic stimulation. *J. Neurophysiol., 28:*1101, 1965.
6. Daitz, H. M., and Powell, T. P. S.: Studies of the connexions of the fornix system. *J. Neurol. Neurosurg. Psychiat., 17:*75, 1954.
7. Gergen, J. A., and MacLean, P. D. The limbic system: Photic activation of limbic cortical areas in the squirrel monkey. *Ann. N.Y. Acad. Sci., 117:*69, 1964.
8. Green, J. D., and Arduini, A. A.: Hippocampal electrical activity in arousal. *J. Neurophysiol., 17:*533, 1954.
9. Jackson, J. Hughlings, and Stewart, P.: Epileptic attacks with a warning of a crude sensation of smell and with the intellectual aura (dreamy state) in a patient who had symptoms pointing to gross organic disease of the right temporosphenoidal lobe. *Brain, 22:*534, 1899.
10. Kinnard, M. A., and MacLean, P. D.: A platinum micro-electrode for intracerebral exploration with a chronically fixed stereotaxic device. *Electroenceph. Clin. Neurophysiol., 22:*183, 1967.
11. Kubie, L. S.: Some implications for psychoanalysis of modern concepts of the organization of the brain. *Psychoanalyt. Quart., 22:*21, 1953.
12. Liddell, H. S.: The nervous system as a whole: The conditioned reflex. In Fulton, J. F.: *Physiology of the Nervous System.* New York, Oxford University Press, 1949, p. 537.
13. MacLean, P. D.: Psychosomatic disease and the "visceral brain." Recent developments bearing on the Papez theory of emotion. *Psychosom. Med., 11:*338, 1949.
14. MacLean, P. D.: Some psychiatric implications of physiological studies on frontotemporal portion of limbic system (visceral brain). *Electroenceph. Clin. Neurophysiol., 4:*407, 1952.
15. MacLean, P. D.: New findings relevant to the evolution of psychosexual functions of the brain. *J. Nerv. Ment. Dis., 135:*289, 1962.
16. MacLean, P. D.: Man and his animal brains. *Mod. Med., 32:*95, 1964.
17. MacLean, P. D.: The limbic and visual cortex in phylogeny: Further insights from anatomic and microelectrode studies. In Hassler, R., and Stephan, H. (Eds.): *Evolution of the Forebrain.* Stuttgart, Georg Thieme, 1966, p. 443.
18. MacLean, P. D.: The brain in relation to empathy and medical education. *J. Nerv. Ment. Dis., 144:*374, 1967.
19. MacLean, P. D.: A chronically fixed sterotaxic device for intracerebral exploration with macro- and micro-electrodes. *Electroenceph. Clin. Neurophysiol., 22:*180, 1967.
20. MacLean, P. D.: Alternative neural pathways to violence. In Ng, L. (Ed.): *Alternatives to Violence.* New York, Time-Life Books, 1968, p. 24.
21. MacLean, P. D.: Ammon's horn: A continuing dilemma. Foreword in Ramon y Cajal, S.: *The Structure of Ammon's Horn.* Translated from the Spanish by Lisbeth M. Kraft. Springfield, Charles C Thomas, 1968.
22. MacLean, P. D.: The internal-external bonds of the memory process. *J. Nerv. Ment. Dis., 149:*40, 1969.
23. MacLean, P. D.: The paranoid streak in man. In Koestler, A., and Smythies, J. R. (Eds.): *Beyond Reductionism.* London, Hutchinson & Co. Ltd., 1969.

24. MacLean, P. D.: A triune concept of the brain and behavior. Lecture I. Man's reptilian and limbic inheritance; Lecture II. Man's limbic brain and the psychoses; Lecture III. New trends in man's evolution, In Boag, T. (Ed.): *The Hincks Memorial Lectures.* Toronto, University of Toronto Press (in press).
25. MacLean, P. D.: The triune brain, emotion and scientific bias. Chapter 33 In *Intensive Study Program in the Neurosciences, Neurosciences Research Program.* New York, Rockefeller University Press, 1970, pp. 336–349.
26. MacLean, P. D., and Cresswell, G.: Anatomical connections of visual system with limbic cortex of monkey. *J. Comp. Neurol., 138:*265, 1970.
27. MacLean, P. D. Horwitz, N. H., and Robinson, F.: Olfactory-like responses in pyriform area to non-olfactory stimulation. *Yale J. Biol. Med., 25:*159, 1952.
28. MacLean, P. D., Yokota, T., and Kinnard, M. A.: Photically sustained on-responses of units in posterior hippocampal gyrus of awake monkey. *J. Neurophysiol., 31:* 870, 1968.
29. Morison, R. S.; Dempsey, E. W., and Morison, B. R.: Cortical responses from electrical stimulation of the brain stem. *Amer. J. Physiol., 131:*732, 1941.
30. Morison, R. S., Dempsey, E. W., and Morison, B. R.: On the propagation of certain cortical potentials. *Amer. J. Physiol., 131:*744, 1941.
31. Penfield, W., and Jasper, H.: *Epilepsy and the Functional Anatomy of the Human Brain.* Boston, Little, Brown & Co., 1954.
32. Pribram, K. H., and MacLean, P. D.: Neurographic analysis of medial and basal cerebral cortex. II. Monkey. *J. Neurophysiol., 16:*324, 1953.
33. Ramón y Cajal, S.: *Studies on the Cerebral Cortex (Limbic Structures).* Translated from the Spanish by Lisbeth M. Kraft. London, Lloyd-Luke Ltd., and Chicago, The Year Book Publishers, Inc., 1955.
34. Rasmussen, G.: Personal communication.
35. Smith, G. Elliot: On the homologies of the cerebral sulci. *J. Anat., 36:*309, 1902.
36. Smith, G. Elliot: The morphology of the retrocalcarine region of the cortex cerebri. *Proc. Roy. Soc. London. 73:*59, 1904.
37. Sudakov, K., MacLean, P. D., Reeves, A. G., and Marino, R. Unit study of exteroceptive inputs to claustrocortex in awake, sitting, squirrel monkey. *Brain Research, 28:*19, 1971.
38. Yokota, T., Reeves, A. G., and MacLean, P. D.: Intracellular olfactory response of hippocampal neurons in awake, sitting squirrel monkeys. *Science, 157:*1072, 1967.
39. Yokota, T., Reeves, A. G., and MacLean, P. D.: Differential effects of septal and olfactory volleys on intracellular responses of hippocampal neurons in awake, sitting monkeys. *J. Neurophysiol., 33:*96, 1970.

DISCUSSION

Dr. Gloor: Have you looked for the receptive field configuration of the cells in the retrosplenial cortex? The single units that you found in this retrosplenial cortex, I understand, must receive their afferents through the geniculate system. Now geniculate cells have a very characteristic receptive field: They are of the concentric type, unlike those of the striate cortex which function as edge detectors, and so forth. Have you looked for the kind of receptive fields these cells have? Do they just respond to change in illumination, as I understand from what you said, or do they have characteristic receptive fields and, if so, how are they organized?

Dr. MacLean: We tried a little bit on that, but these are animals that are sitting in chairs. They are able to move their eyes and look around, so we really do not have any information on receptive fields. We can say about the retrosplenial units that some of them were excited by stimulation only of the contralateral eye as opposed to the units in other areas which responded to stimulation of either eye, and this might suggest that they were activated by the primitive temporal monocular crescent.

Dr. Basmajian: In your exploration, did you stay on any unit long enough to have any conditioning effect as Fetz has reported with cortical units in *Science*? The paper I am referring to is actually a study on operant conditioning of cortical cells.

Dr. MacLean: With our extracellular recording, we can stay with units about as long as we want to, but with intracellular recording, the average time within a unit was six minutes, and the longest that we were ever in a single cell was sixty minutes. I think that to condition cells according to our model, you would need a new animal for every experiment, because after testing first with the medial septum and then with olfactory bulb stimulation, and then pairing them, you would have the animal conditioned, presumably, after a number of such trials. So from the standpoint of experimental design, the model is quite impractical.

Dr. Basmajian: But a variation of this approach might be able to provide a model for operant conditioning in this area, and it sounds like a real possibility.

Dr. MacLean: One of the most important things about the intracellular study, in my opinion, is that it shows that with stimulating the olfactory bulb you are able to generate EPSPs. (We never saw IPSPs, by the way.) With extracellular recording you would never know this. Indeed, one might be tempted to infer from extracellular recording that the cells were unaffected because olfactory volleys never evoked unit spikes.

Dr. Hoffer: Were you ever able to influence on a long-time basis, over a matter of minutes, the spontaneous activity of the cells that you were recording from with any of these stimuli?

Dr. MacLean: We have not looked for subtle changes in the firing rate of cells for prolonged periods following various stimuli. In these particular studies that I was reporting today, we were concerned only with responses that were clearly time-locked to the stimulus. As far as the sustained photic responses were concerned, we tested with periods of up to five seconds with ocular illumination. These cells would show a sustained discharge during that period. In a few instances, we illuminated the eye for longer periods and there was a little adaptation. None of our hippocampal cells responded to photic stimulation. There were 600 units in different parts of the hippocampus that were studied, and none of them responded to photic stimulation. This is opposed to findings in animals anesthetized with choralose in which we did find a few units in the hippocampus responding to photic stimulation. In the awake sitting animal, one of the surprising things is that there is so little convergence on any of these limbic units. One might expect that more than one kind of stimulus would evoke responses in these units, but this has not been our experience.

Dr. French: I was just going to ask that question, Paul. Did I understand you to say that few limbic cells respond to converging stimuli at least from exteroceptive sources or just those in the insular region?

Dr. MacLean: No. In the posterior hippocampal gyrus and the insular region, they all seem to be modality specific cells, as far as we can tell. Now we were *not* looking at the whole gamut of modalities, to be sure, but in these areas they were modality specific and, as I said, we found this a little surprising. In the frontal operculum, however, as I mentioned, we did find a few cells which responded both to auditory and somatic stimulation.

Dr. French: Not very many?

Dr. MacLean: Not very many, no.* The circuits seem "to tighten up" in the awake animal.

Dr. French: Did you ever try interoceptive stimuli—distention of the bladder or something like that?

Dr. MacLean: No, and I am not going to live long enough to do this. That is why it is so terrible to be in one's middle fifties!

Dr. Snider: I don't know how seriously to take your schematized diagram of the hippocampal pyramid, but I judge from it that you mean that the exteroceptive input is the only part of the input that can generate dendritic spikes. Now the reason I bring this up is because it seems to me that the diagram, as I interpreted it, puts a lot of emphasis on the integration of sensory input or data on the pyramidal cell. It may be that this is one way that it does it, because I think that there is fairly good evidence that dendritic spikes do arise in some of these pyramids while the basal dendrites, on the other hand, would have no way of generating such spikes. Would you like to comment? Have you any data on that?

Dr. MacLean: Before publishing this particular paper, we have been trying to find some explanation of why we get EPSPs with about the same range in amplitude † from olfactory bulb stimulation and septal stimulation, yet elicit spikes only with septal volleys. With septal stimulation, contrary to the findings of Kandel and Spencer who observed a fairly constant firing level of about 4 mV upon stimulating the subiculum, our spikes take off anywhere along the rising phase of the EPSP, suggesting, for the reasons I mentioned, that they may be initiated in the basal processes. Why do you say that spikes could not be generated in the basal processes? Anderson also has some evidence for this.[1]

Dr. Snider: Yes, but doesn't Purpura's work contradict that?

Dr. MacLean: I would certainly like to get some discussion on this point because, as I said, this is one of the things that we have been trying to clarify.

Dr. Snider: Well, there is recent work which indicates that dendritic spikes can be obtained from Purkinje cells, and I think that you can get dendritic spikes out of these cells; however, you don't get them from the basal dendrites, only from the large apical dendrites. Isn't that true, Peter?

Dr. Gloor: Yes it is.

Dr. Snider: This might be a partial explanation for your data.

Dr. Gloor: No one has yet shown, as far as I know, that these dendritic spikes in the pyramidal cells of the hippocampus occur under any other conditions than rather excessive stimulation, such as one is dealing with during a seizure or when the hippocampus is close to a seizure discharge. To bring out these dendritic spikes requires repetitive stimulation and, as far as I know, only under conditions of sufficiently strong electrical stimulation capable of generating seizures do these spikes occur. These conditions are not comparable to the natural situation. I am sure that these dendrites can produce spikes, but whether they can produce them without the hippocampus being rather overstimulated, close to or in a seizure state, is questionable.

Dr. Yakovlev: Is there a similar relationship for this question—some analogy in spinal cord anterior horn cell interaction as they mix with the afferents from the reticular formation? Is there some homology or analogue of this relationship in the spinal cord?

Dr. MacLean: Yes, it was originally sug-

* Two of 518 frontal opercular units.

† Statistically, there was no significant difference in peak amplitudes.

gested, I think, by Eccles and by Fadiga and Brookhart in their work on spinal neurons. Terminals causing excitation near the soma were more effective in discharging the cell than those depolarizing distal processes. It seems to me that even in the neocortex people are now beginning to talk about the dendritic origin of the spike. They are not finding the nice constant firing levels that have been reported in the spinal motor neurons.

Dr. Yakovlev: I would like to draw attention to the tectogenesis of these formations making up the "limbic system" in the forebrain, as is currently defined. Their development is very complex. These tectogenetic complexities, particularly in the end brain, have of necessity been somewhat neglected in the construction of the current concept of what this "limbic system" is. Under this broad term the present concept encompasses more than the limbus of the hemisphere proper. It includes also the brain "stuff" between the hemispheres. The limbus of the hemisphere (the mesocortex) is on tectogenetic grounds quite distinct from the allocortical formations in the median core of the end brain. The functional properties of this median telencephalon "impar" and of the borders, or limbi, of the partially paired hemispheres bilaterad from it, must be different. Also, of course, the limbic zone of the hemisphere is different in development, structure and function from the totally paired parts of the two hemispheres which represent the fundi of the paired hemispheres. These three divisions of the end brain are different parts of a single organ. They develop differently. The wall of the median telencephalic "holosphere" of a 4 mm human embryo never shows a clear differentiation into the three layers of His—the matrix, the mantle and the marginal—and never produces a cortical plate. The hippocampus to which we refer as a primitive cortex (archicortex) develops more like a nucleus. If one is willing to accept that the olfactory ("praepiriform") cortex (paleocortex) of the terminal brain is a homolog of the posterior horn, then the hippocampus with its efferent fornix fibers, is comparable to the anterior horn, with that difference that the common efferent path of this median division of the end brain is not "final." The fundamental plan of the reflex arc from the olfactovisceral receptors of the head region via olfactory cortex and thence via medial forebrain bundle, fornix and hypothalamus, to the viscerosomatic effectors is essentially similar to that of the segmental reflex arcs in the brain stem and spinal cord. The limbic mesocortex of the hemisphere is quite a radically different formation from the hippocampal plate of Ammon's horn. The hemispheres have a cortical plate (neocortex) and the limbus of the latter is defined sharply and clearly by the clinoid attenuation of the superficial layers II, III and IV which superlaminate the subiculum and the praepiriform cortex throughout the entire circumference of the limbus of the hemisphere. It seems to me that if one were to take these tectogenetic differences into account, the "limbic system" would become more explicitly definable and would offer a more precise anatomical basis for experimental and electrographic manipulation of its tectogenetically and, therefore, functionally different components.

Dr. MacLean: Well, I have followed you in many things, but I find it hard to look upon the hippocampus as a nucleus. I would like to hear some of the other neuroanatomists here comment on that. I always thought of the primordial hippocampal cortex as first showing up in the reptilian brain, in the dorsomedial part, and then later in phylogeny becoming folded with the development of the other peripheral areas.

Dr. Gloor: Since you injected these phylogenetic aspects into the discussion, I was wondering why you called the limbic system paleomammalian, since it exists at least from the amphibian level up. Amphibians have a hippocampus, they have a large piriform lobe. In the reptilian and amphibian brain the neopallium is practically invisible; it is represented by a little bit of cortex which is wedged between the piriform cortex laterally and the hippocampus medially. If I had to say what is the reptilian brain, I would say it is the hippocampus and the piriform lobe plus the old striatum (that is, the amygdala), and what is really new in the mammalian brain is the neocortex. Of course, what is very special in the reptilian and in the avian brain is the huge striatum. I was therefore wondering why you called the limbic system paleomammalian.

Dr. MacLean: Well, it is a part of the brain which is very well developed in the older mammals, and although you do have what appears to be the beginning of a cortex in the reptilian and amphibian forms, it is a very poorly differentiated cortex compared with the limbic cortex of lower and higher mammals. I raised this question at the first meeting of the International Congress of Phylogeny and Ontogeny of the Forebrain in Frankfurt in 1965. Most of the people there were unwilling "to buy" the reptilian cortex and the amphibian cortex as "good" mammalian cortex.*

Dr. Gloor: In the reptilian hemisphere, the hippocampus is already differentiated into a true hippocampus and dentate gyrus, but it is not enfolded yet as in the mammal. All you have to do is to imagine that the true hippocampus is beginning to curl up and you get a mammalian pattern out of it. There is a huge striatum in the reptilian brain: the posterior, basal part of it, the archistriatum, is the amygdala. Really, when you look at this brain, you can see well-defined separate structures. You have the piriform lobe, the amygdala and the hippocampus, and these make up most of the reptilian hemisphere, which is thus all limbic. The neopallium is still negligible, but there is a rather huge striatum which, of course, does not resemble the mammalian striatum.

Dr. Yakovlev: May I refer back to Pierre's comment? What becomes of the cortex? There is the primordial hippocampus dorsomedially, and there is the so-called paleocortex, the olfactory or "praepiriform" cortex. Now, the cortex means a plate of gray matter covering white matter, as a "bark" would cover some "core" of a different substance, in this instance the white matter. The true cortex must then have white matter under it. The so-called praepiriform cortex (paleocortex) does not have and never had white matter under it. In fact, it has more white matter over it, the thick stratum zonale (not comparable in origin to the lamina zonalis or molecular layer of the true cortical plate over the hemisphere). This so-called cortex blends without any demarcation with the septal area, striatum and amygdala. It is highly significant that in man the true cortical plate is laid down and becomes consolidated throughout the hemisphere some two weeks before the hippocampus and fascia dentata become differentiated. A remarkable breach of Maeckel's law of "biogenetic recapitulation." At ten embryonal weeks the true isocortical plate superlaminates the still inchoate mass of neuroblasts in the wall of the telenceph-

* The mammillo-thalamic-cingulate circuit comprises a large subdivision of the limbic system—a circuit which has hardly any counterpart in this part of the reptilian brain. (Ed.)

alon medium. The clinoid border—the limbus—of the isocortical plate overlaps the paleocortex and archicortex. In the cetacean hemispheres the overlap persists in the adult. In primates and man it becomes obscured but is still clearly recognizable even in the adult in the praesubiculum and along the hemispheric bank of the anterior rhinal sulcus. The clinoid border of the isocortical plate defines the architectonic boundary of the hemisphere and the border of true cortex which covers the paired hemispheres as two caps or mantles (pallia) thrown over them. The term "paleocortex," sanctioned by convention, is a misnomer not a little responsible for the confusion in the interpretation of its probable function. There is a growing body of morphological evidence that the olfactory lobe (paleocortex) is the rostral end of the reticular formation of the brain stem, laid bare here in the end brain, over the foregut and stomadeum.

Dr. Lindsley: My question is a little bit related to the one that Jack French raised. In the very rostral region of the insular cortex, you found only auditory responses. Did I understand you to say that—in the insular region, just at the base of the claustrum?

Dr. MacLean: The auditory units clustered in the posterior part of the insula, the part overlying the posterior part of the claustrum?

Dr. Lindsley: That is very interesting, because Ilan Spector, who did his thesis with Mme Albe-Fessard, found the claustrum to be a polysensory convergence center, and for that reason I was interested to hear you say that you got responses to somatosensory and auditory input in this region. We have found that the pulvinar and other posterolateral nuclei act as polysensory convergence centers, which relates to something you said earlier about the lateral aspect of the ventral lateral geniculate fibers bringing a visual input into this system. We feel that the medial aspect of the optic tract, as it approaches the ventral geniculate, may contribute fibers to the pulvinar. Chuong Huang, working in my laboratory, has done a detailed electrophysiological mapping of responses in the pulvinar to auditory, visual and somatosensory stimuli. We find two kinds of responses: shorter latency ones which are independent of longer latency ones, such as I believe you were speaking about.

Dr. MacLean: Are you recording from awake or anesthetized animals?

Dr. Lindsley: Ours have been done in the unanesthetized brain and under chloralose.

Dr. MacLean: I think one does see much more convergence in the animal under chloralose.

Dr. Abrahams: Are you suggesting that chloralose actually creates a pathway or opens up one that was not functional? Because if you say you are seeing something under chloralose that you did not see in the conscious animal, this poses a very interesting question as to what happens under chloralose. Have you any ideas?

Dr. Abrahams: I have had alpha- and beta-chloralose prepared to look for the differing effects of alpha- and beta-chloralose. The effects of beta-chloralose are pretty close to nil in doses that you would give an animal as a contaminant of alpha-chloralose. I think the attitude that some actions of chloralose are due to high levels of beta-chloralose is an "old canard" which I would like to see dropped. Alpha-chloralose has many interesting actions, and if given to an animal immobilized with Flaxedil, these effects may be both inhibitory and excitatory, depending on the recording site.

Dr. MacLean: The dose, though, is also

very important as Dubner has shown. That is, the deeper the animal is with chloralose, apparently the more convergence you get. This is rather curious, too.

Dr. Dell: I don't believe the only explanation for chloralose convergence is that chloralose is something like a convulsant. No, I believe you see a lot of things under chloralose because inhibitions downstream from the cortex are suppressed.

Dr. Abrahams: Also intraspinal inhibitions are beautifully suppressed.

Dr. Dell: So it is not only because chloralose is a convulsant.

Dr. Abrahams: The point I want to establish is that the connections must be there. You can't get convergence because chloralose creates a new neuronal circuit. What is the significance of the connections which you cannot demonstrate under the conditions of your experiment?

Dr. MacLean: I am just saying that in the awake, sitting animal, the cells seem to be a little more selective in terms of what they respond to—this is as far as I would go. Flaxedil is not without its effects on the resting membrane potential.

Dr. Gloor: I wish to raise the question of the somatic response in the insula. In the next to last of your figures (Fig. 8–7), they seemed to be congregated about the superior part of the caudal insula. Now, this area is very close to the second sensory area, of course, which lies on the upper lip of the Sylvian fissure, and in its inferior part abuts the insula. Now, I wasn't quite clear whether you think that these two areas are identical—the second sensory area and the sensory area you find in the insula—or are they distinct? Is the insular area another system again and not really the second sensory area and, if so, how do you distinguish between them?

Dr. MacLean: The areas seem to be functionally continuous as judged by the plotting of these units in the claustral insula, which in turn seem to be functionally continuous with the frontal operculum.

Dr. French: But, Paul, isn't it true that the operculum also connects with the primary sensory cortex? The superior opercular neurons feed upward into the somatosensory region, whereas you made quite a point out of the fact that the insular cortex feeds into limbic regions, at least into the front part of the limbic area. This I thought was a nice demonstration of the interface between the somatic, on the one hand, and the visceral, on the other. Was I wrong about this?

Dr. MacLean: Yes, if I understand you, that is correct. I have always been interested in the insula as a possible input into the hippocampal formation for auditory or somatic information. Rasmussen has unpublished anatomical material showing projections from the medial geniculate body to the insular cortex. We have indirect evidence of this in some of our own squirrel monkey material; when the auditory radiations are interrupted one can trace degeneration into the cortex overlying the claustrum.

SESSION IV

Chairman: **John I. Lacey**

Chapter 9

Nucleus Fasciculus Solitarius Activity: Visceral Afferents and Somatic Functions

Paul Dell

Although my work is not directly related to the limbic system, it is more than likely that there are inputs from the brain stem to these forebrain regions.

You may recall that many years ago, we described a phenomenon that we called "Adrenalin arousal."[3] The administration of Adrenalin to the cat evoked an arousal at the level of the cerebral cortex which resembled that produced either by external stimuli, by the direct action of epinephrine at a brain stem level or as a consequence of an increase in arterial blood pressure. When we observed this phenomenon, it seemed to us that there must be inputs from another part of the cardiovascular system that subserved a counter-regulatory role. In other words, inputs that might counteract these arousal responses. We were not the first to attempt to investigate this problem. Some of you may remember that Koch[7] studied variations of inputs from the baroreceptors. We did similar experiments in the encéphale isolé preparation using Moissejeff's carotid *cul-de-sac* technique.[6] This allowed us to vary intrasinus pressures, since the spinal cord and vagi were sectioned. When the region of the carotid sinus is distended by changing the pressure from 0 to 160 mm Hg, slow waves appear in cortical recordings—slow spindle waves that persist after distention and, after some time, the cortex again displays the activity pattern seen in the waking state. These experiments are very cumbersome, and the stimulation procedure does not always yield reproducible results over lengthy periods of time. Therefore, a few years ago, we found that we could replicate the results obtained in these experiments by stimulating the central cut-end of the vago-aortic trunk in the encéphale isolé preparation. If, in such a preparation, you repetitively stimulate the central cut-end of the vago-aortic nerve with frequencies of 30 to 50 Hz, the animal's pupils close and, after ten or fifteen seconds, there are huge spindles in the electroencephalogram recorded from the cerebral cortex. This phenomenon can be reproduced many times during an experiment just by stimulating the nerve trunk.

I shall discuss two aspects of these observations: firstly, the kind of afferent input necessary to obtain these sleep-like effects and, secondly, the central mechanisms mediating these effects. We recorded pupillary changes and the EEG from one hemisphere while stimulating with higher and higher intensities. Pupillary diameter was recorded indirectly by using a very simple device. We recorded the electroretinogram, the b wave of the electro-

Note: This chapter was abstracted from Professor Dell's presentation by the Editor.

retinogram, the amplitude of which is proportional to the quantity of light falling on the retina, and this amount, of course, depends on the diameter of the pupil. In order to stimulate only the large afferents, we used a square wave pulse with a narrow width (20μ to 50μ seconds). When the vago-aortic and sympathetic trunk was stimulated at the cervical level, the pupil closed, and spindles appeared in the EEG record. If the stimulus intensity was then increased from 1 to 3 volts, the contralateral pupil remained closed while the ipsilateral pupil was widely dilated due to stimulation of sympathetic afferents.

The aortic nerve in the cat can be easily dissected free, and as you know, it carries fibers from the baroreceptors and chemoreceptors of the aortic arch. As Agostoni and his colleagues [1] showed, this nerve contains a group of large, fast conducting fibers (8μ to 12μ) and, in general, this is the group that we stimulated in these experiments. We also found that it is not necessary to prepare the aortic nerve but that we could stimulate the aortic and vagus nerves together and excite only the large baroreceptor fibers. With higher intensity stimuli, one also activates the smaller chemoreceptor fibers, and this evokes an arousal.

My next point is concerned with the mechanism by which these effects are induced. When we speak about sleep, we think about "passive sleep" and "active sleep": "passive sleep" being a state induced by the suppression of all external stimuli and "active sleep" suggesting that there are, somewhere in the brain, mechanisms that are capable of inducing sleep. During the past twenty years, there have been a number of excellent studies on ascending inhibitory effects, particularly at a medullary level. The data from our experiments are directly related to the work of Moruzzi and his group [8] and that by Bonvallet and Allen.[2] As you know, the nucleus fasciculus solitarius receives primary afferents from the ninth and tenth nerves. We recorded from this region of the medulla with microelectrodes (at the level of the obex). In the animal with a transection at D-2, we electrically stimulated the afferents of the vago-aortic nerve, and we observed a closing of the pupils, a reduction in respiration, but the main effect was an increase in firing recorded from a small population of cells at the level of the nucleus fasciculus solitarius. This discharge builds up until a maximum is reached and decreases at the end of stimulation. An unexpected observation was that the same response occurred in spontaneous sleep: a closing of the pupils and a reduction in respiration indicating that the latter is not due to stimulation of afferent pulmonary fibers. However, the most interesting observation made during spontaneous sleep was the augmentation in activity at the level of the nucleus fasciculus solitarius. When the animal was aroused from sleep, this discharge was suppressed completely. We have observed the spontaneous appearance of this activity in the encéphale isolé preparation after sectioning both vagus nerves.

I would like to say a few words about the work in which Bonvallet and Allen destroyed this region of the nucleus fasciculus solitarius. If, prior to coagulation of this region, a brief stimulus is delivered to the mesencephalic reticular formation in such a way as to produce a negligible arousal response, the activity recorded from the Edinger-Westphal nucleus is inhibited for a brief period of time. After coagulation of the region of the nucleus fasciculus solitarius, the same stimulus now evokes a prolonged cortical arousal, an opening of the pupils and a prolonged inhibition of the activity of the Edinger-Westphal nucleus that persists for the duration of the stimulus. This would suggest that this region exerts a continuous inhibitory effect upon mechanisms which generate arousal. The building up of inhibition during arousal would suggest that we have to look for a mechanism by which the nucleus fasciculus solitarius exerts this control. These experiments suggest that the input to the nucleus fasciculus solitarius during stimulation probably triggers the synchronizing thalamic recruiting system and that this likely produces a diminution in reticular activity. If we think about some mechanism that would recontrol this activity, it would seem that we have a recontrol of activity during arousal in the sense of an inhibition from some part of the reticular formation. Our hypothesis is that in some part of the reticular formation, a presynaptic inhibitory effect is exerted at the level of the nucleus fasciculus solitarius.

We then stimulated the nucleus fasciculus solitarius and recorded antidromic potentials from the aortic nerve. When a stimulus to the nucleus fasciculus solitarius was preceded by stimulation of the nucleus gigantocellularis, we observed a marked increase in the amplitude of the antidromic potential. This suggests that if such connections do exist, they act in such a way as to inhibit presynaptically the cells of the nucleus fasciculus solitarius. While this is only preliminary work, these results give some justification for the proposal for such a feedback loop.

In other experiments, we found that there are many areas in the brain stem at the bulbar and mesencephalic levels from which unit recordings indicate increased activity at the moment when the organism goes to sleep. We also observed an increase in unit activity from these regions when the vago-aortic trunk was stimulated. When we moved the recording electrode approximately ½ mm away from some of these regions, we observed the opposite—that is, inhibition of activity. Recording throughout the brain stem suggests to us that there is a system which still remains to be worked out—a system which is indicated by the fact that each time you induce stimulation, you observe an augmentation in activity. This system projects to the Edinger-Westphal nucleus and from there most likely to the intralaminar thalamic region involved in recruiting.

As a final point, I would like to mention another aspect of this sleep-like effect. This may not only be an "active sleep" but also a sleep due to the suppression of afferent input. When we record at the level of the nucleus cuneatus, we pick up spontaneous activity, activity triggered by stimulation of the radial nerve or activity elicited by natural stimulation of the feet of the cat. If, at the same time, we stimulate the vago-aortic afferents (with the same stimulus parameters that produced the sleep-like effects), the activity at this first synapse in the somatic system is inhibited. If we employ the technique that I described earlier [9]—that is, stimulate the nucleus cuneatus while recording antidromically from primary sensory afferents —we observe that the antidromic potential is increased in amplitude if preceded by vago-aortic stimulation. These results would suggest that the vago-aortic afferents exert presynaptic inhibitory effects on transmission at the level of the nucleus cuneatus. Much work remains to be done before we learn precisely by which mechanisms these afferents act and before we understand teleologically why baroreceptor afferents produce these effects. It should be pointed out that in our earlier work,[4,5] we showed that visceral afferents of these systems have ascending effects on the reticular formation, on the thalamic synchronizing recruiting system, as well as descending effects, which we demonstrated a number of years ago, probably acting via the bulbar inhibitory region.

Although one of the main roles of the vegetative input is the maintenance or regulation of activities of the internal milieu, it also influences somatic functions, generally in the same direction.

REFERENCES

1. Agostoni, E., Chinnock, J. E., Daly De Burgh, M., and Murray, J. G.: Functional and histological studies on the vagus nerve and its branches to the heart, lungs and abdominal viscera in the cat. *J. Physiol. (London)*, *135:*182, 1957.
2. Bonvallet, M., Dell, P., and Hiebel, G.: Tonus sympathique et activité électrique corticale. *Electroenceph. Clin. Neurophysiol.*, *6:*119, 1954.
3. Bonvallet, M., and Allen, M. B., Jr.: Prolonged spontaneous and evoked reticular activation following discrete bulbar lesions. *Electroenceph. Clin. Neurophysiol.*, *15:* 969, 1963.
4. Dell, P., and Olson, R.: Projections thalamiques, corticales et cérébelleuses des afférences viscerales vagales. *Compt. Rend. Soc. Biol.*, *145:*1084, 1951.
5. Dell, P., and Olson, R.: Projections "secondaires" mésencephaliques, diencéphaliques, et amygdaliennes des afférences viscerales vagales. *Compt. Rend. Soc. Biol.*, *145:*1088, 1951.
6. Heymans, C.: *Introduction to the Regulation of Blood Pressure and Heart Rate.* Springfield, Charles C Thomas, 1950.
7. Koch, E.: Die Irradiation der pressorezeptorischen Kreislaufreflexe. *Klin. Wschr.*, *2:*225, 1932.
8. Magnes, J., Moruzzi, G., and Pompeiano, O. Synchronization of the EEG produced by low-frequency electrical stimulation of the region of the solitary tract. *Arch. Ital. Biol.*, *99:*33, 1961.
9. Wall, P. D.: Excitability changes in afferent fibre terminations and their relation to slow potentials. *J. Physiol. (London)*, *142:*1, 1958.

DISCUSSION

Dr. Lacey: One of the more important things involved in modulating the effectiveness of the baroreceptor feedback system is the thickness, the rigidity of the wall of the carotid sinus itself. This is variable, as Lyle Peterson has shown with strain gauge measurements, so that sympathetic contributions, for example, to the carotid sinus have been implicated. Dr. Reis also has some evidence of peripheral contributions to the wall of the sinus which reduce its elasticity. If the wall of the carotid sinus stiffens, input variations aren't as effective in stimulating the mechanoreceptors.

Dr. Calaresu: What is this stiffness change due to?

Dr. Lacey: This was never very clear. There has been implicated an unknown variable sympathetic contribution. Dr. Reis has some data on that. Let us call on him for a moment.

Dr. Reis: There has always been a question about the sympathetic innervation of the carotid sinus. Recently, Fuxe and I have shown by fluorescent histochemistry that there is indeed an adrenergic innervation of the sinus wall. Furthermore, by electrical stimulation of the cervical sympathetic nerve or by topical application of reserpine, the stores can be depleted showing that there is local release of amines. Now, whether or not the sympathetic innervation of the sinus has any function is another matter. However, the fact is established that noradrenalin is being released at the sinus, and we know that noradrenalin can act upon mechanoreceptors not only by indirectly constricting the smooth muscle matrix in which they are embedded but also directly. It seems reasonable, therefore, to consider that the receptor sensitivity may be modified by the sympathetic barrage.

I would like to make a few comments about Professor Dell's most interesting paper. Over the past several years, we have been trying to trace the central projections of the carotid sinus nerve in the cat. One of the features of the carotid sinus reflexes that has intrigued me (as it obviously has Dr. Dell) is that the carotid sinus not only influences blood pressure and heart rate but also has a far-ranging repertoire of autonomic, somatic and behavioral effects. For example, it is evident in Dr. Dell's work that carotid sinus stimulation can induce slow wave sleep. Now, as Jouvet has shown, the main nuclei involved in the production of slow wave sleep are the raphe nuclei in the brain stem. The question then arises, What are the connections between the nucleus of the solitary tract where the sinus nerve is reputed to terminate and the nuclei of the raphe? During this past year in New York, Dr. Mitsuhiko Miura and I have attempted to trace the central projections of the carotid sinus nerve. This has been accomplished by electrically stimulating the nerve and recording evoked unit activity and field potentials in the brain stem with microelectrodes. Our findings have been summarized in Figure 9–1. What we have found is that on entering the brain, the carotid sinus nerve apparently bifurcates. One portion terminates in the nucleus of the tractus solitarii at around the level of the obex. The other descends directly into the medial reticular formation at the same level to terminate in the large part within the confines of the paramedian reticular nucleus. In the nucleus tractus solitarii, carotid sinus fibers are in a region termed the "intermediate portion of the nucleus." This is a region which Cottle, on anatomical grounds, considered the most likely site of termination of cardiopulmonary fibers. It is interesting to find that activity cannot be found in the more rostral or caudal portions of the nucleus. More fascinating is that there is a monosynaptic pathway directly into the paramedian reticular nucleus. This nucleus is an important cerebellar relay, and within its confines we have been able to show an interaction between afferent fibers from the carotid sinus nerve and a projection from the fastigial nucleus of the cerebellum. Secondary projections from the carotid sinus nerve are restricted to several nuclei of the lower brain stem. After entering the nucleus tractus solitarii, local activity seems to be set up within local nerve nets, presumably through disynaptic and trisynaptic relays. Responses of longer latency, presumably reflecting more complex pathways, are found in three specific nuclear groups of the reticular formation of the medulla and pons: one is localized to the raphe nuclei in the medulla and pons possibly relayed from the lateral regions. This may be the pathway by which the carotid sinus nerve activity induces sleep. A second area of projection is localized to the dorsolateral reticular formation corresponding to an area which Rothballer finds very active in inducing the secretion of ADH and conceivably could be the region through which the carotid sinus nerve effects on the release of this hormone are mediated. Finally, there is a long latency activity within the paramedian reticular nucleus. In the pons, there

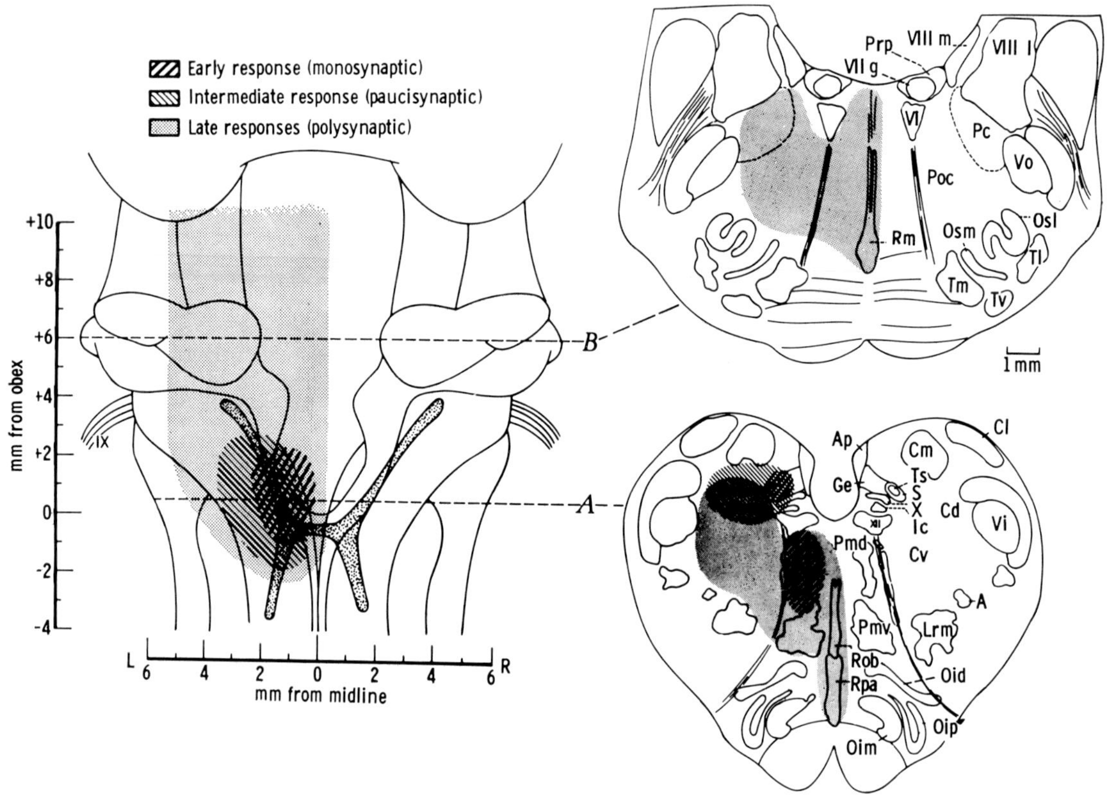

Figure 9–1. (*Left*) Distribution of monosynaptic and polysynaptic activity evoked by electrical stimulation of carotid sinus nerve in cat in medulla and pons projected onto the floor of the IVth ventricle. Stippled bilateral structure represents nucleus tractus solitarii. (*Right*) Summary of nuclear distributions in representative sections through medulla (*A*) and pons (*B*). *Abbreviations:* A (nucleus ambiguus); Ap (area postrema); Cd (nucleus medullae oblongatae centralis, subnucleus dorsalis); Cl (nucleus cuneatus lateralis); Cm (nucleus cuneatus medialis); Cv (nucleus medullae oblongatae centralis, subnucleus ventralis); G (nucleus gracilis); Gc (nucleus gigantocellularis); Ge nucleus tractus solitarii, subnucleus gelatinosus); Ic (nucleus intercalatus); Lrm (nucleus lateralis reticularis, subnucleus magnocellularis); Lrs (nucleus lateralis reticularis, subnucleus subtrigeminalis); Oid (nucleus olivaris inferior accessorius dorsalis); Oim (nucleus olivaris inferior accessorius medialis); Oip (nucleus olivaris inferior principalis); Osl (nucleus olivaris superior lateralis); Osm (nucleus olivaris superior medialis); Pc (nucleus parvocellularis); Pmd (nucleus paramedian reticularis, subnucleus dorsalis); Pmv (nucleus paramedian reticularis, subnucleus ventralis); Poc (nucleus pontis centralis caudalis); Prp (nucleus praepositus hypoglossi); Pyr (tractus pyramidalis); Rm (nucleus raphe magnus); Rob (nucleus raphe obscurus); Rpa (nucleus raphe pallidus); S (nucleus tractus solitarii); Tl (nucleus trapezoidalis lateralis); Tm (nucleus trapezoidalis medialis); Ts (tractus solitarius); Tv (nucleus trapezoidalis ventralis; V (nucleus nerve trigemini); Vi (nucleus tractus spinalis trigemini interpolaris); Vo (nucleus tractus spinalis trigemini oralis); VI (nucleus nervi abducentis); VII (nucleus nervi facialis); VIIg (genu nucleus nervi facialis); VIII 1 (nucleus vestibularis lateralis); VIIIm (nucleus vestibularis medialis); X (nucleus nervi vagi dorsalis motorius); XII (nucleus nervi hypoglossi). (From Miura, M., and Reis, D. J.: *Amer. J. Physiol., 217:* 142, 1969.)

are no monosynaptic connections. All are polysynaptic and localized to the central tegmental region and also to the nuclei of the raphe. This is as far rostral as we have traced activity.

We have not studied in detail the projections of the aortic depressor nerve. However, several years ago, Dr. Crill and I studied the projections of both the carotid sinus and aortic depressor nerves by an antidromic technique very similar to the one described by Dr. Dell. With antidromic stimulation, we found that the carotid sinus and aortic depressor nerves could be excited from within the nucleus tractus solitarii and the paramedian reticular areas, findings subsequently confirmed by our orthodromic study with Dr. Miura. One interesting finding, however, was that the aortic depressor nerve, but not the carotid sinus nerve, could be excited from punctate stimulation within the cuneate nucleus. We have speculated that one of the possible functions of this projection is to keep cuneate cells firing "spontaneously." This would have an advantage in allowing cuneate neurons to change their activity either upward or downward as a device for coding sensory information. It might explain the phenomenon described by Amassian and others that these cells are spontaneously active.

To continue, it is known that the pain theory of Wall speculates that the presynaptic inhibition of primary afferents in the spinal cord required for pain transmission is mediated by small neurons in the substantia gelatinosa, and Dr. Nauta will correct me on this if I am in error, but I believe that it is histologically almost identical with the substantia gelatinosa of the spinal cord. This raises the interesting possibility that a similar mechanism of gating of information from C and A fibers from chemoreceptors and baroreceptors may be operating within the nucleus of the tractus solitarii.

Dr. Nauta: Yes, Olszewski and Meesen in their atlas of the rabbit brain describe a small-celled dorsomedial nucleus of the solitary tract which really makes the impression of being a gelatinosa-like cell group associated with the larger-celled lateral subdivision of the nucleus of the solitary tract. It is confined to the caudal half or so of the solitary nucleus complex. There is an enormous afferent supply of sensory vagus fibers to this small-celled nucleus which you do not see with routine staining techniques but can be demonstrated by the Fink-Heimer method. We have been unable, so far, to find any comparable afferent supply from the glossopharyngeal nerve. Whether or not this parvicellular subdivision of the nucleus of the solitary tract really can be regarded as a viscerosensory substantia gelatinosa will, of course, have to await physiological proof.

The other remark I should like to make is that the apparent distribution area of ascending fibers in the pons would agree rather well with Morest's findings.

Dr. Reis: Yes, it is interesting that Morest made lesions of the nucleus tractus solitarii and found degeneration only in the dorsal lateral reticular formation, but none medially. The question then is, Since we know that the depressor area lies medially, how does information from the carotid sinus nerve get into this area? I believe that our findings of a monosynaptic shortcut indicates that there is a "maximal security route" directly into the medial depressor area.

Dr. Nauta: He also identified a longer ascending path that appears to be distributed to the central gray substance of the midbrain. Looking at Morest's illustrations, I have been tempted to think that it might to some extent involve the nuclei of Gudden and thus lead into what I like to see as part of the limbic circuitry. Once in the central gray, of course, fibers could very easily—but without proof you can't be sure—link up with the ascending bundle of Schutz leading into the thalamic midline. This could be one of the routes of conduction into the anterior thalamic territory.

Dr. Reis: One of the mysteries, one that maybe Dr. Dell can comment on, is that the body goes to an enormous extent to reproduce with incredible fidelity the pulse wave, the pulse contour and all the information on the cardiovascular system, and yet when you get into the brain stem, it is damn hard, if not impossible, to find the neuron which gives you a signal which is in any way replicating the pulse. It is wiped out immediately.

Dr. Abrahams: Is it wiped out?

Dr. Lacey: Well, it loses its original form, and we do not understand the new code.

Dr. Dell: Yes, we tried very hard each time we had the microelectrode in position to see if some of the cells were not synchronous with the input. We found only one locus. Available computer techniques might reveal some regularity, but this hasn't been done.

Dr. Lacey: Hellner and von Baumgarten said that, in their experience, in up to 80 percent of their penetrations they detected cardiac synchrony. Does that correlate with your experience?

Dr. Dell: Just in one very small area. I know the paper very well.

Dr. Reis: Were they in cells or fibers?

Dr. Dell: Probably fibers.

Dr. Hoffer: I would like to ask Dr. Reis for an opinion. Swedish investigators have done a number of catecholamine histochemistry studies in the medulla of the rat. I was wondering if the region that they call A-1 in the medullary reticular formation is coexistent with that region which you find in the cat to which the baroreceptor afferents project?

Dr. Reis: A-1 cells are the cells of origin, aren't they? The reason they called them an A-1 group is that they didn't correspond to any well-defined nucleus in the brain, so that they finally had to name it themselves. You find a few cells running here and there, running into the nuclei. It is the terminals that I am talking about, going into the nucleus tractus solitarius.

Dr. Dell: As you know, there is some discussion on these points. People who have worked in this area are perfectly sure that all of the area postrema is full of endings, and they speak as if the entire fasciculus solitarius has such a heavy innervation.

Dr. Reis: I know that in the cat that it does in this region.

Dr. Hockman: Dr. Dell, a number of years ago, you indicated in your evoked response studies that there was a probable diffuse projection to various forebrain areas, including the amygdala and orbital cortex. Would you like to relate or speculate on how this might tie in with your present work—in terms of possible limbic system effects?

Dr. Dell: The boys in the lab don't like to study projections and point-to-point anatomy, and so we have not correlated our present studies with the earlier work on the various projections. I mentioned to someone the other day that all the work on central vagal projections showed, for instance, projections to some of the regions of the intralaminar nuclei. I have been thinking of reopening these investigations using the technique which I have just described. I would not use the evoked potential method but would record with microelectrodes from different regions to find out if there is sustained and integrated activation and then, with single or double shocks, study the evoked activity and calculate latencies. But this hasn't been done yet, and it surely should be done. I would like to add one more thing in relation to what you said. We have done part of this work but not in detail, and of course, we found projections to the raphe nuclei at the pontine level.

Dr. Lacey: Exercising my prerogative as chairman, I'm going to call on a visitor. Dr. Smyth has some extremely relevant information in man that I think you might be interested in hearing about.

Dr. Smyth: We have been hearing chiefly about the effects of baroreceptor input on arousal, and our work concerns the obverse of this—that is the influence of alteration of arousal on baroreceptor activity. Some of this work was recently published with Sir George Pickering, who was concerned with the control of arterial pressure during sleep. This first slide may give confirmatory evidence of the theory that Dr. Dell is working with. Figure 9–2 is a plot of the alpha rhythm of the electroencephalogram in a resting human, in a subject lying in bed ready to go to sleep for the night, who had his blood pressure acutely elevated by small increments with intravenous injections of angiostin. The pressure rose, and the beat-by-beat pressure rise was followed while the alpha rhythm was plotted for the same 4-second interval. The alpha rhythm slowed proportionately as the pressure rose. This is an indirect study because it was carried out in intact man. You can't get any closer

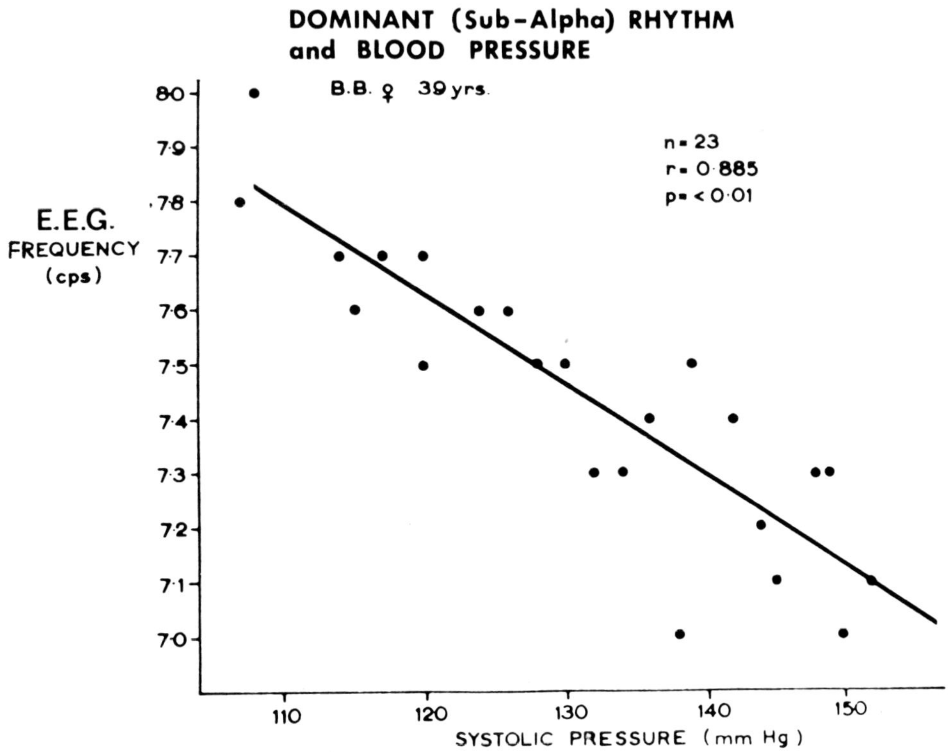

Figure 9–2. Relationship between systolic blood pressure and simultaneous frequency of prevailing rhythm (sub-alpha) in a resting wakeful subject during pressor response to an intravenous injection of 0.25μg of angiotensin.

to a correlation than that. This corroborates the inhibitory effect of rises in blood pressure on the dominant rhythm of the brain at rest.

Dr. Lacey: May I ask why you chose systolic blood pressure to plot rather than mean pressure or diastolic?

Dr. Smyth: The inputs that the baroreceptor afferent impulses represent are mean pressure, pulse pressure and rate of rise of pressure. These are all difficult to measure in man, but we thought that the systolic pressure was an adequate representative measure of these three different components in the input system.

Dr. Lacey: Did you use an arterial catheter?

Dr. Smyth: This is with an indwelling ar-

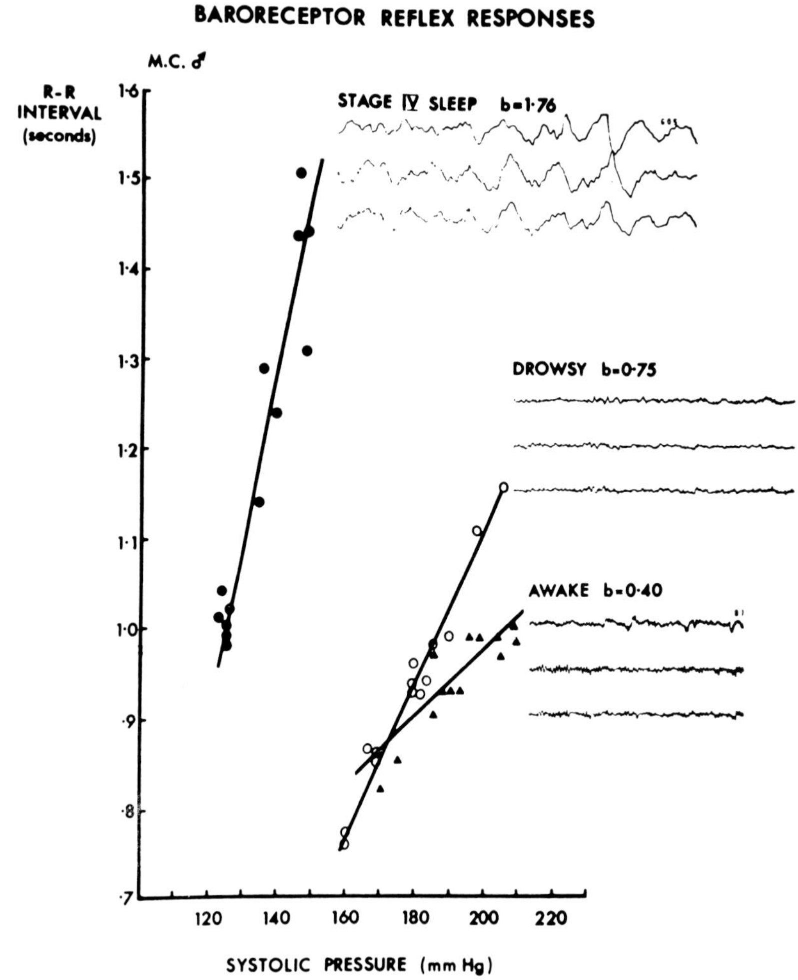

Figure 9–3. Plots describe beat-by-beat cardiac slowing per unit rise of systolic pressure during responses to intravenous administration of angiotensin to a subject awake, drowsy and, in stage IV (slow wave), sleep. The slope of each line, *b*, indicates reflex sensitivity in the respective states (corresponding EEGs were sampled from intervals synchronous with the development of each pressor reflex response; channels, from above downward, were recorded from frontocortical, temporo-occipital, and centro-occipital leads.)

terial catheter during a normal night's sleep.

Dr. Lacey: A normal night's sleep?

Dr. Smyth: During the third of three nights' sleep in the lab, after which time the EEG pattern of sleep was stable and normal. Figure 9–3 deals with an effect of the alteration of level of arousal on the responsiveness of the heart-rate reflex which I would anticipate might relate to the next paper. Here, a study was made of the individual, awake, drowsy and in the first cycle of deep slow wave sleep (stage four). Three channels of the electroencephalogram are seen beside the plotted results of a reflex response. The reflex is measured simply by plotting successive R-R intervals of the electrocardiogram against the value of the systolic pressure of the preceding beat, so that one has a beat-to-beat measure of the reflex sensitivity at any time. It is a rapidly repeatable test for study under changing conditions of arousal. This was a hypertensive subject, the degree of blood pressure rise being shown on the abscissa and the slowing of the heart on the ordinate. As the alpha rhythm waxes in amplitude and then fragments and disappears in the early stage (Ib) of sleep, there is a small increase in reflex sensitivity. Then there is a major increase during stage four sleep so that in some way, it seems that there is an alteration in the sensitivity, at least of the cardiac elements receiving baroreceptor inputs. During sleep, they seem more sensitive to what is even a lower input. A lower pressure stimulus gives rise to a greater baroreceptor reflex response.

Dr. Lacey: This is downstream sensitivity. We don't know yet whether upstream sensitivity would do the same thing.

Dr. Smyth: Yes, that's right. In other words, we didn't do any experiments lowering the pressure because that wakens the patient. But this reflex change results in a "clamping" of the arterial pressure at a lower mean level. There is thus less tolerance to a rise in pressure during sleep than there is to that same rise in pressure during waking. Figure 9–4 shows the difference between subjects whom we have studied who have so-called normal arterial pressures (dotted lines), and the subjects who have elevated arterial pressures (solid lines). This subject had diminished reflex sensitivity. A group of hypertensives studied showed a much diminished reflex sensitivity both awake and at rest. In other words, they were less able to cope with rises in blood pressure. However, this hypotensive subject enjoyed both a normal blood pressure and a normal regulation of that blood pressure, comparable to the normal subject shown when he went to sleep. So that this man who was hypertensive with renal disease was able to regulate his blood pressure normally during sleep. He not only had a normal pressure, but he also had a normal reflex sensitivity.

Dr. MacLean: How are you recording pressure?

Dr. Smyth: We are recording pressure with an extremely sensitive transducer from a brachial arterial cannula and measuring the peak pressure of each systolic pulse.

Dr. Calaresu: I would like to make one comment and then ask a question. It is very interesting, as Dr. Reis has shown, that there are catecholamine-containing fibers ending in the general area of the carotid sinus. On the other hand, Floyd and Neil stimulated the cervical sympathetic while recording from carotid baroreceptor fibers, and they failed to show any effect due to the stimulation. The question that I am asking is, Do you find catecholamine-containing fibers in all species? Is there any difference in density?

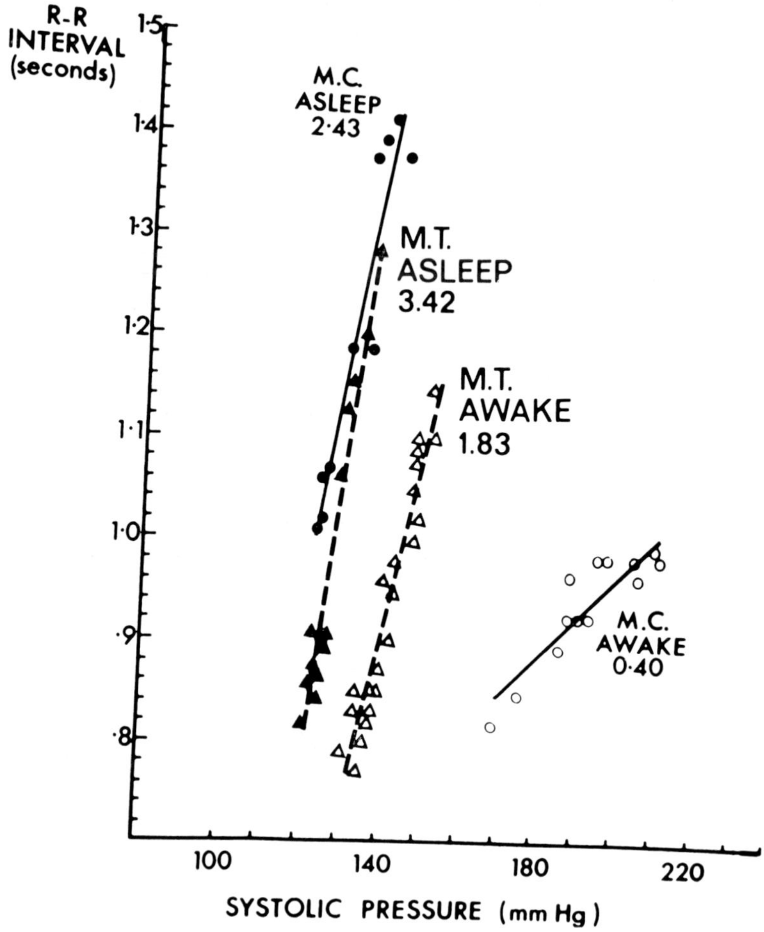

Figure 9–4. Baroreceptor reflex responses plotted (as in Fig. 9–3) in a subject with normal blood pressure (M.T.) and in a subject with renal hypertension (M.C.) The latter showed reversion to both normal blood pressure and normal reflex regulation of pressure with the onset of sleep.

Dr. Reis: No, it is species specific. You couldn't see it in the rat. You see it in the rabbit and in the cat, and the point was merely that there is an anatomical substrate for anyone who wants to make an argument that there is sympathetic control of baroreceptors—there are sympathetic fibers there. This has been questioned before. I don't know what the functional significance is, except that it may be the modulation of the receptor by the sympathetic division which can, in turn, act upon the reflex arc. All I can say is that catecholamines are released.

Dr. Calaresu: I have two questions for Dr. Dell. The first one is, did you mention that you had some data on intracellular recordings from the nucleus of the tractus solitarius cells or was it extracellular?

Dr. Dell: No, it was extracellular.

Dr. Calaresu: Then the obvious thing to do is to get intracellular data. The second question is a minor one: do you get such nice amplitude evoked responses—antidromic responses from the vagus—while you are stimulating the nucleus of the tractus solitarius?

Dr. Dell: Yes, I have to explain the technique. These are not single responses, but the average of twenty or fifty responses from the CAT and written out on an X-Y recorder.

Dr. Calaresu: What is the amplitude of the response. I did not see a calibration.

Dr. Dell: The amplitude is not very high. It is in the order of 100 μV.

Dr. Andy: I would like to hear Dr. Dell's comments on this last figure in which the hypertensive patient does not have the adjustment in this system in the awake state that he has in sleep. How do Dr. Dell and Dr. Reis explain this in relation to their hypothesis as to the function of this system?

Dr. Dell: There is a control before the first synapse in the nucleus fasciculus solitarius, and the synapse that he is talking about is in the medial region of the medulla. All the vasomotor centers have to be considered, and each would have to be studied with all its interactions.

Dr. Reis: The possibility that there is a central neural regulation of baroreceptor reflexes was demonstrated by Dr. Cuenod and myself in Dr. MacLean's laboratory several years ago. There are very powerful effects on the carotid sinus reflex exerted by the brain. Another possibility is that changes in sensitivity of the carotid sinus mechanism may occur at the level of the receptor itself. Some years ago, McCubbin, in Page's lab, produced renal hypertension in dogs and showed that after several months of renal hypertension that the sensitivity of the carotid sinus had been modified.

Dr. Lacey: One question to ask is, What is the mechanism of this change in sensitivity from sleep to waking? This is a question for which we presently have no answer.

Dr. MacLean: I wanted to ask Dr. Dell what happens if one stimulates the carotid sinus nerve in an intact, freely moving animal? Has this been done?

Dr. Dell: We have just prepared some animals, but not with the carotid sinus nerve which would be very difficult. We placed an electrode on the aortic nerve, but I cannot tell you about the results at this time. Anyway, these can only be preliminary experiments because you are working under conditions similar to those under which Koch worked. If you have intact animals, you have to cope with variations in pressure. You then must re-do these chronic experiments in preparations with the spinal cord transected at C-7, let us say.

Chapter 10

Supramedullary Modulation of Autonomic Reflexes

CHARLES H. HOCKMAN, KENNETH E. LIVINGSTON AND JAIME TALESNIK

THE RESULTS from a number of investigations [27] indicate that in the somatic sphere, central nervous system mechanisms regulate incoming traffic from the level of the receptor through all major relay stations up to and including the cortex, and similarly modulate motor outflow all the way to the effector organ. Such regulation is indispensable for the adaptive adjustments inherent in all purposive behavior. If the organism's responsiveness to events in the *outer world* is thus characterized by continuous modulation of neural activity, it would seem probable than an analogous system of central controls regulates the *inner visceral* world of which we are normally less aware.

In an earlier publication,[18] we alluded to the voluminous literature, covering a period of almost one hundred years, which has shown that autonomic or visceral effectors can be profoundly influenced by activity in structures at all levels of the central nervous system. However, it is still not clear how different regions of the brain modulate autonomic reflex mechanisms.

There have been few reported studies in which peripheral and brain stem autonomic reflex activity has been analyzed by the introduction of central interventions, such as limbic system activation. In an early report in 1937, Morison and Rioch [31] showed that stimulation of the orbital cortex inhibited reflexly induced contraction of the nictating membrane. A few years later, Freeman and Krasno [15] reported that electrical stimulation in the head of the caudate nucleus inhibited both sweating and contraction of the urinary bladder in the cat. In 1956, Wang and Brown [38] showed that the galvanic skin reflex could be inhibited by electrical stimulation of the frontal cortex, caudate nucleus, bulbar ventromedial reticular formation and the anterior lobe of the cerebellum. Writing at that time, Wang and Brown drew attention to the paucity of research on inhibitory control of autonomic reflexes. For instance, they were able to find but one report on modulation of autonomic brain stem reflexes by a region of the brain other than the medulla. In the study to which they referred, Moruzzi [32] had shown in vagotomized cats with a precollicular transection that the rise in blood pressure produced by carotid artery occlusion and the fall elicited by electrical stimulation of the depressor nerve were both inhibited by simultaneous stimulation of the paleocerebellar cortex. Since then, there has appeared a short report by Hilton [17] indicating that hypothalamic stimulation inhibits the blood pressure component of the baro-

Note: All experiments from our laboratory that are discussed in this chapter were supported by grants from the Ontario Alcoholism and Drug Addiction Research Foundation, and the Medical Research Council of Canada.

ceptor reflexes. More recently, Reis and Cuénod[35] demonstrated that the pressor response to carotid artery occlusion could be potentiated by stimulation of regions of the brain rostral to the medulla, and they drew attention to the fact that this reflex could be so altered independently of changes in systemic blood pressure. Covian[10] also reported an interplay between septal stimulation and the blood pressure reflex. In cats, he demonstrated that the reflex response elicited by bilateral carotid artery occlusion was inhibited during septal stimulation and for varying intervals of time after the stimulus was withdrawn.

It will be recalled that in 1927, Hering[16] demonstrated the existence of two separate cardiovascular reflexes. He produced a cardiodepressor response in the dog by mechanical stimulation in the region of the carotid sinus and found that after administration of atropine, systemic hypotension still occurred without a change in heart rate. Since the studies that we have just discussed indicated that the blood pressure reflex was subject to modulation by regions of the brain other than the medulla, it seemed reasonable to assume that the cardiac reflex was similarly regulated. Besides, a number of investigators[4-6,8] have shown that alterations in impulse activity in baroceptor nerves induces a number of effects in various regions of the brain. For example, Bonvallet *et al.*[6] showed that distention of the carotid sinus produces a slowing of the EEG with frequencies that resembled those seen during sleep. Chase and his colleagues[8] demonstrated that stimulation of the central end of the cervical vagus produces cortical desynchronization or synchronization, depending upon the afferent fiber systems activated by different stimulus parameters. Inhibitory effects, other than cortical synchronization, were convincingly demonstrated by Zanchetti and his colleagues[4,5] who showed, in acutely decorticate cats, that both the autonomic and motor manifestations of sham rage could be suppressed by stimulation of either the carotid sinus or aortic depressor nerves. Furthermore, Dell[11] has just told us about the exciting experiments he is doing in this area. In assessing this work, Lacey[26] drew a rather important conclusion when he pointed out that "the neurophysiological investigations so far have examined only the effects from the carotid sinus forward and have treated higher integrating mechanisms as passive recipients of whatever inhibitory influx is allowed to enter." Little attention has been directed to the possibility that these neural regions might exert reciprocal influences upon baroceptor reflex mechanisms.

We began our investigation with adult cats anesthetized with alpha chloralose and found, in a first series of experiments, that reflex vagal bradycardia elicited by electrical stimulation of the carotid sinus nerve (CSN) could be enhanced if a concurrent stimulus were delivered to loci in either the central gray substance of the midbrain (CG) or the posterior hypothalamus (Hp).[19,20] This is illustrated in Figure 10–1.

In an attempt to rule out peripheral effects due to changes in systemic blood pressure, low-intensity stimuli were applied to the brain. In a number of animals, we experienced some difficulty in replicating our findings, in that we observed only reflex inhibition but no augmentation. We assumed that the depressant effects of the anesthetic were causing this variability.

At this point, we decided to ascertain whether or not the inhibition and facilitation of the bradycardic reflex response was in any way related to peripheral sympathetic events. Accordingly, we anesthetized an animal with ether and, after transecting

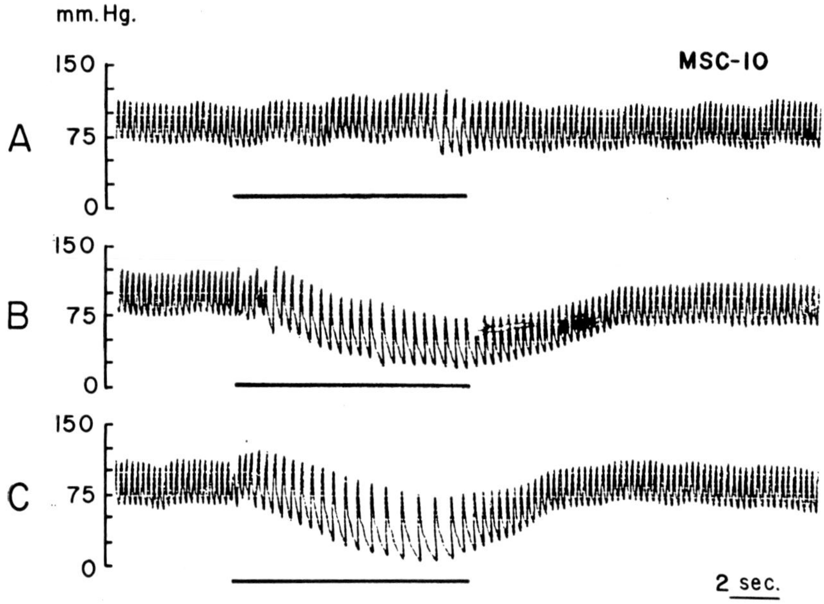

Figure 10–1. (*A*) Elicited response to stimulus of 0.1 ma delivered to gray substance of midbrain (CG). (*B*) Cardiac slowing was produced by stimulating carotid sinus nerve (CSN) with an intensity of 0.4 ma. (*C*) Stimuli to CG and CSN were applied simultaneously. Horizontal lines beneath each tracing indicate stimulus duration of 10 sec. (From Hockman, C. H., Talesnik, J., and Livingston, K. E.: *Amer. J. Physiol., 217:* 1681, 1969.)

the spinal cord at the first cervical vertebra, withdrew the anesthetic, taking great care to keep all incision margins infiltrated with procaine. In this preparation, the facilitatory effect on the reflex was not only reproducible, but was more marked. This is illustrated in Figure 10–2. It was now possible to study this central phenomenon without the depressant action of anesthetics.

In these experiments, our attention was drawn to the onset of the facilitatory effect in both the anesthetized and encéphale isolé (unanesthetized) animal. When compared with the reflexly-elicited response (see Figs. 10–1 and 10–2), the augmentation of bradycardia was somwhat delayed in onset; in fact, with concurrent stimulation of the CG and CSN, an initial inhibition of the reflex was quite evident. We found that this inhibitory phase could be lengthened by increasing the intensity of central stimulation. With a strong stimulus, the bradycardic reflex response could be completely suppressed. In this manner, we were able to choose stimulus parameters that would inhibit the reflex. Then, by progressively delaying the interval between the delivery of the stimuli to the CG and CSN, a separation between the two stimuli was reached at which facilitation failed to occur. This is illustrated in Figure 10–3. We observe that the enhancement of reflex bradycardia appears when the CSN stimulus is delayed by two seconds and that this potentiation increases gradually to reach a peak with a ten-second delay—that is, when the CSN is stimulated at the end of CG stimulation.

Since the choice of stimulus parameters appeared to play such an important role in both inhibition and facilitation of reflex

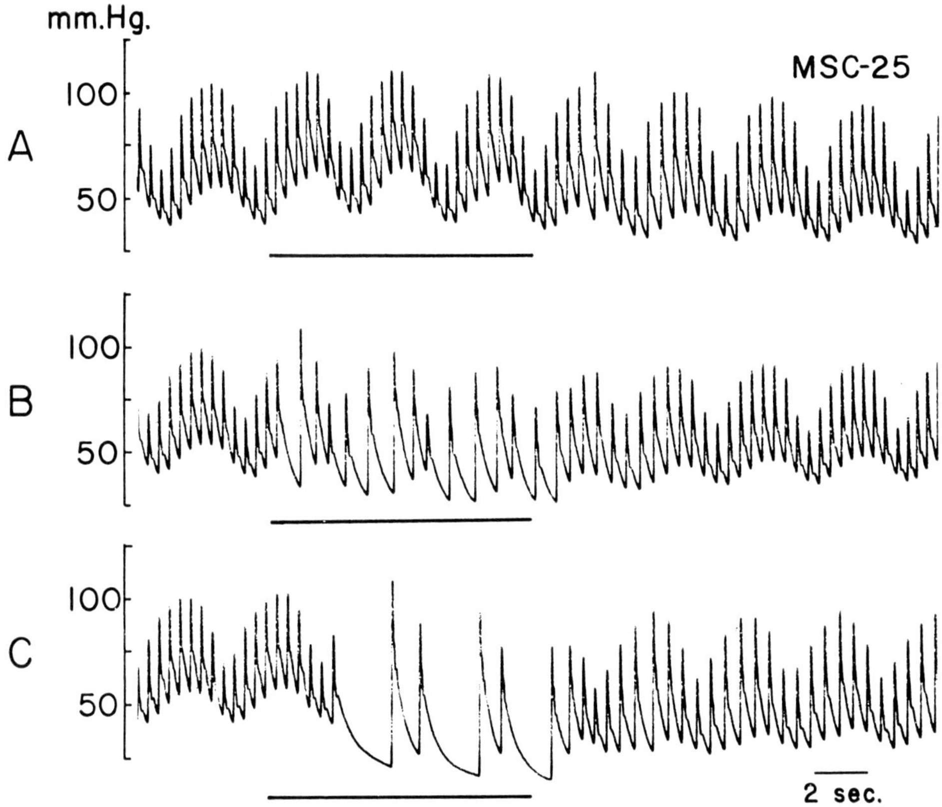

Figure 10–2. (*A*) Stimulus of 0.7 ma delivered to central gray substance of midbrain. (*B*) Stimulus of 0.02 ma applied to carotid sinus nerve. (*C*) Response evoked when stimuli were delivered to brain and nerve simultaneously. Horizontal lines beneath each tracing denote 10-second duration of stimulus. (Encéphale isolé preparation.) (From Hockman, C. H., Talesnik, J., and Livingston, K. E.: *Amer. J. Physiol., 217:*1681, 1969.)

vagal bradycardia, this aspect was subjected to further study. In another series of experiments, the intensity of a stimulus applied to the CSN was held constant, while that delivered to the CG was gradually increased. An example in which stimuli either followed one another or were delivered concurrently is given in Figure 10–4. Such experiments show that when a stimulus to the CSN follows the termination of one delivered to the brain, a gradual increase in intensity of the CG stimulus results in a progressive enhancement of the reflex (Fig. 10–4a). They also demonstrate that there is a progressive inhibition of the reflex with increasing intensity of the CG stimulus when both stimuli are applied simultaneously (Fig. 10–4b).

We see clearly, from the example in Figure 10–5,(*a*), that reflex vagal bradycardia elicited by electrical stimulation of the CSN is dependent upon the strength of the stimulus; however, a response level is soon reached following which additional increments in stimulus intensity appear to have but little effect. We observe in Figure 10–5,(*b*), that a constant stimulus delivered to the CG results in a progressive reduction in the degree of inhibition when the CSN is stimulated simultaneously with

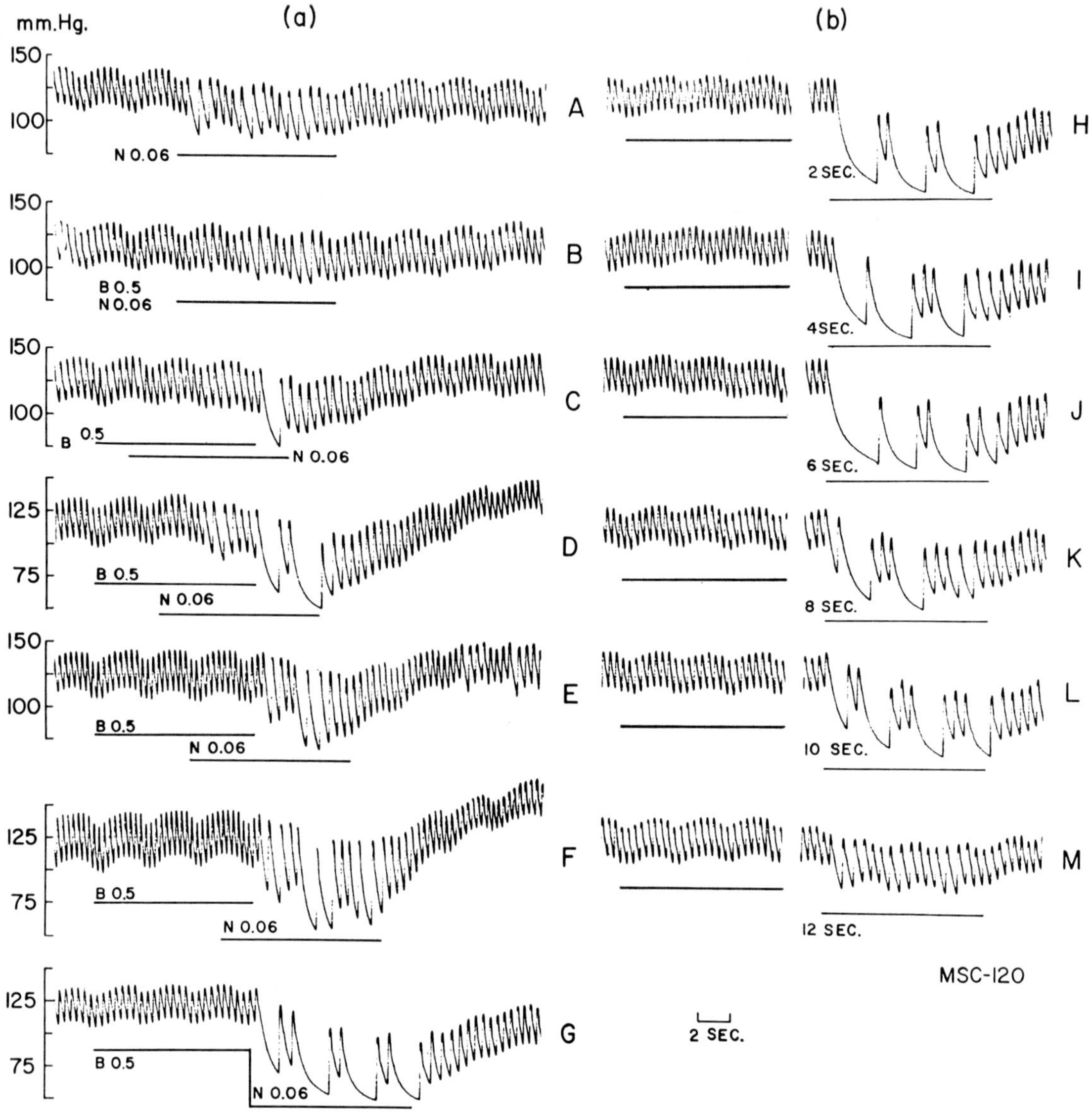

Figure 10–3. (*a*) Effect of overlapping stimuli delivered to central gray substance of midbrain (CG) and carotid sinus nerve (CSN). *A:* shows reflex response elicited by electrical stimulation of CSN. *B:* both stimuli are applied simultaneously and response is inhibited. In *C, D, E* and *F*, onset of stimulus applied to CSN is delayed for 2, 4, 6 and 8 seconds, respectively, following onset of stimulus delivered to CG. *G:* stimulus to CSN is applied at the end of CG stimulation. (*b*) Stimulus to CSN was delivered 2, 4, 6, 8, 10 and 12 seconds, respectively, following termination of CG stimulation. Intensities (ma) delivered to brain (B) and nerve (N) are indicated in each tracing, and horizontal lines denote 10-second period of stimulation. (Encéphale isolé preparation.) (From Hockman, C. H., Talesnik, J., and Livingston, K. E.: *Amer. J. Physiol., 217:* 1681, 1969.)

increasing current intensities. The inhibitory effect is illustrated in the stimulus-response curve. In both Figures 10–4 and 10–5, the stimulus-response curves were prepared by measuring the area under the curves of the beat-to-beat cardiotachograms.

Having shown that activation of cell populations in the CG and Hp could modulate the bradycardic reflex, we decided to assess the role of forebrain regions in the mediation of these central influences. We decerebrated animals in such a manner as to leave the diencephalon intact (thalamic preparations). It is noteworthy that in these preparations all modulatory influences on the baroceptor reflex, both inhibitory and facilitatory, were abolished. The results shown in Figure 10–6 are from a cat twenty-four hours after a high decerebration. We should point out that the reflex bradycardic response elicited by electrical stimulation of the CSN was unaltered after decerebration.

In another group of animals loci in the ventral hippocampus were stimulated, and we found that the cardiac reflex could be either inhibited or facilitated. This is illustrated in Figure 10–7.

Since the baroceptor reflex could be modulated by structures in the mesencephalon, diencephalon and telencephalon, it seemed to us that these regions of the brain must receive information from the baroceptors. A number of years ago, Dell and Olson [12,13] demonstrated that visceral afferents in the vagus projected to different levels of the brain, including regions stimulation of which has influenced the cardiac reflex in the present investigation. In exploratory experiments,[21] we found that single-shock stimuli delivered to the central cut-end of the CSN evoke short latency slow potentials in the midbrain and forebrain, as shown in Figure 10–8. Parallel recordings on a storage oscilloscope revealed little variability.

In exploratory studies, we have also found that reflex vagal bradycardia elicited by stimulation of the aortic depressor nerve can be modulated in a manner identical to that demonstrated in the foregoing experiments, and these central influences can also be seen when loci in the amygdala and midbrain reticular formation are stimulated.

Existing neuroanatomical [9,25] and electrophysiological [3] evidence indicates that primary afferents from the ninth and tenth nerves terminate in the nucleus of the tractus solitarius and results from recent experiments suggest that baroceptive influences likely reach regions of the brain rostral to the medulla via reticular relays. Following lesions in the regions of the nucleus of the tractus solitarius that receive primary glossopharyngeal and vagal afferents, Morest [30] found degenerated axons in the dorsal and lateral reticular formation of the medulla. In addition, electrophysiological data reported by Miura and Reis [28] demonstrated a direct projection from the CSN into the medial reticular formation. This collateral input would provide the basis for a multisynaptic relay system transmitting information from baroceptors (and probably chemoceptors) to supramedullary regions of the brain.

It is interesting that the paramedian nucleus of the reticular formation (that has been shown to receive collateral baroceptor fibers) should also play an important role in mediating pressor responses elicited by electrical stimulation of the fastigial nucleus of the cerebellum.[29]

We have recently demonstrated that stimulation of the fastigial nucleus can also influence the cardiac reflex.[22] In these experiments, the fastigial nucleus was explored until electrical stimuli elicited a

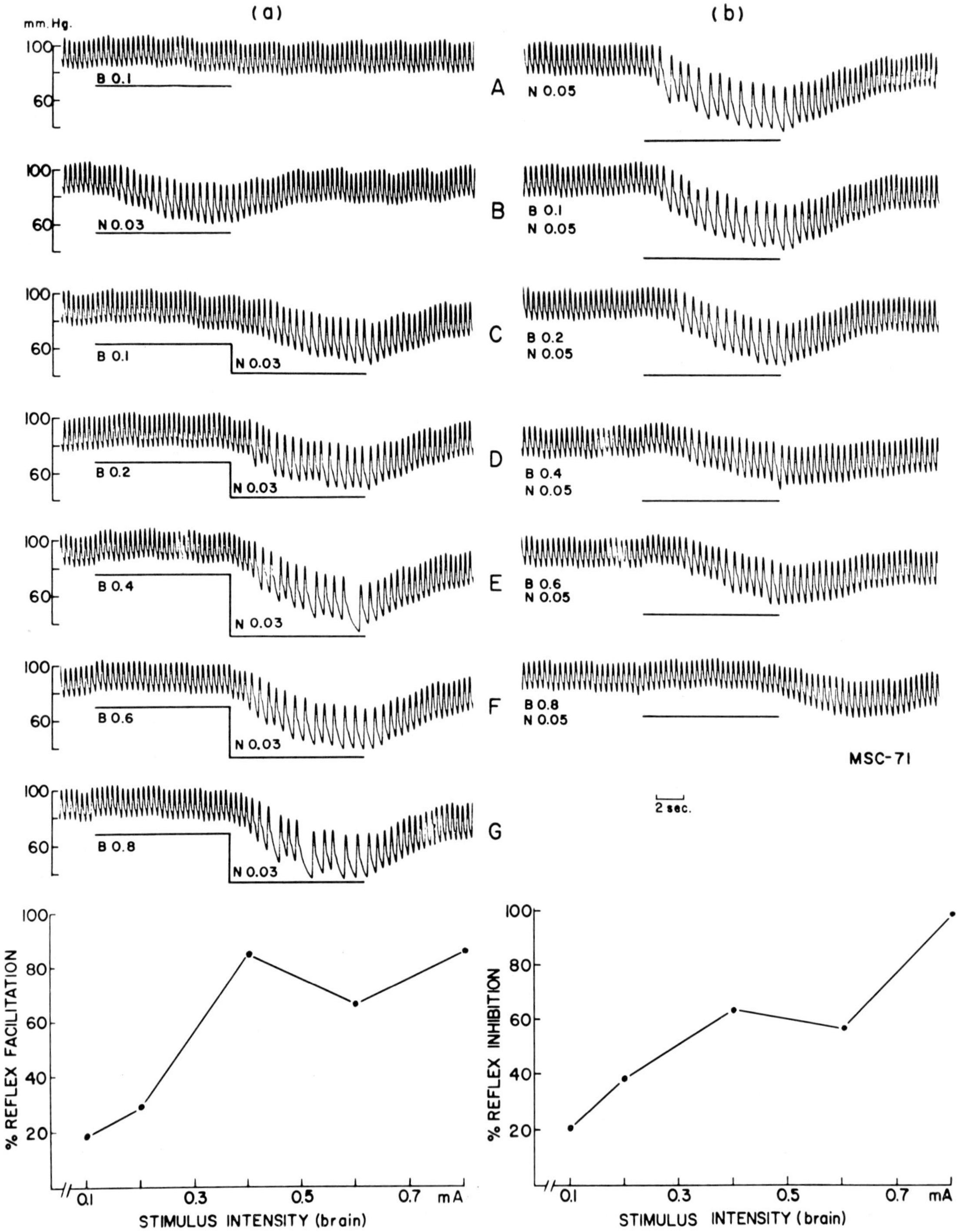

Figure 10–4. (*a*) Electrical stimuli were delivered to carotid sinus nerve (CSN) at end of a 10-second stimulus applied to central gray substance of midbrain (CG). *A* and *B* show results of stimulation of CG and CSN, respectively. In *C*, *D*, *E*, *F* and *G*, intensity of CSN stimulus was held constant, while that delivered to CG was gradually increased from 0.1 to 0.8 ma. Reflex facilitation as a function of stimulus intensity is shown in graph. (*b*) A stimulus of 0.05 ma to CSN elicited rsponse in *A*. In *B*, *C*, *D*, *E*

→

pressor response. After spinal transection to abolish sympathetic outflow, we observed that stimulation of the cerebellum inhibited the reflex produced by stimulation of the CSN. This is illustrated in Figure 10–9.

We also induced reflex vagal bradycardia by clamping the aorta for a ten-second period. In these experiments, simultaneous aortic clamping and cerebellar stimulation also inhibited the reflex, as we see in Figure 10–10,A. As in our earlier investigation,[20] when we decerebrated the animal, leaving the diencephalon intact, inhibition of the reflex failed to occur (Figure 10–10,B). We should point out that facilitation of the bradycardic reflex was not observed in this cerebellar study.

Although Moruzzi [32] demonstrated cerebellar inhibition of vasomotor reflexes in the precollicular cat, it would appear that modulation of the cardiac reflex requires an intact forebrain. This hypothesis receives some support from the experiments that we have been describing, as well as from studies that have demonstrated reciprocal avenues of communication between the cerebellum and limbic system structures.[2,14] It should be mentioned that Dell and Olson [12] recorded evoked responses in the cerebellum to stimulation of vagal afferents. Since the paramedian nucleus of the reticular formation receives projections from both the fastigial nucleus and the CSN,[28,29] it may well be that the reticular formation establishes the link in this intercommunication.

The possibility exists that inhibition of the vagal reflex may be caused by presynaptic inhibition of baroceptor impulses at a medullary level. This suggestion receives support from recent work by Weiss and Crill,[39] who showed that the antidromic response recorded from the CSN to stimulation in the nucleus of the tractus solitarius could be augmented by a prior conditioning stimulus delivered to the Hp. The depolarization of these primary afferents is presented by Weiss and Crill as evidence for presynaptic inhibition of this baroceptor input. It is also possible that similar events are operating when inhibition of reflex vagal bradycardia is produced by electrical stimulation of other regions of the brain. Poststimulus potentiation of the reflex could be the result of a rebound phenomenon following a period of inhibition of baroceptor input.

The time course of these central effects is, in some ways, similar to those events reported by Bronk and his colleagues [7] a number of years ago. These investigators observed that a poststimulus depression of sympathetic activity following delivery of stimuli to the hypothalamus that *did not* produce any alteration in blood pressure. They hypothesized that activation of the hypothalamus to altered sympathetic and parasympathetic mechanisms at a brain stem level that the latter became dominant and inhibited tonic discharge in the cardiac nerves. In his recent study, Covian [10] suggested that impulses originating in the septal area "at least partially inhibit the bulbar vasomotor center, thus blocking the action of the reflex mechanisms of the baroceptor nerves."

Activation of the CG, Hp, as well as

---

and *F*, stimuli to CSN and CG were delivered simultaneously. While stimulus applied to CSN was held constant, that to CG was gradually increased from 0.1 to 0.8 ma. Reflex inhibition as a function of stimulus intensity is shown in graph. Stimulus intensities (ma) to both brain (B) and nerve (N) are indicated on each tracing, and horizontal lines denote 10-second stimulation period. (Encéphale isolé preparation.) (From Hockman, C. H., Talesnik, J., and Livingston, K. E.: *Amer. J. Physiol., 217*:1681, 1969.)

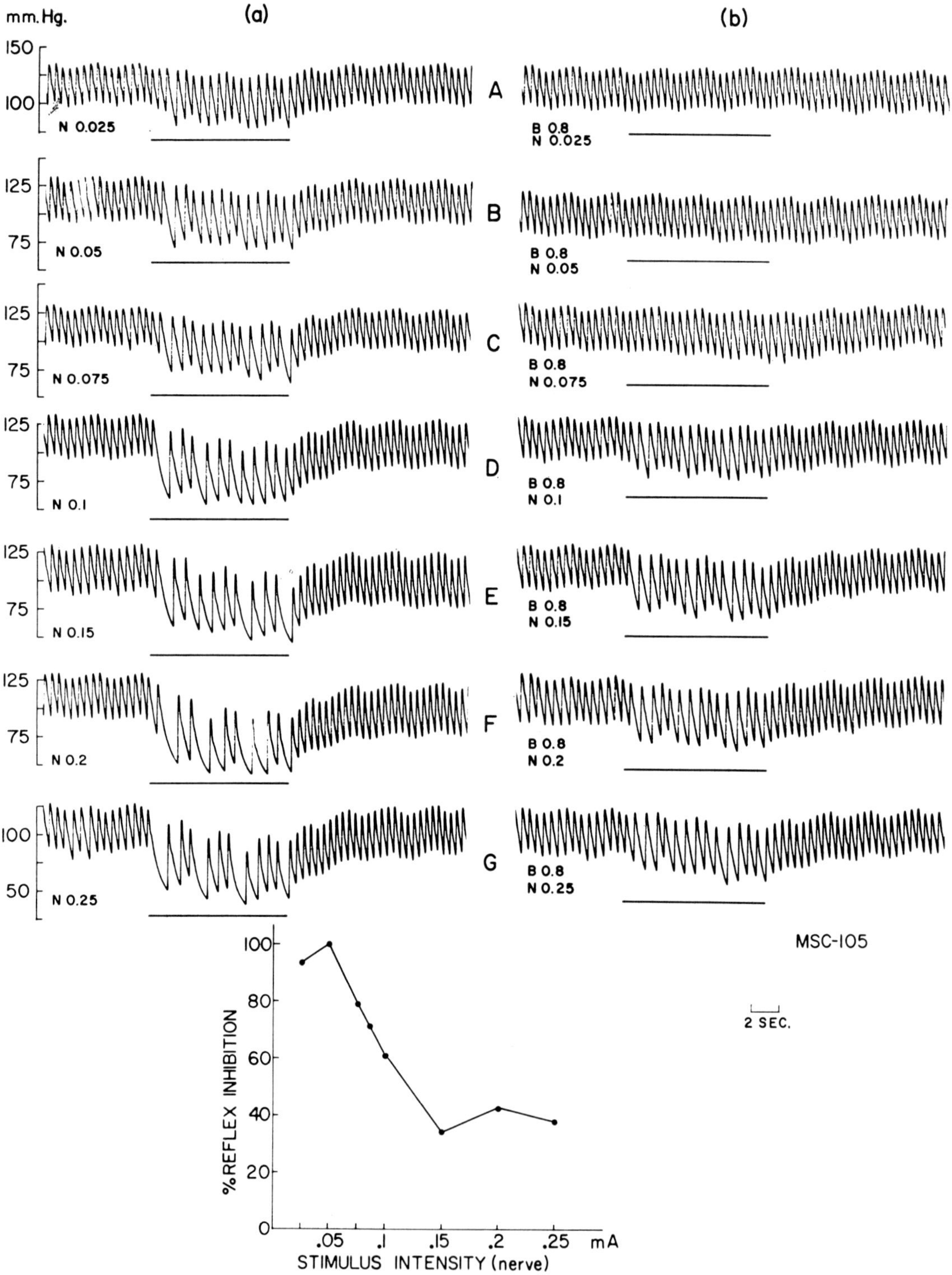

Figure 10–5. (*a*) From *A* to *G* shows reflex response as stimulus applied to carotid sinus nerve (CSN) is gradually increased from 0.025 to 0.25 ma. (*b*) Stimulus delivered to central gray substance of midbrain is held constant and both stimuli are delivered simultaneously; in tracings *A* to *G*, intensity of stimulus applied to CSN is gradually

→

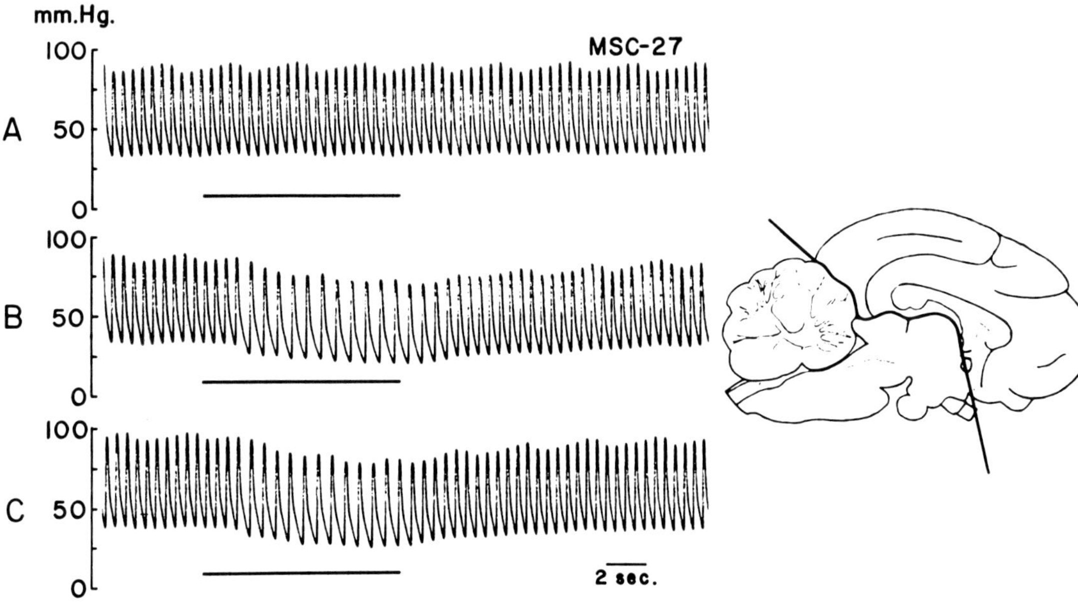

Figure 10–6. (*A*) Results of stimulus of 1.2 ma delivered to central gray substance (CG) of decerebrate cat (24 hours after truncation), as illustrated in drawing. (*B*) Intensity of stimulus applied to carotid sinus nerve (CSN) was 0.15 ma. Stimuli delivered to both CSN and CG were superimposed in (*C*). Horizontal lines beneath each tracing indicate duration of stimulation period. (Encéphale isolé preparation.) (From Hockman, C. H., Talesnik, J., and Livingston, K. E.: *Amer. J. Physiol., 217*:1681, 1969.)

other regions of the brain, may excite elements at both the level of the vagal motor neuron pool and the nucleus of the tractus solitarius. In the latter case, the depolarization of baroceptor afferent terminals would inhibit reflexly induced bradycardia. When the inhibitory stimulus is withdrawn, reverberating activity at the level of the vagal motor neuron pool would lead to potentiation of reflexly elicited bradycardia. The persistence of a central excitatory state is suggested by delayed potentiation of the reflex following brain stimulation (see earlier discussion of this).

On the basis of these experiments, we can unequivocally state that the cardiac component of the baroceptor reflexes is subject to inhibitory control by regions of the brain other than the medulla. Furthermore, the expression of these central influences appears to require an intact forebrain. To our knowledge, this is the first demonstration of centrifugal modulation of the cardiac baroceptor reflex.

The limbic system has been shown to play a very important role in many processes, including learning, motivation and emotion.[24] When electrical stimuli are delivered to limbic regions in the unanesthetized, freely moving, animal, one observes

increased from 0.025 to 0.25 ma. These results are also shown in graph, with inhibition of reflex plotted as function of intensity of stimuli delivered to CSN. Stimulus intensities to brain (B) and nerve (N) are indicated on each tracing, and horizontal lines denote 10-second stimulation period. (Encéphale isolé preparation.) (From Hockman, C. H., Talesnik, J., and Livingston, K. E.: *Amer. J. Physiol., 217*:1681, 1969.)

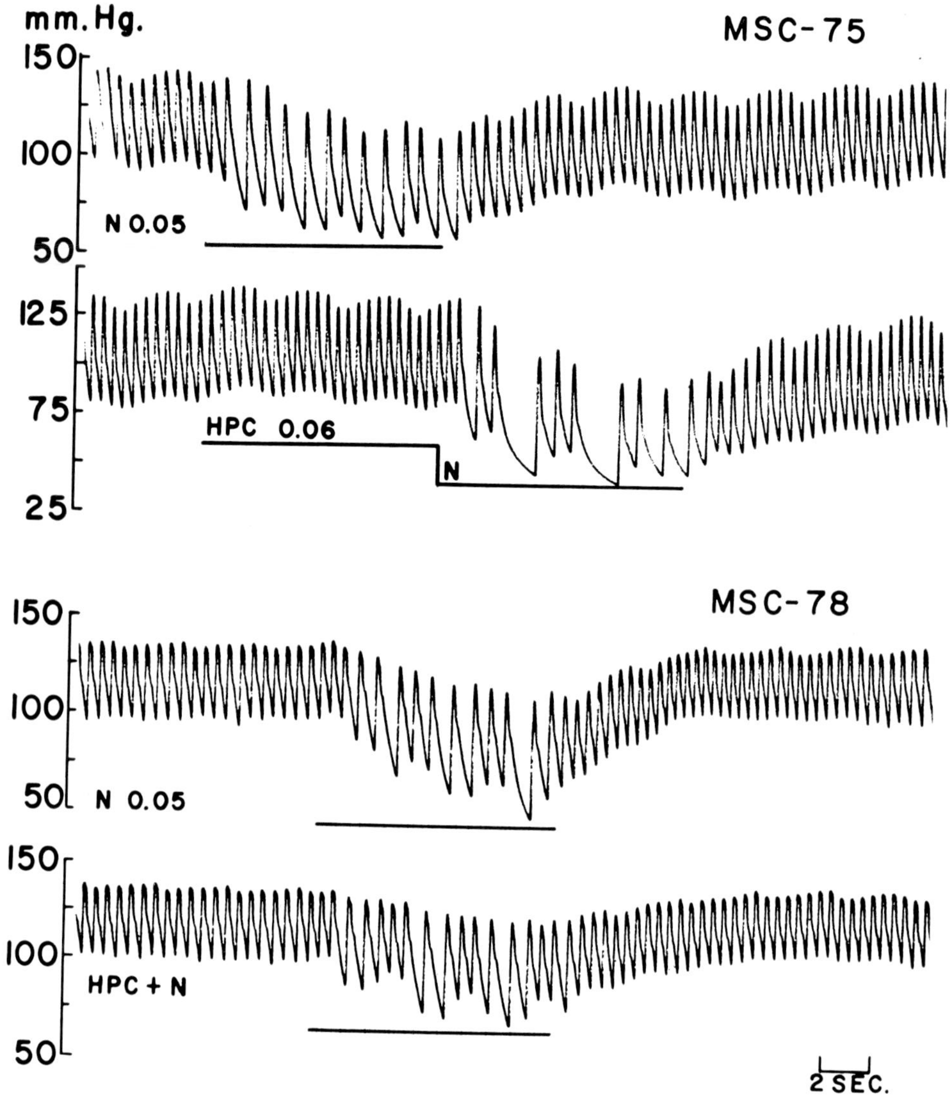

Figure 10–7. Two upper tracings show reflex response elicited by stimulation of carotid sinus nerve (CSN) and enhancement of that response when CSN stimulus is preceded by one to ventral hippocampus (HPC). In two lower tracings, from another animal, electrical stimulation of CSN evokes cardiodepressor reflex, which is inhibited when stimuli are delivered to HPC and CSN concurrently. Intensity of stimuli delivered to nerve (N) and brain (HPC) are indicated on tracings, and horizontal lines indicate stimulus duration. (Encéphale isolé preparation.) (From Hockman, C. H., Talesnik, J., and Livingston, K. E.: *Amer. J. Physiol.*, *217*:1681, 1969.)

that alterations in behavior are usually accompanied by pronounced and widespread influence on somatic and autonomic effectors.[23] The complexity of these response patterns often makes it very difficult to assess autonomic components separately, especially when we possess so little knowledge regarding the manner by which these regions of the brain receive and transmit information to visceral effectors.

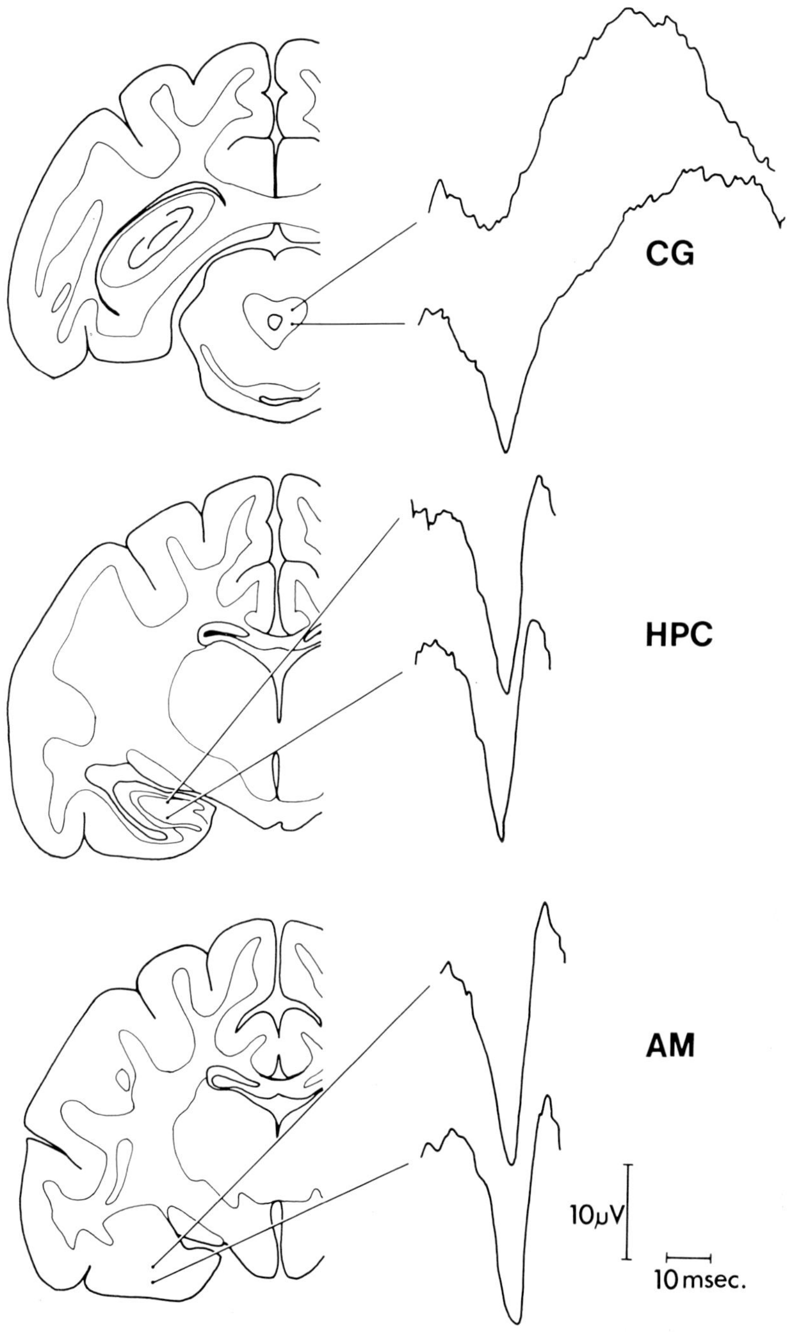

Figure 10–8. Each tracing represents 25 responses (computer-averaged) evoked in the ventral hippocampus (HPC), amygdala (AM), and central gray substance (CG) of the midbrain to single-shock stimuli (0.1 msec) delivered to the central cut-end of the carotid sinus nerve. Positivity is downward. Drawings were made from projections of stained sections, and loci identified by the Prussian blue method. (Encéphale isolé preparation).

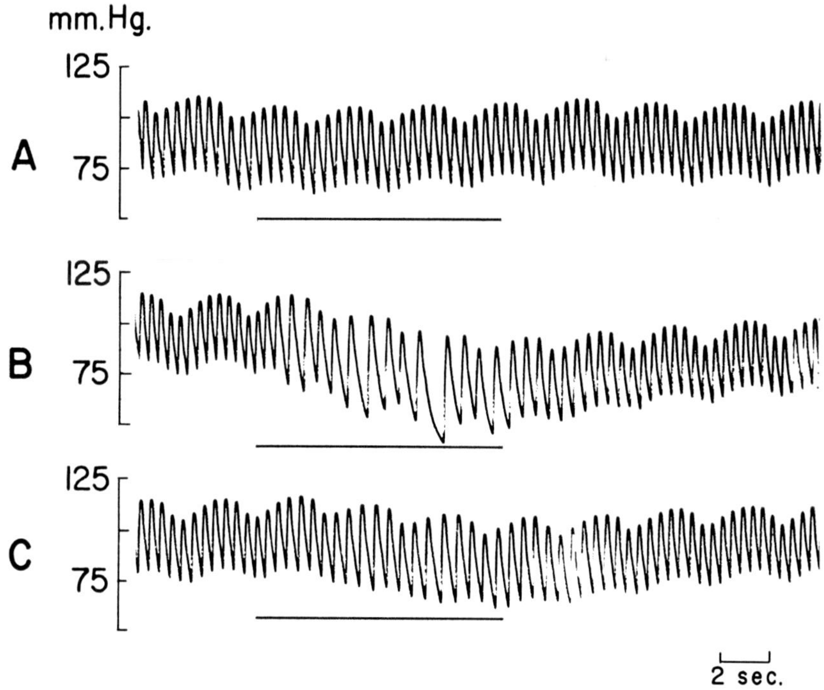

Figure 10–9. (*A*) Stimulus of 0.5 ma delivered to the fastigial nucleus of the cerebellum in the encéphale isolé preparation. (*B*) Cardiac slowing elicited by stimulating the carotid sinus nerve (CSN) with an intensity of 0.05 ma. (*C*) Stimuli were applied concurrently to CSN and cerebellum. Horizontal lines beneath each tracing indicate the stimulus duration of 10 seconds. (From Hockman, C. H., Livingston, K. E., and Talesnik, J.: *Brain Res., 23*:101, 1970.)

As mentioned earlier, visceral afferents are known to project to structures at different levels of the central nervous system (see earlier discussion), and activation of these fiber bundles can alter activity in various regions of the brain (see earlier discussion of this). Results from such studies raise a number of questions regarding the role of forebrain-midbrain circuits in the integration of autonomic mechanisms. A few years ago, Stuart *et al.*[36] reported that hypothalamic unit activity could be altered by bladder distention and sciatic stimulation, many units responding to both somatic and visceral stimuli. In a subsequent study,[37] they showed that hypothalamic units that were responsive to visceral inputs could also be influenced by electrical stimulation of limbic system structures. When they paired central and peripheral stimuli, they found that the direction of the effect of firing rate was similar for "central-visceral and central-somatic stimulation procedures." They also found that units that responded in a different direction to central as opposed to peripheral stimuli "tended to reflect the peripheral influence when the stimuli were paired." Stuart and his associates interpreted their data as favoring the concept that the afferent input to the hypothalamus might play an important role in determining the sign of forebrain influences on somatovisceral and endocrine mechanisms, drawing attention to the interaction between the somatic and autonomic systems.

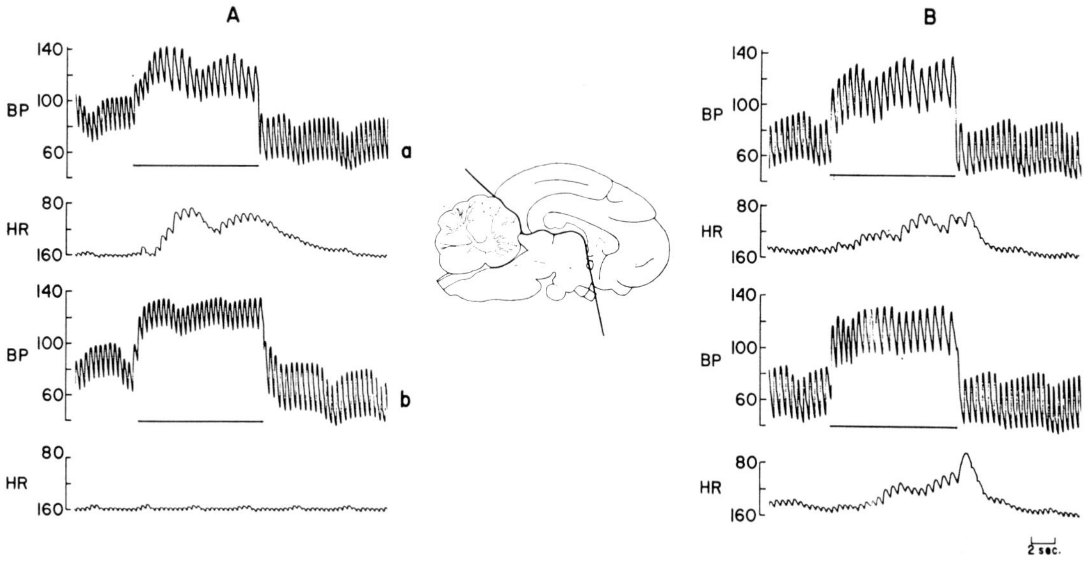

Figure 10–10. (*A*) Blood pressure (BP) and heart rate (HR) in the encéphale isolé preparation. In (*a*) the aorta was clamped and in (*b*) a stimulus of 0.5 ma was delivered to the cerebellum simultaneously with aortic clamping. The tracings in (*B*) were recorded after this animal was decerebrated and represent in (*c*) aortic clamping and in (*d*) concurrent cerebellar stimulation and aortic clamping. The heavy line in the drawing shows that the truncation was performed so as to leave the diencephalon intact. Horizontal lines beneath each tracing indicate clamping and stimulation periods. (From Hockman, C. H., Livingston, K. E., and Talesnik, J.: *Brain Res.*, *23*, 101, 1970.)

The complexities of these interacting variables has been given emphasis by Akert and Gernandt,[1] who demonstrated that limbic and vestibular influences converge on vagal motor neurons and compete for access to these cells.

Although centrifugal modulation of the cardiac reflex appears to require an intact forebrain for its expression, it is probable that an afferent "bias" on hypothalamic cells determines both the extent and sign of forebrain influences on autonomic integrative mechanisms. The intimate interrelationships between the hypothalamus and limbic forebrain-midbrain circuits,[33,34] are such as to provide the anatomical substrate for widespread limbic influences on both visceral and somatic reflexes.

Much more information is needed before any attempt can be made to draw a parallel between the central mechanisms that control incoming afferent traffic from the external world and those that regulate information from the internal world. Certainly, the interaction between behavioral, visceral and somatic components in affective response patterns adds a dimension which does not yield readily to existing probes. Data from the many studies which we have been discussing so far during this conference, however, do permit us to state, with some degree of confidence, that information from our *inner visceral world* is indeed subject to modification by structures at all levels of the central nervous system.

REFERENCES

1. Akert, K., and Gernandt, B. E.: Neurophysiological study of vestibular and limbic influences upon vagal outflow. *Electroenceph. Clin. Neurophysiol., 14:*904, 1962.
2. Anand, B., Malhotra, C. L., Singh, B., and Dua, S.: Cerebellar projections to limbic system. *J. Neurophysiol., 22:*451, 1959.
3. Anderson, F. D., and Berry, C. M.: An oscillographic study of the central pathways of the vagus nerve in the cat. *J. Comp. Neurol., 106:*163, 1956.
4. Baccelli, M., Guazzi, M., Libretti, A., and Zanchetti, A.: Pressoceptive and chemoceptive aortic reflexes in decorticate and decerebrate cats. *Amer. J. Physiol., 208:*798, 1965.
5. Bartorelli, C.; Bizzi, E., Libretti, A., and Zanchetti, A.: Inhibitory control of sinocarotid pressoceptive afferents on hypothalamic autonomic activity and sham rage behavior. *Arch. Ital. Biol., 98:*308, 1960.
6. Bonvallet, M., Dell, P., and Hiebel, G.: Tonus sympathetique et activité electrique corticale. *Electroenceph. Clin. Neurophysiol., 6:*119, 1954.
7. Bronk, D. W., Pitts, R. F., and Larrabee, M. G.: Role of the hypothalamus in cardiovascular regulation. *Res. Publ. As. Res. Nerv. Ment. Dis., 20:*323, 1939.
8. Chase, M. H., Sterman, M. B., and Clemente, C. D.: Cortical and subcortical patterns of response to afferent vagal stimulation. *Exp. Neurol., 16:*36, 1966.
9. Cottle, M. K.: Degenerative studies of primary afferents of the IXth and Xth cranial nerves in the cat. *J. Comp. Neurol., 122:*329, 1964.
10. Covian, M. R.: Studies of the neurovegetative and behavioral functions of the brain septal area. In Adey, W. R., and Tokizane, T. (Eds.): *Structure and Function of the Limbic System, Progress in Brain Research.* Amsterdam, Elsevier, 1967, Vol. 27.
11. Dell, P.: Activity of the nucleus fasciculus solitarius: visceral afferents and somatic functions. In Hockman, C. H. (Ed.): *Limbic System Mechanisms and Autonomic Function.* Springfield, Charles C Thomas, 1972.
12. Dell, P., and Olson, R.: Projections thalamiques, corticales et cerebelleuses des afferences viscerales vagales. *Compt. Rend. Soc. Biol., 145:*1084, 1951.
13. Dell, P., and Olson, R.: Projections "secondaires" mesencephaliques, diencephaliques, et amygdaliennes des afferences viscerales vagales. *Compt. Rend. Soc. Biol., 145:*1088, 1951.
14. Fox, S. S., Liebeskinde, J. C., O'Brien, J. J., and Dingle, R. D.: Mechanisms for modification of cerebellar and cortical afferent information. In Adey, W. R., Tokizane, T. (Eds.): *Structure and Function of the Limbic System, Progress in Brain Research.* Amsterdam, Elsevier, 1967, Vol. 27, pp. 254–280.
15. Freeman, G. L., and Krasno, L.: Inhibitory functions of the corpus striatum. *Arch. Neurol. Psychiat., 44:*323, 1940.
16. Hering, H. E.: *Die Karotissinusreflexe auf Herz und Gefasse.* Dresden und Leipzig, Steinkopff, 1927.
17. Hilton, S. M.: Inhibition of baroreceptor reflexes in hypothalamic stimulation. *J. Physiol. (London), 165:*56, 1963.
18. Hockman, C. H., Mauck, H. P., Jr., and Hoff, E. C.: Experimental neurogenic arrhythmias. *Bull. N.Y. Acad. Med., 43:*1097, 1967.
19. Hockman, C. H., Talesnik, J., and Livingston, K. E.: Central nervous system modulation of cardiovascular reflexes. In *Proc. Int. Congr. Physiol. Sci.,* Vol. VII, No. 586, 1968.
20. Hockman, C. H., Talesnik, J., and Livingston, K. E.: Central nervous system modulation of baroceptor reflexes. *Amer. J. Physiol., 217:*1681, 1969.
21. Hockman, C. H., Livingston, K. E.: Carotid sinus nerve projections to the forebrain and midbrain of the cat. *Fed. Proc., 29(2):*837, 1970.
22. Hockman, C. H., Livingston, K. E., and Talesnik, J.: Cerebellar modulation of reflex vagal bradycardia. *Brain Res. 23:*101, 1970.
23. Kaada, B. R.: Somato-motor, autonomic and

electrocorticographic responses to electrical stimulation of rhinencephalic and other structures in primates, cat and dog. *Acta. Physiol. Scand., 23 (Suppl.)*:83, 1951.
24. Karli, P.: Systeme limbique et processus de motivation. *J. Physiol. (Paris), 60*:3, 1968.
25. Kerr, F. W.: Facial, vagal and glossopharyngeal nerves in the cat. Afferent connections. *Arch. Neurol., 6*:264, 1962.
26. Lacey, J. I.: Somatic response patterning and stress: Some revisions of activation theory. In Appley, M. H., and Trumbull, R. (Eds.): *Conference on Psychological Stress, Toronto 1965*. New York, Appleton, Century, Crofts, 1967, pp. 14–42.
27. Livingston, R. B.: Central control of receptors and sensory transmission systems. In *Handbook of Physiology. Neurophysiology*. Washington, D. C.: *Amer. Physiol. Soc.*, 1960, Vol. 1, Sect. 1, Chapt. 31, pp. 741–760.
28. Miura, M., and Reis, D. J.: Termination and secondary projections of the carotid sinus nerve in the cat brain stem. *Amer. J. Physiol., 217*:142, 1969.
29. Miura, M., and Reis, D. J.: Cerebellum: A pressor response elicited from the fastigial nucleus and its efferent pathway in brain stem. *Brain Res., 13*:595, 1969.
30. Morest, D. K.: Experimental study of the projections of the nucleus of the tractus solitarius and the area postrema in the cat. *J. Comp. Neurol., 130*:277, 1967.
31. Morison, R. S., and Rioch, D. McK.: The influence of the forebrain on an autonomic reflex. *Amer. J. Physiol., 120*:257, 1937.
32. Moruzzi, G.: Paleocerebellar inhibition of vasomotor and respiratory carotid sinus reflexes. *J. Neurophysiol., 3*:20, 1940.
33. Nauta, W. J. H.: Hippocampal projections and related neural pathways to the midbrain in the cat. *Brain, 81*:319, 1958.
34. Nauta, W. J. H.: Limbic system and hypothalamus: Anatomical aspects. *Physiol. Rev., 40 (Suppl. 4, Part II)*:102, 1960.
35. Reis, D. J., and Cuenod, M.: Central neural regulation of carotid baroceptors in the cat. *Amer. J. Physiol., 209*:1267, 1965.
36. Stuart, D. G., Porter, R. W., Adey, W. R., and Kamikawa, Y.: Hypothalamic unit activity. I. Visceral and somatic influences. *Electroenceph. Clin. Neurophysiol., 16*:237, 1964.
37. Stuart, D. G., Porter, R. W., and Adey, W. R.: Hypothalamic unit activity. II. Central and peripheral influences. *Electroenceph. Clin. Neurophysiol., 16*:248, 1964.
38. Wang, G. H., and Brown, V. W.: Suprasegmental inhibition of an autonomic reflex. *J. Neurophysiol., 19*:564, 1956.
39. Weiss, G. K., and Crill, W. E.: Carotid sinus nerve: primary afferent depolarization evoked by hypothalamic stimulation. *Brain Res. 16*:269, 1969.

DISCUSSION

Dr. French: It's a matter of considerable interest that these autonomic inputs to the brain are so prominent. Perhaps we are only beginning to find out how prominent they are and that they can elicit responses which are capable of being potentiated by other parts of the brain is equally impressive. I presume that Dr. Hockman is aware of the work that Dr. Porter has been doing in our laboratories. This involves stimulation of the vagus nerve and, at the other end of the neuraxis, of the bladder, another mechanoreceptor. This work is impressively similar, in many ways, to the demonstrations that Porter has reported. Dr. Porter has recorded primarily from the hypothalamus and the hippocampus and found that distension of the bladder elicits very prominent increases in unit firing patterns in different regions of the hypothalamus. Upon stimulation of the same hypothalamic regions, he finds remarkable changes in the conduction patterns of the ECG, up to and including complete heart block. The cardiographic effect can be potentiated, as Dr. Hockman has pointed out, by concurrent stimulation of hypothalamic loci and carotid sinus nerve. The urinary bladder almost certainly has a great deal to do with the vascular system, too, and this information comes from different sources. Anyone who has seen patients with a transected spinal cord is aware of the fact that when they get into bladder difficulties, when their bladder becomes distended, they get the most frightful bouts of hypertension which is indeed a serious threat to their lives. This observation, and many more like it, suggest that visceral inputs, about which we are just beginning to learn a little, certainly have as much to do as environmental stimuli with physiological control of function.

Dr. Hockman: A few years ago, Baccelli and his colleagues, in commenting on the frequent mention in the literature of the central influences on sign and extent of autonomic reflexes, spoke of a stereotyped central excitability which they attributed to the use of anesthetics. Would you like to comment on this, Dr. French?

Dr. French: Many suggestions have been made to explain the effects of anesthetics on the nervous system, particularly in connection with autonomic responsiveness. In one of his studies, Dr. Porter found that by changing the level of excitability of the reticular formation by the administration of anesthetics in increasing amounts, the loss of inhibitory control exerted over these visceral mechanisms, presumably about which you spoke, reached a point where the cardio-inhibitory reflex could be easily elicited, and the heart thrown into ventricular fibrillation and ventricular arrest. Not only anesthetic agents but also differences in the environment, such as anoxia, will produce the same effect.

Dr. Hockman: Your mention of the work done on the bladder in California is extremely pertinent, especially since Dr. Snider spoke yesterday of cerebellar modulation of the distended bladder. I wonder if Ray would like to make any comments in the light of Dr. Porter's work?

Dr. Snider: Paul Dell has very modestly concealed the fact that he has done a conclusive job in demonstrating a projection of visceral afferents to the cerebellum. Quite apart from that, the question comes up repeatedly about the anesthetic effects of chloralose. We have published two papers contrasting the effects of chloralose and Flaxedil in the decerebrate and encephalon preparations. Now let me go on record in saying this: If one studies evoked responses from the somatic system to the cerebellar cortex, there is a very diffuse projection. If one gives Nembutal to the animal, localized foot, arm and face areas can be seen. I like to think of this as a type of chemodissection method in which certain systems are dissected away, allowing other systems to show through. Some good work has been done on the circulatory system of chloralose-treated animals, and this has its advantages. Regarding chloralose and cerebellar systems, this drug is a depressant and not an excitant. If one does test and conditioning stimulations of the tactile system while studying cerebellar activity, a 400 msec recovery period between stimuli can be observed. It only takes 100 msec if the animal is under Flaxedil, and it only takes about 40 msec in an encephalon preparation. So these anesthetics do make a difference, and we can use them to our advantage to help dissect out certain systems.

Dr. Dell: I'd like to address a first question to Dr. Hockman. Under what conditions have you studied evoked potentials, under chloralosane?

Dr. Hockman: No. In the encéphale isolé preparation.

Dr. Dell: I'd like to clarify this because it is very important. Dr. Snider has alluded to the cerebellum. I remember very well working in Chicago, and for a period of six weeks, we used chloralose (one of the few times in my life that I have used this anesthetic) and Nembutal, and I never found one vagal projection to the brain stem. I was working with Olson at the time, and since he didn't believe that I would find any projections, he left for his vacation. This was at the beginning of August, and during the entire month, I did these studies in the encéphale isolé preparation, and I found the projections very beautifully. So the anesthetic state is very important, at least for visceral projections. Then I have another point concerning your very interesting observations. In your high decerebrate, thalamic decerebrate preparations, these baroreceptive reflexes are much less well developed if you combine central stimulation with stimulation of baroreceptors. Your effect is much less.

Dr. Hockman: While reflex vagal bradycardia can still be elicited by stimulation of the baroreceptor nerves, the central modulatory influences are abolished entirely.

Dr. Dell: Yes, and this is very interesting because there is a paper by Mlle Bonvallet who has studied the effects of central stimulation on increases in blood pressure. She stimulated the hypothalamus and, very curiously, she observed that if you increase the intensity of the stimulus continuously (Hugelin developed such a system), the blood pressure augments continuously almost in a parallel manner, as seen in the case of the diencephalic preparations, as if there were no counterregulation. If you repeat the experiment, however, in an animal with the cortex intact, you observe a very rapid counterregulation. It's not parallel at all—the carotid sinus works again. We were always very astonished that, in a preparation with the thalamus but without the cortex, these reflexes didn't work as well as in a preparation with the cortex.

Dr. Jasper: Perhaps Dr. Nauta would answer my question. I couldn't resist the temptation, with Doctors Green, Nauta and Hockman here, to raise the question as to whether there really is any direct information passing into this midline system from the more recent rapidly conducting pathways at all. Now Albe-Fessard's work and some others have shown that if you're careful in the stimulation of peripheral nerves to excite only the larger fibers, the large Type I afferents, for example, you don't get evoked potentials in midline structures at all. I'm wondering if the more highly differentiated rapid lemniscal-type pathways to the cortex have any direct connections with midline "nonspecific" systems or whether they are relayed back from the cortex via corticofugal pathways to the midline "nonspecific" systems.

Dr. Nauta: In general, it seems true that certain major lemniscal pathways such as the medial lemniscus have few if any direct connections with thalamic cell groups outside the specific sensory nucleus in which they terminate. A question I could not answer is whether visceral afferent systems have access to such "closed" conduction pathways. Alternatively, one could speculate that there may exist some neurons in the brain stem reticular formation that project exclusively to specific thalamic cell groups and that might be accessible to ascending viscerosensory impulses. Kuypers and I, for example, found evidence of axons ascending from the rhombencephalic tegmentum to the ventrobasal nucleus of the thalamus. The tegmental lesions that led to the degeneration of such fibers invariably also caused fiber degeneration in the intralaminar cell groups, and we therefore could not say whether or not there are reticuloventrobasal connections independent of the reticulo-intralaminar pathway.

Dr. Killam: I'd like to make a comment about the use of chloralose in the general practice of neurophysiology. Chloralose, in the eyes of the pharmacologist, particularly the neuropharmacologist, is both a sedative and a convulsant. It produces a convulsive state similar to centrencephalic "petit mal" that lasts for long periods of time. There are several other compounds that fall into the same category. There is no question that the limbic system is extraordinarily sensitive to anesthetic agents, and perhaps more so than the reticular formation. For example, 5 mg/kg of any of the barbiturates will completely block the arousal response from the reticular formation, but it will also block a modulatory effect attributed to the limbic system, besides being a convulsant within the limbic system. This is also true of ether and any of the other conventional anesthetic agents. The mesage that I have for all, and to my senior colleagues here who have used these anesthetic agents for years, is not meant to negate the kind of work that they have done. I think that they have, in fact, laid down the type of wiring diagram that is possible within the system, but how these things interact in the generation of behavior is something else, and under these conditions, you must begin working with unanesthetized preparations and preferably with chronic animals.

Dr. Basnajian: What would the influence of alcohol or various other agents such as nicotine be in this model that you demonstrated, Dr. Hockman?

Dr. Hockman: In preliminary studies, we have observed that alcohol has a tendency to inhibit these modulatory influences. So far, we haven't looked at the effects of nicotine or other compounds.

Dr. Lacey: I'd like to ask a question of both of our speakers and one of Dr. French. Is my recollection correct that the studies by Clemente and his colleagues showed that stimulation of the vagus had a synchronizing effect on cortical EEG? Or is splanchnic stimulation tapping the other afferent systems and producing either excitation or synchronization on the cortex?

Dr. French: Sorry, I can't remember. Do you know, Don?

Dr. Dell: In connection with what you say, I'd just like to mention that there have been studies in California by Chase, Sterman and Clemente.

Dr. Lacey: Yes, that is the paper that I was referring to.

Dr. Dell: Showing synchronization from vagal stimulation.

Dr. Lacey: I thought that vagal stimulation unequivocally produced synchronization, whereas splanchnic stimulation produced either excitation or synchronization. The reason I bring this up is to suggest that we must remind ourselves that we're concerned with more than one visceral afferent system and that we can't state that the inhibitory effects are produced by all visceral afferent systems. The gut may have very different effects on higher levels than the cardiovascular system does.

Dr. Reis: I wonder if I can make one more comment about receptors in the brain itself which may be of importance in cardiovascular regulation. There is a well-known phenomenon of which neurosurgeons are well aware called the Cushing response. This is the acute rise of systemic blood pressure consequent to a sudden increase in intercranial pressure. Dr. Julian Hoff and I have made a very interesting observation that the Cushing response appears to be mediated by structures highly localized to the floor of the fourth ventricle. We have found this by mapping the brain with a small pressure probe and thus discovering that pressure over a very small region of the caudal end of the fourth ventricle lying nearly over the nucleus tractus solitarius will produce a rise in systemic blood pressure. Such effects are not evoked by pressure anywhere else on the dorsum or ventrum of the brain stem.

Dr. Lacey: You're just pressing?

Dr. Reis: We have a probe of ½ mm in diameter mounted on a strain gauge mounted on a micromanipulator. Pressure and displacement are well controlled. The floor of the fourth ventricle is the only place in the brain from which a rise in blood pressure can be elicited by local pressure. There are some segmentally specific regions of the spinal cord, however, from which a rise in blood pressure can also be elicited. These responses from the brain seem to be under supramedullary control, because when you decerebrate the animal, the responses are markedly facilitated. Thus there is another order of cardiovascular receptors lying within the substance of the brain itself which seem to run in the same region of the nucleus tractus solitarii which Dr. Dell has been talking about today.

Dr. Jasper: Dr. Reis' comment concerning localized pressure reminded me of an accidental observation that we made on the motor cortex in studying monkeys with Parkinson-like tremor. A very light local pressure on the motor cortex, which was accidental, stopped this tremor immediately, within seconds. We never thought about mechanoreceptors in the cortex to arrest the tremor by pressure. I was wondering how you can rule out a local ischemia?

Dr. Reis: Well, I think the mechanism of this is not known. It could be a local hypoxia although the latency seems too short (less than 2 seconds).

Dr. Jasper: I wasn't thinking of a chemoreceptor, but rather of ischemic effects on the cells in the area. I was thinking of the reflex.

Dr. Reis: And you think that this would produce the effect on the blood pressure that rapidly?

Dr. Jasper: Oh, yes.

Dr. Reis: That may well be. The threshold, incidentally, is about equal to the systolic blood pressure.

Dr. Calaresu: May I ask Dr. Reis a question? Is bradycardia the only response you can get or can you get other changes—or would you say that you're only stimulating baroreceptors?

Dr. Reis: No, because you're getting a rise in blood pressure and a slowing of the heart rate.

SESSION V

Chairman: Donald B. Lindsley

Chapter 11

Some Cardiovascular Correlates of Sensorimotor Behavior: Examples of Visceral Afferent Feedback?

JOHN I. LACEY

IS THE IMPACT of the environment on the autonomic functions of the organism really as diffuse as traditional doctrine would suggest? The opinion was advanced repeatedly in this symposium that it could not possibly be and that there had to be much more delicate modulation of the effects of internal and external events on autonomic functions. I agree with this opinion, and I plan to present experimental data demonstrating that autonomic effectors show different patterns of activity during different kinds of ongoing behavior. I will come to focus on differential responses of heart rate and blood pressure, and I will offer, as a provocative working hypothesis, the notion that explanations for the data are to be found in the mechanisms of feedback from the cardiovascular system that Dr. Dell and Dr. Hockman talked about in previous chapters.

We have found it increasingly useful to classify behaviors along an hypothetical continuum that ranges from pure attention to external stimuli, on the one extreme, to motivated inattention, on the other. Let me expand on the nature of this continuum. Some behaviors, it is clear, require primarily responses to external environmental cues. In driving a car or piloting a plane, we must note and detect external environmental events, and we must make prompt, precise and preprogrammed responses. For other behaviors, the importance of external environmental cues is either absent or minimal, or, in the extreme, attention to the environment may degrade performance. For example, external stimuli disturb me when I engage in internalized cognitive work—such as doing mental arithmetic, marshalling logical arguments or solving a problem in circuit analysis. If I can, I may shut my eyes, the better to think; this is a not uncommon response of one who desires to reject and eliminate unwanted visual intrusions. A somewhat different example of motivated inattention is also not an uncommon experience: when unavoidable pain or discomfort exists, many of us are quite successful in being inattentive to the undesired sensory input, by using means and resources that are by no means clear to the student of behavioral physiology. One easily can conceive of behaviors in which the demands for attentiveness fall between these two hypothetical polar extremes. These would be tasks that involve simultaneously both attention to the external environment and the kind of cognitive work in which such attention degrades performance. Consider, for example, an

Note: This study was supported by grants MH000623 and FR00222 from the National Institute of Mental Health and the National Institutes of Health, United States Public Health Service.

artificial laboratory task to which I will refer a bit later. The subject listens to the rules of a nonsensical card game, under the instructions that as soon as the verbal recital is over he will be required to answer questions about the game. The subject is required to attend closely to incoming auditory information, but he simultaneously is engaged in organizing and re-organizing the incoming information and is storing it for retrieval.

This classification of behaviors is not the result of an idle exercise in armchair speculation. Our experimental work has consistently led to a striking autonomic differentiation of behaviors that are classifiable along this continuum. Our first clear demonstration of this was made some years ago,[7] in an experiment whose main results, for our present purposes, are shown in Figure 11–1.

This figure shows some results for three groups of subjects who were engaged seriatim in a number of tasks that had been chosen a priori to fall on our hypothetical continuum. The figure shows, separately for each of the three groups, the percentage of subjects showing increases and the percentage showing decreases in five simple physiological variables, recorded simultaneously during the performance of each of the tasks. The tasks are arranged roughly in order from those in which on the one hand, the subject's primary task was to attend to environmental inputs, like photic flashes at 10 Hz, white noise or a dramatic recitation with which he was asked to empathize, to tasks, on the other hand, like doing mental arithmetic, comprehending words spelled in reverse, making up sentences all the words of which begin with a named letter and withstanding noxious stimulation (the cold pressor test). In the last four tasks, there is warrant for assuming that external environmental inputs are disruptive to the organism's task performance or are aversive.

In this and the next two figures, abbreviations are used along the X-axis to symbolize these tasks. The abbreviations are "Se" for the make-up sentences task; "Ar" for mental arithmetic; "Sp" for reverse spelling; "Co" for the cold pressor test; "Ru" for rules of the game, the task earlier described as requiring simultaneously attention to incoming auditory information and organization and storage of the material; "Dr" for the dramatic recitation; "No" for white noise fluctuating in intensity; and "Fl" for photic flashes.

The bottom panel shows the results for electrodermal responses. Practically 100 percent of the subjects showed increases in electrodermal activity in all the tasks except for "rules of the game." It is clear that there was no distinction among these tasks by the so-called galvanic skin response.

The figures for the incidence of cardiac acceleration and cardiac deceleration are in marked contrast. At the right end of the figure, which presents the results for tasks in which environmental events are important and relevant, there is a predominance of the occurrence of cardiac slowing. At the left side of the figure are presented results for tasks in which environmental events were unimportant, deleterious or aversive. Here there is a predominance of cardiac acceleration. Heart rate, then, does discriminate among the tasks, whether we evaluate heart rate changes by sampling the twelve highest beats in a minute (indicated in the figure as data for "Maximum" sympathetic-like activity) or by sampling the twelve slowest beats in a minute ("Minimum"). Heart rate variability, the difference between the average of the twelve fastest and the twelve slowest beats ("Spread" in the

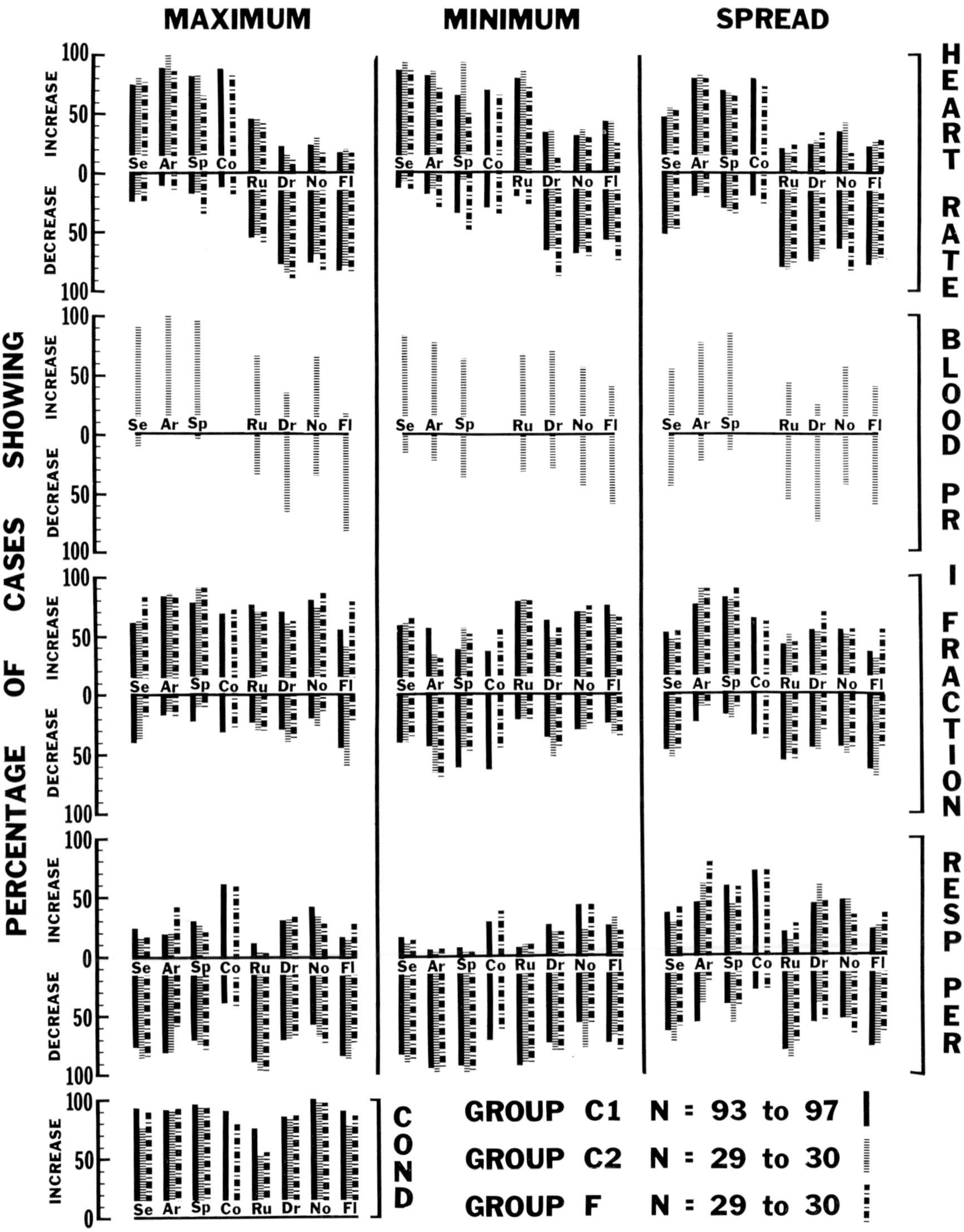

Figure 11–1. Percentages of subjects showing increases and percentages showing decreases in heart rate, blood pressure, I-fraction (ratio of inspiratory duration to total cycle time), respiratory period and palmar conductance, in eight different stimulus situations, for three groups of subjects. The stimulus situations are indicated by symbols on the abscissae (see text). (From Lacey, J. I., and Lacey, B. C.: In Black, P. (Ed): *Physiological Correlates of Emotion.* New York, Academic Press, 1970, p. 213.)

figure) also seems to discriminate the tasks. Noting and detecting environmental events produces a decrease in variability; doing mental work or withstanding pain produces an increase.

Digitally recorded systolic blood pressure also discriminates among the tasks. On the left side of the figure we see predominantly increases in blood pressure; on the right side of the figure there is a more frequent occurrence of depressor responses.

Inspiratory fractions (the ratio of inspiratory duration to total cycle time) and respiratory periods are like the electrodermal responses; they do not differentiate the tasks.

The results for "rules of the game" are remarkable. This task requires the attentive behavior that seems to be correlated with cardiac deceleration and the cognitive work that seems to be correlated with cardiac acceleration. The results seem to strike a balance between these opposing physiological demands. Approximately 50 percent of the subjects show acceleration

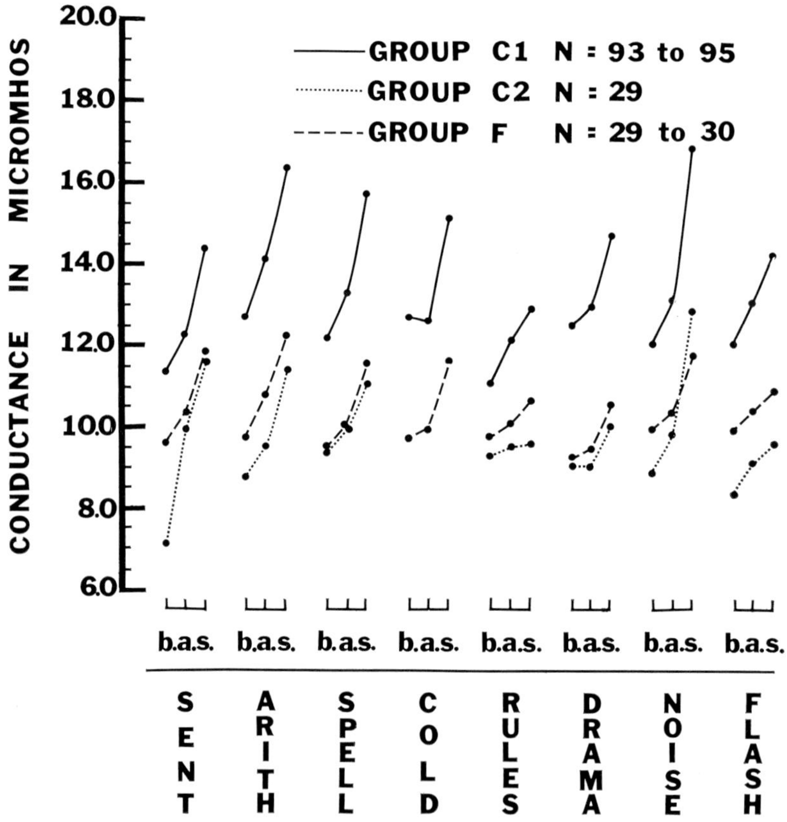

Figure 11–2. Average palmar conductance response curves for three groups of subjects, in eight different stimulus situations. The stimulus conditions are described in the text and are indicated in the figure by single words or abbreviations. Each graph consists of three points: "b," for base level, is the average prestimulus or resting value; "a," for alerted level, is the average value during one minute of anticipation of the stimulus condition; "s," for stress or stimulus level, is the average value during the administration of the stimulus condition. (From Lacey, J. I., and Lacey, B. C.: In Black, P.: (Ed.): *Physiological Correlates of Emotion.* New York, Academic Press, 1970, p. 211.)

and 50 percent deceleration. Blood pressure response for this task is also intermediate between the responses elicited during purely attentive behavior (such as merely noting photic flashes) and pure cognitive work (such as mental arithmetic). The results suggest that blood pressure and heart rate are like vectorial resultants of contrary psychophysiological demands.

The white noise situation had also been planned to impose opposing physiological demands. While the subjects were asked to pay close attention to the noise, which fluctuated in intensity, the stimulation became aversive, for it reached peak intensities in excess of 100 db above threshold. As can be seen, blood pressure, but not heart rate, reflected the intermediate status of this task along our hypothetical continuum.

Figure 11–2 shows average palmar conductance response curves for the same experiment. Skin conductance clearly increases for all tasks for all groups. The amount of increase differs for the tasks, but not in any way clearly related to our behavioral continuum.

Figure 11–3 shows the average heart rate curves. There is a dramatic difference among the tasks. Compare the acceleration accompanying the mental arithmetic test, the intermediate response of "rules of the game" and the deceleration while the subject paid attention to photic flashes. The decelerations seen during flash, noise and the dramatic recitation carry the heart rate to significantly lower levels than seen while the subject was recovered from the previous task and was resting quietly seated in a comfortable armchair!

In all subsequent experiments, we have continued to find, without exception, that when the prime requirement of the task is to note and detect external environmental events, the response of the heart is to decelerate. Under the same conditions, blood pressure either drops or trivially increases. Other simultaneously recorded variables continue to give the sympathetic-like effects so commonly seen in psychophysiological investigations in the laboratory. The most recent example from our laboratory is presented in Figure 11–4, which shows some results from a study just completed by Dr. Libby, Mrs. Lacey and myself, on autonomic response patterns while subjects looked at pictorial patterns exposed on slides. There were thirty-four subjects, each of whom looked for fifteen seconds at each of thirty slides. Before and after each exposure of interesting pictorial material, the subject looked for fifteen seconds at a control pattern of five dots. As the figure shows, looking at the interesting and provocative pictorial slides produced cardiac deceleration—a parasympathetic-like response—and pupillary dilation—a sympathetic-like response. The response to the control dot patterns shows primarily a recovery from the previous pictorial slide followed by a stabilization.

The pictorial materials used for the slides were subjected to elaborate rating scales filled out by an independent sample of subjects. One of the attributes that was rated was the attention-provoking value of the slides. We divided the slides into three groups, those high, low or intermediate in attention value, and determined the average response curves. The results are shown in Figure 11–5. It is clear—and statistical analyses showed the differences to be significant—that the slides higher in attention value elicited greater and better-sustained cardiac decelerations and greater pupillary dilations.

We have been concerned in our laboratory for years with such phenomena as I have just reported, and we continually ask,

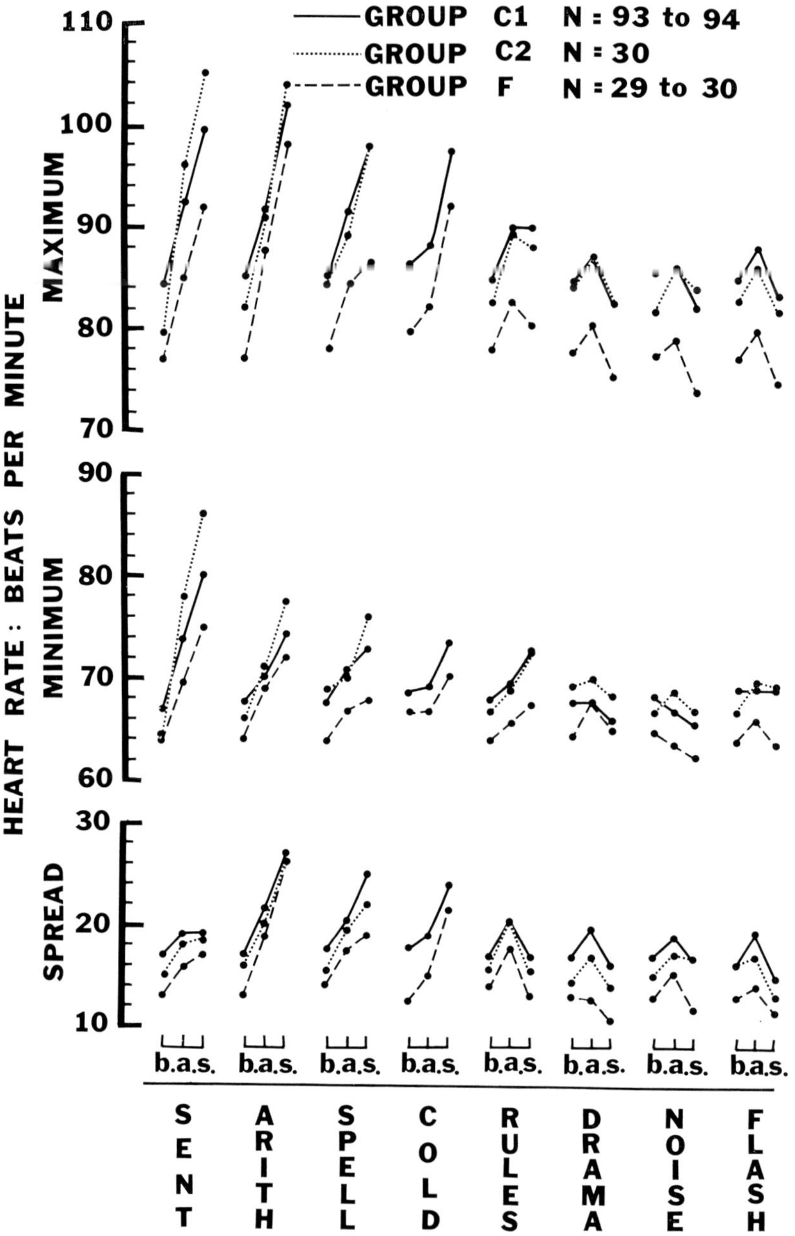

Figure 11–3. Average heart rate response curves for three groups of subjects, in eight different stimulus conditions. Abbreviations have the same meaning as in Figure 11–2. (From Lacey, J. I., and Lacey, B. C.: In Black, P. (Ed.): *Physiological Correlates of Emotion*. New York, Academic Press, 1970, p. 212.)

Why does the heart decelerate during attention and accelerate during motivated inattention? Why does blood pressure either drop during attention or show insignificant changes? Why do these parasympathetic-like effects occur while other simultaneously recorded measures, such as pupillary diameter or electrodermal re-

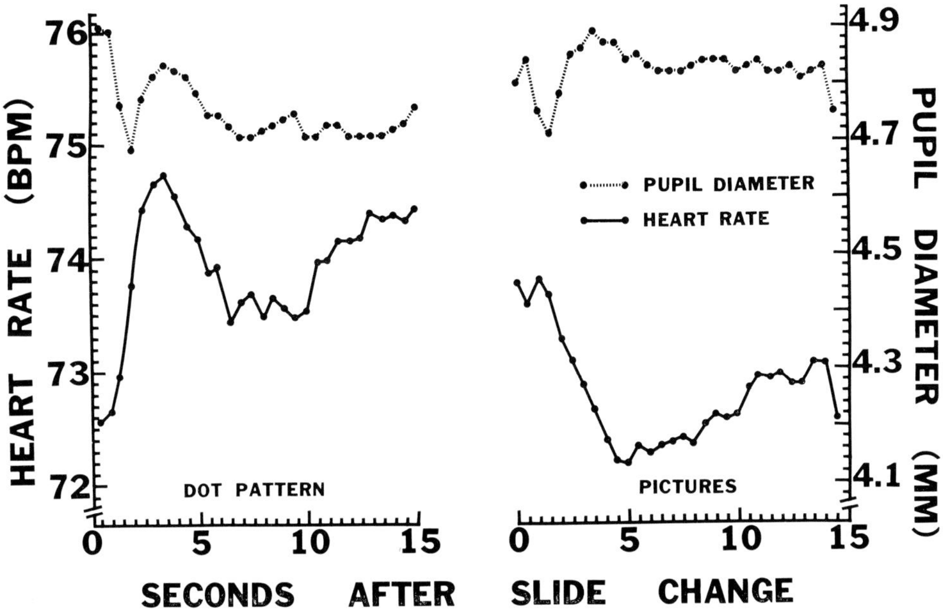

Figure 11–4. Average curves for heart rates and pupillary diameters, for 34 subjects, as they looked at interesting pictures (N = 30) and at repeated uninteresting control slides of patterns of five dots. Pictures were exposed for 15 seconds and were alternated with 15-second exposures of dot patterns. The early part of the response to dot patterns, then, represents recovery from the pupillary dilatation and cardiac deceleration exhibited in response to the pictures.

sponses, show sympathetic-like effects? Do the decelerations and hypotensions convey any behavioral advantage? If so, how shall we explain these advantages? I need not say that no decisive answers exist yet to these questions, but the recent neurophysiological studies of the relationship of cardiovascular function to brain function serve to provide the beginnings of an explanatory framework. Much of this basic material has been mentioned already in this conference.

We know that changes in blood pressure are detected by mechanoreceptors in the aortic arch, carotid sinus, and elsewhere, and are fed back, in a negative feedback loop, to the central nervous system. We know that this visceral afferent feedback loop has functions that go further than the maintenance of physiological levels of heart rate and blood pressure. Years ago Dr. Dell and his colleagues demonstrated that increases of pressure within the carotid sinus produce elevations in the threshold for the evocation of simple reflex movements.[4,5] In Chapter 9, Dr. Dell presented evidence that increased impulse traffic into the head of the nucleus of the solitary tract results in decreasing receptivity to an afferent volley over the radial nerve. Bonvallet and Allen showed that minute coagulations of this area—presumably the area receiving impulses from the baroceptors of the carotid sinus and aortic arch—result in a prolongation of the central, muscular and autonomic effects of input stimulation. Increased impulse traffic into this area, produced by increased heart rate and blood pressure, could be expected then to result in

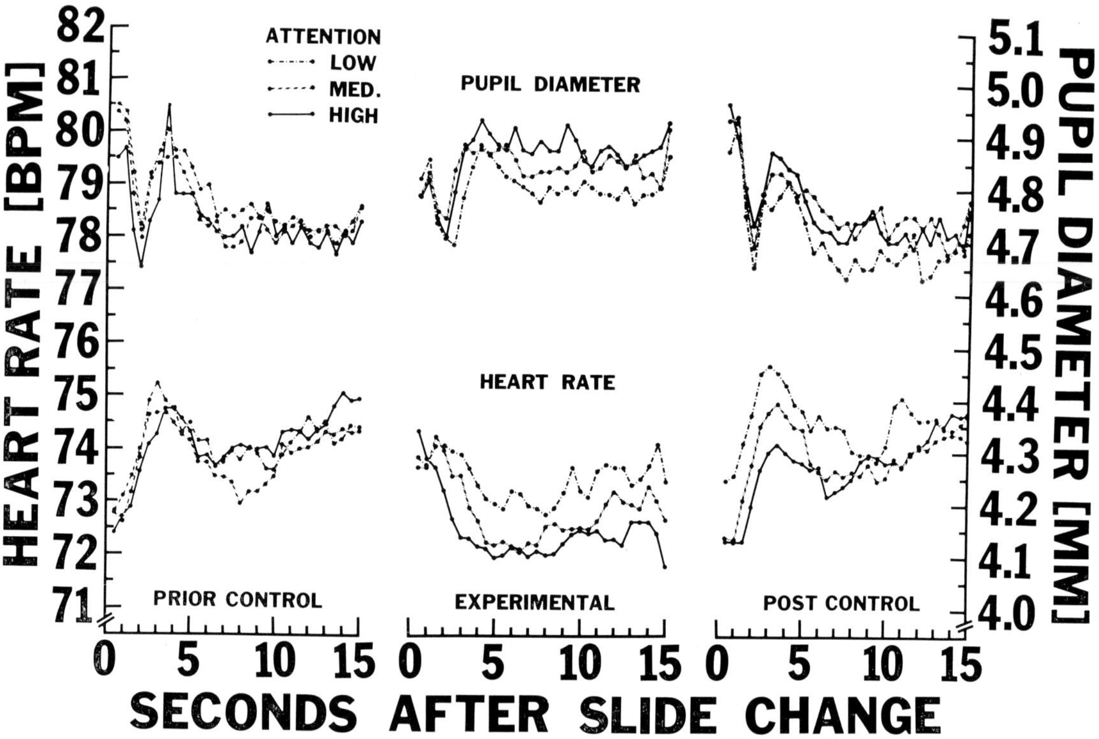

Figure 11–5. Average heart rate and pupillary responses of 34 subjects looking at interesting pictorial slides (N = 30 "experimental" slides), preceded and followed by control slides of five dots. The responses are shown separately for experimental slides rated independently for attention value.

prompter termination of input effects; decreased heart rate and blood pressure would result in more prolonged effects of input stimuli. The dramatic results of Zanchetti and his colleagues [1,2] have similar implications. They found that the autonomic and motor manifestations of sham rage in the acutely decorticated cat could be terminated promptly by stimulation of the large pressoreceptive fibers in either the aortic depressor nerve or Hering's nerve. Finally, we know that the sensitivity of the feedback system from the carotid sinus is frequency dependent. Increases in heart rate increase the vigor and briskness of the depressor responses mediated by the carotid sinus; [6] decreases in heart rate decrease the "gain" and the "phase shift" of the carotid sinus control loop.[10]

These are remarkable facts to the psychophysiologist. They imply that an increase in heart rate and blood pressure may be assumed, under as yet unspecified circumstances, to have the potential of producing a number of *inhibitory* effects on brain function and behavior, whereas decreases in heart rate and blood pressure might have the potential of producing *excitatory* effects. Such effects would be quite unpredictable from current doctrines concerning autonomic function and "arousal." I say "have the potential of producing" because it is clear that all changes in heart rate and blood pressure need not be effective in modifying the function of higher levels of the central nervous system. For one thing, we have already heard in this symposium, and will undoubtedly hear again, that baroceptor reflexes are modulated and controlled by a variety of central structures. For another, as Peterson has shown,[9] the carotid sinus (and presumably the aortic arch) is not a passive organ, inevitably and uniformly responding to changes in heart rate and blood pressure. It is instead a reactive organ. The walls of the sinus may become acutely stiffer or more flaccid. If the sinus is stiffened, increments in pressure and rate cannot be communicated upwards along the visceral afferent feedback pathways, for a rigid pipe is not distended and stretched in response to changes in the head of pressure. Because such control mechanisms exist, we must accept as one very important task the specification of the exact circumstances in which the intact organism will exhibit predictable sequences of changes in cardiovascular activity followed by changes in brain and behavior.

Do the neurophysiological demonstrations provide an explanation for the bradycardia of attention? Does the organism *instrumentally use* his cardiovascular system to increase or decrease feedback to the central nervous system because such feedback affects brain function and behavior? The statements implied by these questions seem teleological. It is entirely possible, however, that higher centers, serving as the structural substrate of attentive behavior, also serve to initiate those cardiovascular changes we have described as being correlated with such behavior. Moreover, the neurophysiological studies suggest that the observed decrements in heart rate and blood pressure truly might convey a behavioral advantage, perhaps strong enough to ensure selection of the underlying mechanism during evolution. For example, extrapolation from the neurophysiological demonstrations that increased intrasinusal pressure elevates the threshold for the evocation of a monosynaptic reflex and that a diminution of cardiovascular feedback to the *nucleus tractus solitarius* leads to a prolongation of the central "arousing" effects of afferent stimulation suggests that the decreased heart rate (and blood pressure) seen in attentive states might serve the function of improving both the organism's receptivity to afferent stimulation and the organism's readiness to make effective responses to such stimulation.

These are brave and perhaps foolhardy questions and speculations, but they have proved to be heuristically fruitful, for they provoked us to generate some suggestive parallels with the neurophysiological demonstrations, in experiments with intact normal human subjects. The classical reaction-time experiment seems ideally suited to the study of sensorimotor integration suggested at the end of the last paragraph, for the experiment makes it possible objectively to measure "the organism's receptivity to afferent stimulation and the organism's readiness to make effective responses to such stimulation."

Figure 11–6 shows extracts from cardiotachometric and respiratory tracings of three subjects working in a fixed foreperiod simple visual reaction-time experiment. The moment of occurrence of the ready signal—onset of a green lamp—is indicated by the letter *R* in the figure. The subject is then required to depress a telegraph key conveniently located near his right hand, to stare intently at a point in space where the imperative stimulus—a white light—will occur and to release the key as rapidly as possible when the imperative stimulus does occur. The onset of the imperative stimulus is indicated

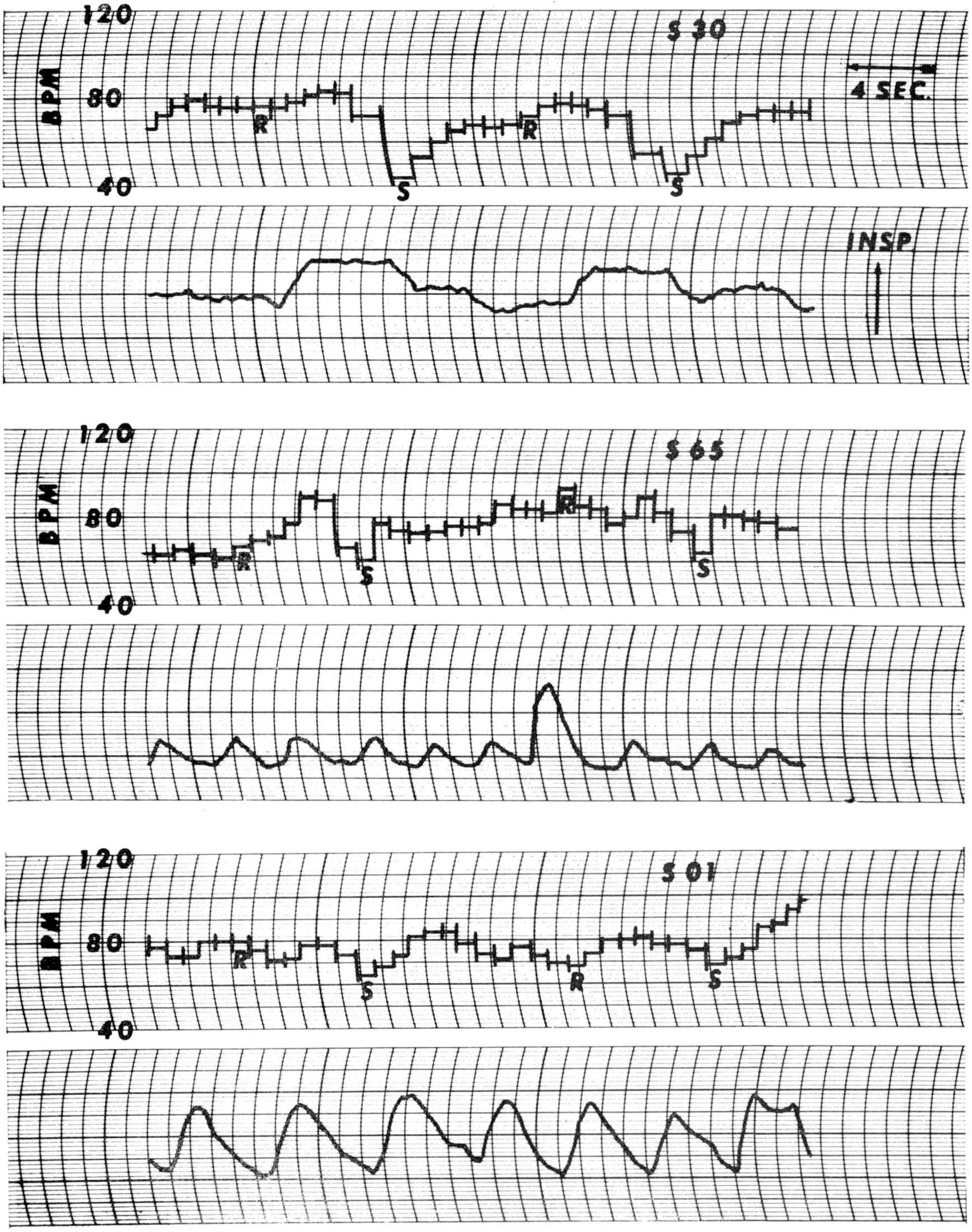

Figure 11–6. Excerpts from simultaneously recorded cardiotachometric and respiratory curves of three subjects in a simple visual reaction experiment. R shows the time of occurrence of the ready signal, S the time of occurrence of the imperative stimulus. (From Lacey, J. I., and Lacey, B. C.: In Black, P. (Ed.): *Physiological Correlates of Emotion*. New York, Academic Press, 1970, p. 215.)

by the letter S in the figure. Upon the completion of the response, the subject simply quietly awaits the next ready signal. Each subject had one hundred and eight trials. The elapsed time between the onset of the ready signal and the onset of the imperative stimulus was four seconds.

The figure shows two consecutive trials for each subject. As you can see, a cardiac *deceleration* occurs in the latter part of the foreperiod, sometimes preceded by an acceleration in the early part of the foreperiod and sometimes not. The deceleration continues, beat-by-beat until the imperative stimulus and the subsequent motor response occur. This remarkable anticipatory deceleration can be quite large. It amounts to almost forty beats per minute for the topmost subject in the figure. The deceleration occurs in the face of diverse respiratory patterns. Other data from this experiment show that the decelerations are not explainable as the reflex consequence of elevation of blood pressure. Blood pressure, we found, under the circumstances of this experiment, sometimes went up and sometimes down. In most instances, the changes were small, amounting to three to five mm Hg. Nowlin and his colleagues [8] studied blood pressures recorded from indwelling arterial cathethers, a more conclusive technique than ours. (We used the digital systolic follower.) They found that both systolic and diastolic pressure decreased modestly during the foreperiod. The diastolic pressure decrease was more marked and was attributed to the greater time available for the drainage of blood from the arterial system that is available with the decreased heart rate.

The anticipatory deceleration is highly reliable. It occurs both early and late in the experiment and in an overwhelming majority of subjects and trials. If the subject is especially motivated to respond as quickly as possible and shows this by highly significant decreases in reaction time, both the early acceleratory and the late deceleratory components of the cardiac response are increased. This is shown in Figure 11–7, which summarizes the results of an experiment by Mrs. Lacey and myself. In this experiment, timing of the foreperiod began only when the subject depressed the telegraph key after the ready signal, thereby signalling that he was ready to anticipate the next imperative stimulus and that, according to instructions, his eyes were fixated on the white lamp. The figure shows group averaged cardiac response curves for twenty-eight subjects, for twenty "motivated" and twenty "unmotivated" trials. "Motivated" trials were trials in which the subject was told his reaction time after each response and was under special instructions to maintain very quick responses. Statistical analyses showed that the subjects responded unequivocally with faster reaction times and that the increase of the early acceleration was algebraically smaller and statistically less significant than the increase of the later cardiac deceleration. Both increases were significant. So, in its response to the special motivating conditions, the anticipatory cardiac deceleration seems well qualified, despite its parasympathetic-like nature to be considered an "activation" response.

The presence of the early acceleratory limb is difficult to interpret in terms of our theory. It cannot be considered to be the primary "arousal" response, which would make the subsequent deceleration into a secondary rebound; for, if this were true, why is the acceleratory limb not sustained until the imperative stimulus? Moreover, why is the cardiac deceleration so time locked to the imperative stimulus? Dr.

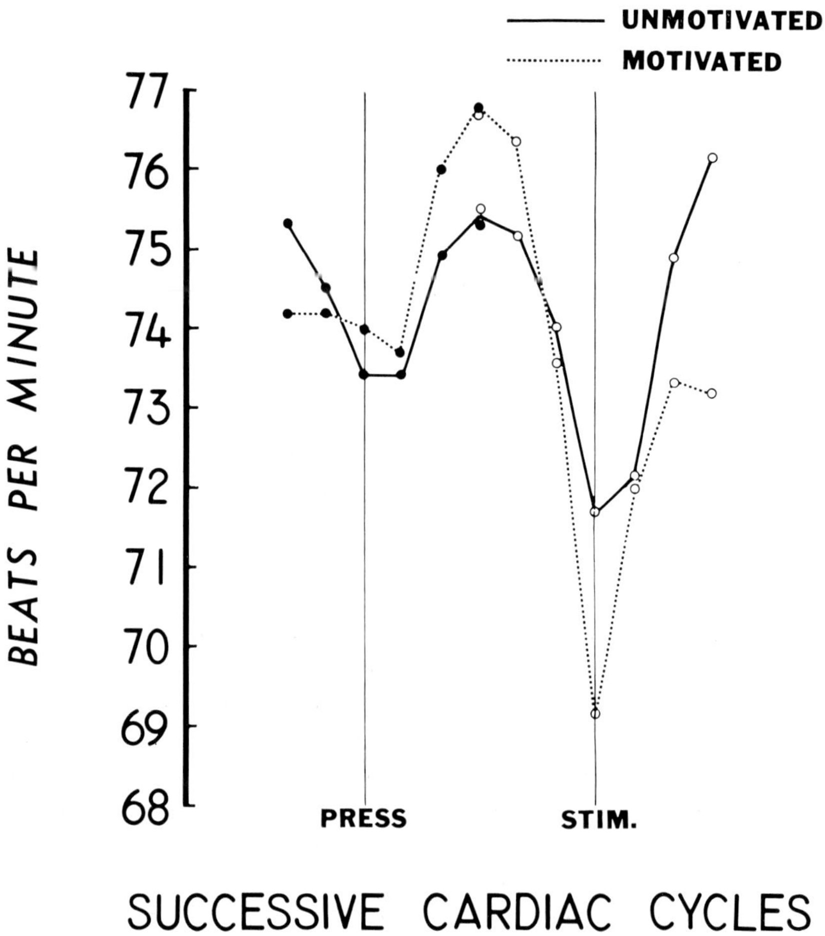

Figure 11–7. Group averages of median cardiac response curves for 28 subjects to 20 "unmotivated" and 20 "motivated" trials (see text). (From Lacey, J. I., and Lacey, B. C., In Black, P. (Ed.): *Physiological Correlates of Emotion.* New York, Academic Press, 1970, p. 217.)

Coquery felt that the early acceleration might be a response to the key press required of the subject after the onset of the ready signal. Accordingly, he and I performed an experiment in which no preparatory key press was required. Either four or ten seconds after the onset of the ready signal, the imperative stimulus occurred, and the subject responded, not as in earlier experiments with a key release but with a key press. Foreperiods of ten seconds were used, in addition to those of four seconds, to insure that, in the earlier experiments, we had not been seeing merely a response, evoked by the ready signal, with a time course adventitiously coincident with the four-second duration of the foreperiod. Trials with four- and with ten-second foreperiods were presented in blocks. Two subgroups of subjects were used to counterbalance the order of presentation of the two foreperiods. The results for twenty-six subjects, each of whom executed one hundred trials, are shown in Figure 11–8. Clearly, the development of the obtrusive de-

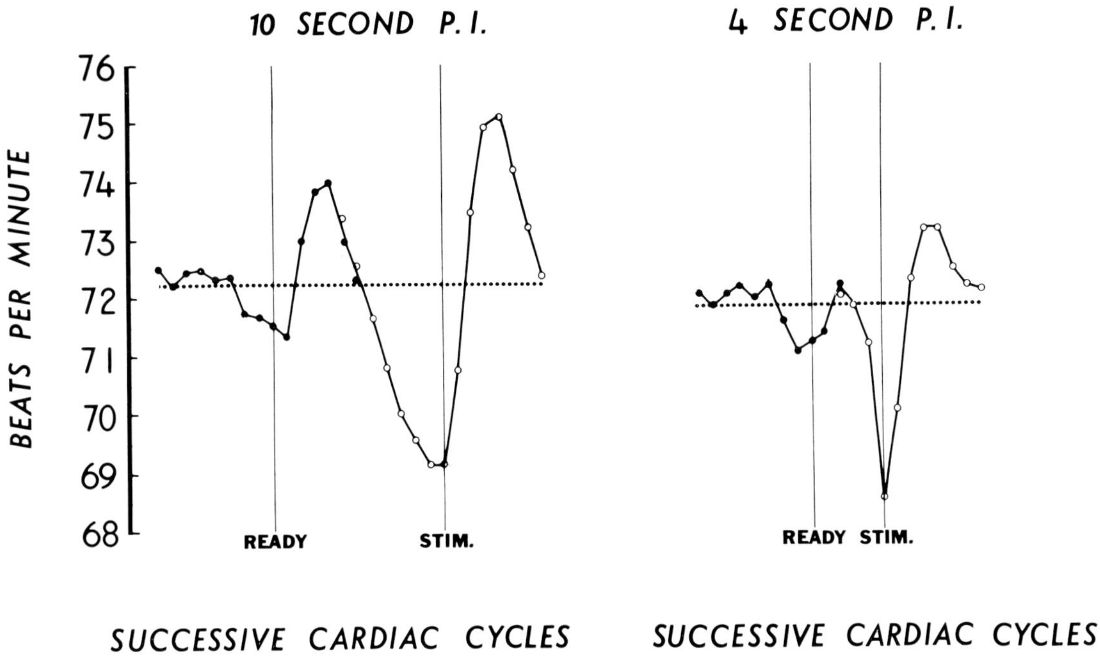

Figure 11–8. Group averages of the median cardiac response curves for 26 subjects for 100 trials, half with a 10-second and half with a 4-second preparatory interval. Successive cardiac cycles were oriented with respect to both ready signal (*solid circles*) and imperative stimulus (*open circles*). (From Lacey, J. I., and Lacey, B. C.: In Black, P. (Ed.): *Physiological Correlates of Emotion*. New York, Academic Press, 1970, p. 218.)

celeratory response is not restricted to a four-second preparatory interval; rather it is time locked to the presentation of the imperative stimulus. Despite the six-second difference in duration of the two preparatory intervals, the heart decelerates to almost identical levels at the time of the imperative stimulus. Dr. Coquery, moreover, was partially right. As the results for trials with four-second foreperiods show, elimination of the preparatory key press did markedly diminish or eliminate the early acceleratory response. This was not true for trials with foreperiods of ten seconds. We do not have a ready explanation yet for the role of the early acceleration.

The next figure shows a rather dramatic effect, discovered by Mrs. Lacey, concerning the consequence of the omission of the imperative stimulus at the expected time. The subjects had been performing a simple visual reaction-time experiment with a fixed four-second foreperiod. On about 10 percent of the trials, the imperative stimulus was not presented at the end of four seconds. Instead, the elapsed time since the preparatory key press was extended by one second, and then the ready signal was turned off. These are so-called catch trials, used to prevent the subject from responding prematurely, in the absence of the imperative stimulus, simply because he anticipates the end of the foreperiod. As Figure 11–9 shows rather dramatically, the heart continues to decelerate—searching for the missing stimulus—until the trial is terminated.

In all the experiments so far described, we used either a single foreperiod or two foreperiods which were employed in

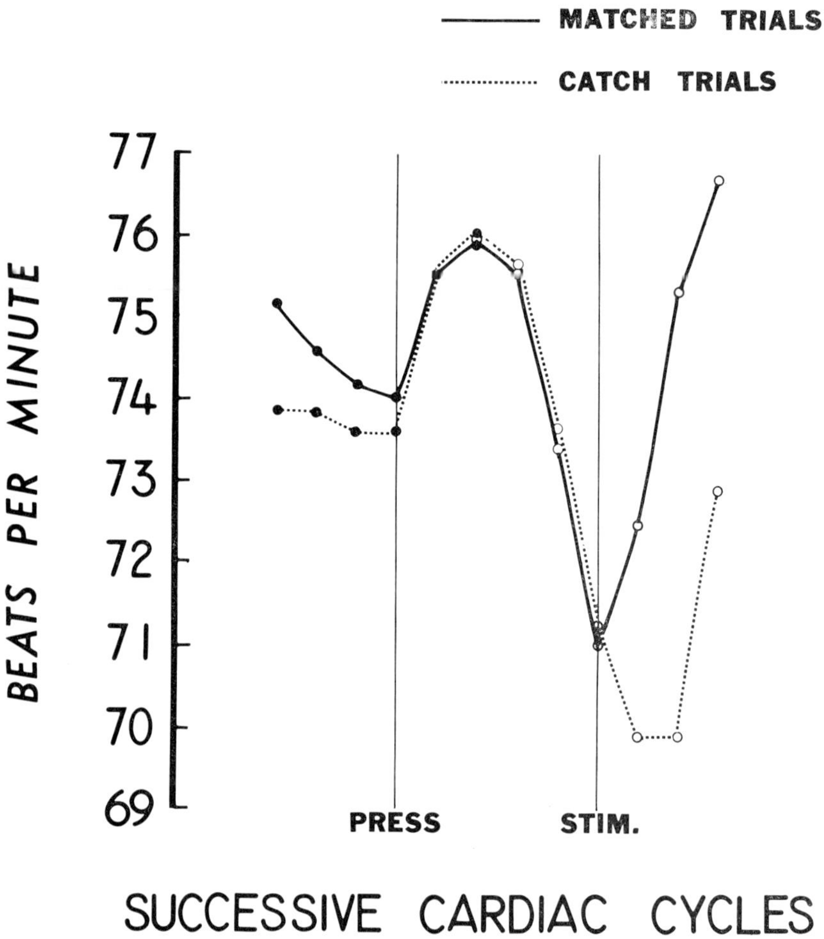

Figure 11–9. Group averages of the median cardiac response curves of 66 subjects for 12 regular reaction-time trials and 12 temporally contiguous "catch trials" in which the imperative stimulus was omitted. Successive cardiac cycles are oriented as in Figure 11–8.

blocks, so that the subject was able to anticipate the moment of onset of the imperative stimulus. In the next experiment I am going to talk about, we used a preplanned, apparently haphazard order of presentation of foreperiods of three, four and five seconds. Each foreperiod preceded all foreperiods, including itself, equally often. The subject was unable to predict when the imperative stimulus was going to occur. Under such circumstances, as is well documented in experimental psychology, there seems to occur a temporal growth and decay of response-readiness; the subjects seem to prepare to respond most effectively at the expiration of the *average* foreperiod. As a consequence, two functions are generated by such an experiment, the current foreperiod effect and the preceding foreperiod effect.

Let us deal first with the current foreperiod effect. Reaction time on a given trial will be a function of the length of the preparatory interval. The reaction time tends to be quicker at the end of preparatory intervals of average duration than of shorter than average duration. Presumably because response-readiness reaches its peak at a time equal to the elapsed time of the average foreperiod, the subject is "caught short" if the imperative stimulus occurs at an earlier time, and hence he responds more slowly. The reaction times secured at preparatory intervals longer than average do not differ as much from those secured at average foreperiods; the readiness-to-respond decays slowly after it has reached its peak or is even increased a bit.

In our variable preparatory interval experiment, forty-six subjects were used. The median amount of cardiac deceleration shown by each subject was determined. Two subgroups of subjects were then formed; one of subjects whose individually determined median deceleration was greater than the group median of medians and one of subjects who showed less than the group median deceleration. Because of a tie, there were twenty-two cases classified as below average in the magnitude of cardiac deceleration and twenty-four cases classified as above average. Average curves of reaction time as a function of the preparatory interval are shown for these two groups in Figure 11–10. The broken line shows the results for subjects who showed greater than average anticipatory cardiac decelerations; the solid line shows results for subjects with less than average anticipatory decelerations. At all foreperiods, and whether we look at the first or second halves of the experiment ("Work 1" and "Work 2," respectively, in the figure), or the whole experiment ("Work All"), we find that *the greater the cardiac de-*

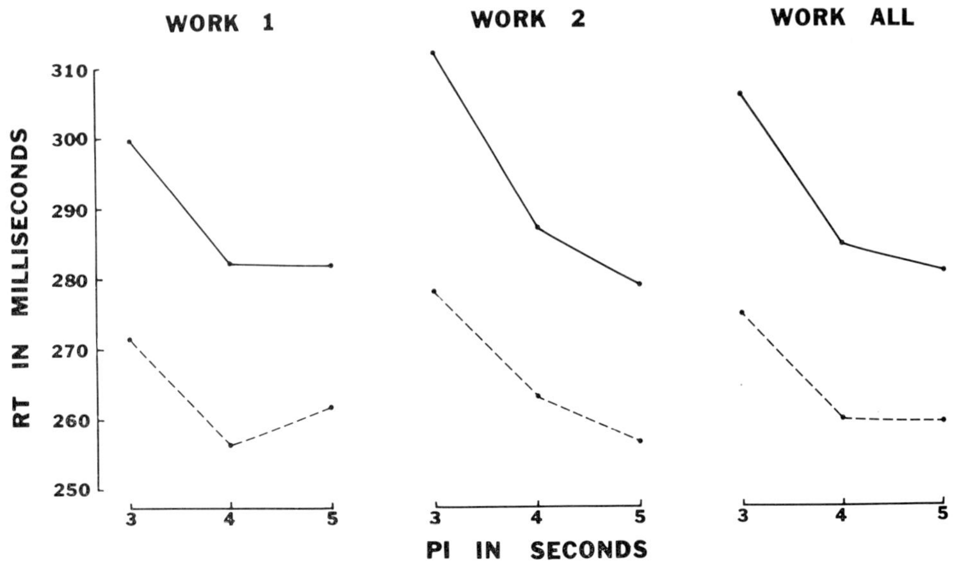

Figure 11–10. Average curves of simple visual reaction time, for 46 subjects, as a function of the duration of the preparatory interval, in an experiment in which preparatory intervals of 3, 4 or 5 seconds were used in prearranged apparently haphazard sequence. Thirty-six trials were given at each preparatory interval. The solid line shows the function for subjects showing less than the median cardiac deceleration for the group; the broken line is for subjects whose cardiac deceleration was above the median. Results are shown separately for the first 54 trials (WORK 1), the second 54 trials (WORK 2) and all trials (WORK ALL).

celeration the faster the reaction time and the less drastically is the reaction time modified by the duration of the preparatory interval. Statistical analyses show that both parts of this statement are based on significant differences. The fact that reaction time is faster the greater the cardiac deceleration was found also in the fixed foreperiod experiments earlier described. The correlation is not very high: it seems to vary around an average of .30 to .40. It is the *direction* of the relationship that is so theoretically meaningful: cardiac deceleration is related to quicker reaction time was predictable with some degree of certainty from considerations of visceral afferent feedback; clearly, however, the opposite effect would be predicted by traditional "arousal" theory.

Let us now turn to the preceding foreperiod effect. Reaction time is a function both of the foreperiod on the Nth trial—the just described current foreperiod effect—and of the foreperiod on the (N–1)th trial or, more accurately stated, of the relationship between the two foreperiods. If one takes all trials with a foreperiod of a given duration and classifies them according to the foreperiod used on the previous trial, one generates groups of paired trials. One now finds that for a given foreperiod duration, reaction time is slowed if the preceding foreperiod was longer than the current one and quickened if the preceding foreperiod was shorter than the current one. In a single phrase, reaction time is a monotonically increasing function of the foreperiod used on the preceding trial. Short preceding foreperiods accelerate the temporal growth of readiness-to-respond on the next trial; long preceding foreperiods slow down the growth of response-readiness. The subject seems to adjust his notion of the "average foreperiod," at which he strives to be optimally ready to respond, on the basis of the foreperiod of the just-completed trial. Does the magnitude of cardiac deceleration relate to this effect? The answer to this question is shown in Figure 11–11, for the two subgroups of subjects previously described. The above-average decelerators, shown by the broken line, again are seen to be more rapid in their responses and are *significantly less prone to the preceding foreperiod effect.* The correlation of deceleration with the preceding foreperiod effect was —.50, significant at better than the 0.1 percent level. Cardiac deceleration seems to be correlated with a more stable, more rapid, less easily influenced, temporal growth of response-readiness during the foreperiod interval. Those who decelerate more are primed to act rapidly to simple afferent stimuli.

Now let us turn to the relationship of cardiac deceleration to electroencephalographic events. In our most recent experiment, we recorded DC potentials from vertex to mastoid to measure the now-familiar Expectancy Wave or Contingent Negative Variation first reported by Gray Walter and his colleagues.[11] The subjects executed a simple visual reaction-time experiment with fixed foreperiods of four seconds. The foreperiod timing did not begin until the subject had his eyes fixated on the locus of the imperative stimulus and was ready to inhibit blinks for the duration of the trial; he signalled his readiness to begin the trial by depressing a telegraph key. The response to the imperative stimulus was release of the key. Each subject received forty-five trials. Trials were segregated into those in which the subject had shown minimum cardiac deceleration (lower third of the individual's distribution of decelerations) in anticipation of the imperative stimulus and those in which he demonstrated maximum

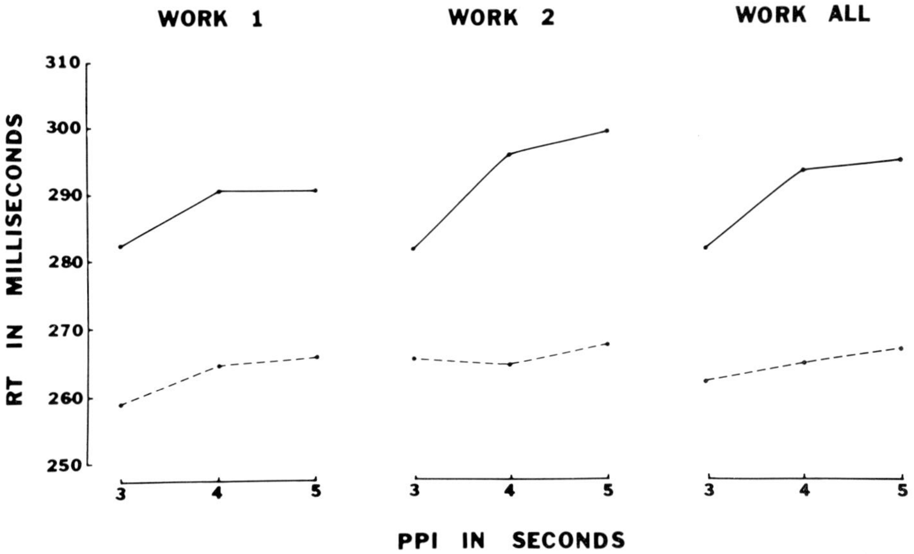

Figure 11–11. Average curves of reaction time as a function of the duration of the preceding preparatory interval (PPI) and the median magnitude of the cardiac deceleration during the preparatory interval. The solid line is for subjects whose median cardiac deceleration was below the overall group median; the dotted line is for subjects with greater cardiac decelerations. See text and legend for Figure 11–10 for experimental details. (From Lacey, J. I., and Lacey, B. C.: In Kimble, D. P. (Ed.): *Readiness to Remember.* New York, Gordon & Breach, 1969, Vol. 2, p. 583.)

deceleration (upper third). The EEGs for these groups of trials were averaged separately by a Computer of Average Transients (Model 400B), digitized and then reanalyzed by an IBM 360/44 digital computer which regrouped the scalp potentials by half-second intervals and provided average group curves. The results are shown in Figure 11–12. The solid lines show results for those trials in which there was minimal cardiac deceleration and the broken lines for trials with maximal cardiac decelerations. Results are shown separately for the first and second halves of the experiment. The base line or reference level from which measurements were made was taken as the level of the potential after the response evoked by the ready signal and key press were over; this level was commonly much more negative than the base level existing before the ready signal. As you can see in the figure, if the subject is engaged in trials in which he minimally decelerates (solid line), there is an increasing positivity of the vertex in the early part of the foreperiod, followed by a weak shift towards greater negativity at the end of the foreperiod. If, on the other hand, the subject is executing trials in which he shows large anticipatory decelerations, there is an early termination of the positive limb, followed by a marked increase in vertex negativity. The relationship between the magnitude of cardiac deceleration and the magnitude of increased vertex negativity was statistically significant.

Let me now turn to the final topic of this chapter.

It is clear to us, as it must be to you, that the phenomena we have reported so far are only suggestive parallels with the neurophysiological fact that the cardiovascular system has controlling effects on brain function which are mediated by visceral afferent feedback mechanisms. Parallels based on far-from-perfect correlations, however, are not proof. We are attempting to provide proof by chronic experiments in cats. We hope to be able to demonstrate, in the cat, the same kind of correlation between cardiac function and behavior that we have demonstrated in man and then to augment and diminish that correlation by suitable experimental manipulations.

As a first step, Dr. Galin and I pursued reaction-time experiments with five cats

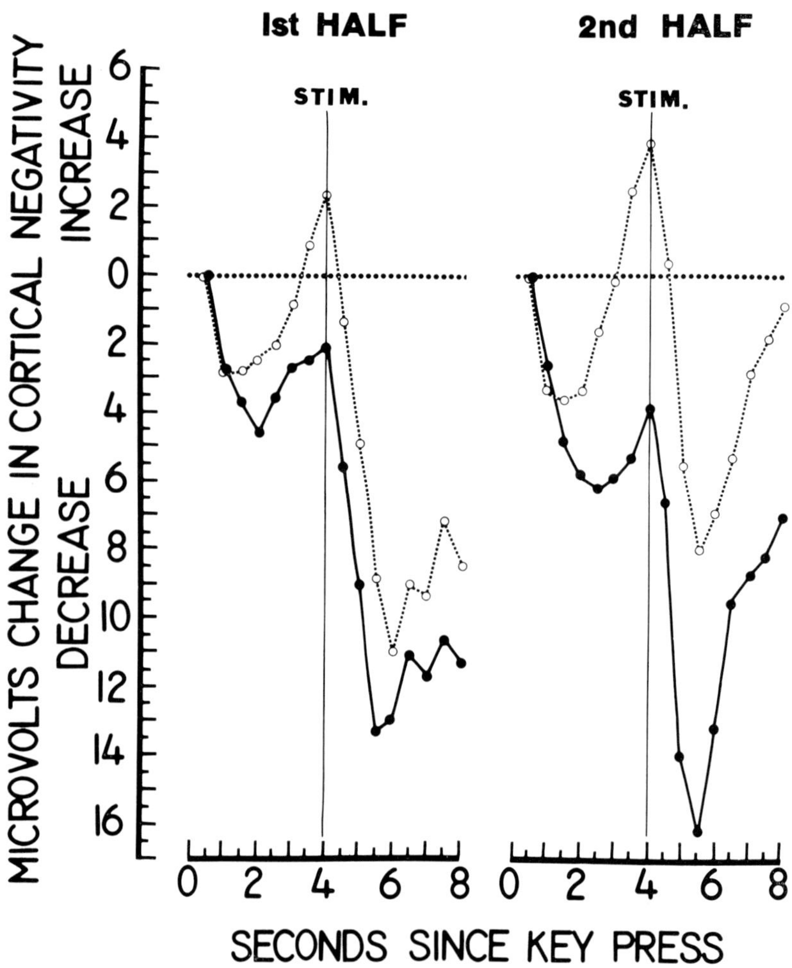

Figure 11–12. Average group curves (N = 22) showing changes in vertex negativity by half-second intervals during a 4-second foreperiod that was initiated by a key press as a function of the magnitude of cardiac decelerations and of whether the data were from the first half or the second half of the experiment. There were 56 trials in each half of the experiment. The solid line shows results for the trials in which there was minimal cardiac deceleration (lower third of distribution for the individual subject) and the broken line shows results for trials with maximal cardiac deceleration (upper third of distribution). (From Lacey, J. I., and Lacey, B. C.: In Black, P. (Ed.): *Physiological Correlates of Emotion.* New York, Academic Press, 1970, p. 221.)

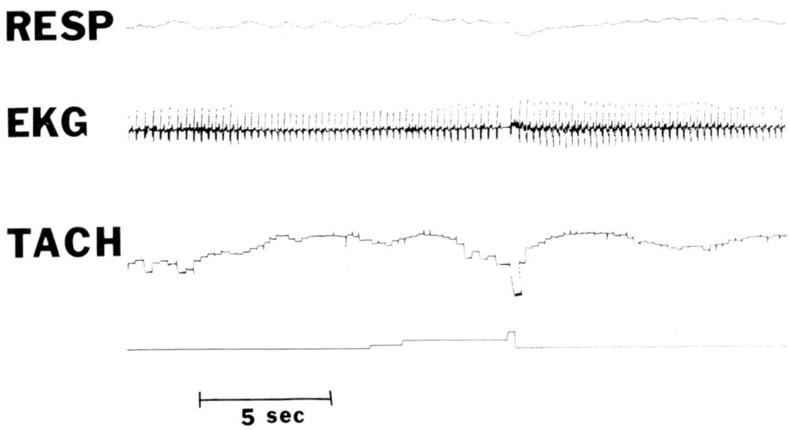

Figure 11–13. Extract of recording of respiratory and cardiac changes in a cat performing a simple auditory reaction time experiment with a fixed 4-second preparatory interval. "RESP" shows respiration recorded via implanted electrodes; "EKG" shows the electrocardiogram picked up from implanted electrodes; "TACH" is the cardiotachometric record derived on-line from the EKG. The heart rate change is from 360 beats per minute at the top of the "TACH" tracing to 120 beats per minute at the bottom. The bottom channel is the event marker (see text).

chronically implanted with electrodes for the recording of heart rate, respiration and electroencephalograms and for the stimulation of the mesencephalic reticular substance. Our first questions were (a) do cats, like humans, show cardiac deceleration during the preparatory interval in a reaction-time experiment and (b) is the magnitude of deceleration accompanied by speedier reaction time in cats as it is in humans? The two questions are critical ones, because a positive answer is necessary if the chronic cat experiment is to be useful in providing proof or disproof of our hypotheses.

Figure 11–13 is an extract from the polygraph recording of a cat working in a simple auditory reaction-time experiment with a fixed five-second foreperiod. He has been well trained to press a bar when it is presented to him, to maintain the press until he hears a tone and to release the bar immediately upon the onset of that tone. He receives a small portion of liquified cat food upon the appropriate bar release. The cat receives his entire daily ration of food and water, day after day, in this situation. The bottom trace in Figure 11–13 is an event marker. The first small elevation begins when the bar is presented. The second elevation ensues during the bar press. The third elevation occurs at the onset of and is sustained during the tone. The tone is turned off by the bar release. As you can see, the small acceleration followed by the larger beat-by-beat deceleration that we saw in humans is also clearly seen in this cat. This massive deceleration was seen in trial after trial, day after day, for as many as fifty days. He and one other cat demonstrated this pattern; two other cats, however, showed acceleration just as consistently; and one cat was variable. This was a severe disappointment; indeed, almost a setback. We have never seen humans consistently accelerate during foreperiods. As I will show later, we have a partial explanation for this contrary finding in the cat, but only a partial one. For the moment, let us continue to describe the phenomenon of deceleration in the cats who do show it and show it with extreme consistency.

Figure 11–14 shows median heart rate response curves for successive daily sessions for a cat who was being trained to longer and longer preparatory intervals. The curve for the two-second foreperiod shows a massive deceleration time locked to the presentation of the tone ("S" in the figure, for "stimulus"). This deceleration is preceded by a small acceleration following the initial bar press ("P" in the figure). When the foreperiod was lengthened in successive sessions, to four, six and eight seconds, the major deceleration still took place in the early part of the foreperiod, but the low heart rate was sustained until the imperative stimulus. The point at which the maximal deceleration was first reached is shifted forward in time as the cat is exposed to longer foreperiods. After the cat became more experienced with fixed four-second foreperiods, the median curves showed a smooth deceleration that reached its minimum at the time of the imperative signal. It is obvious that the time course of deceleration in the cat is subject to modification by learning.

The fact that two cats showed consistent

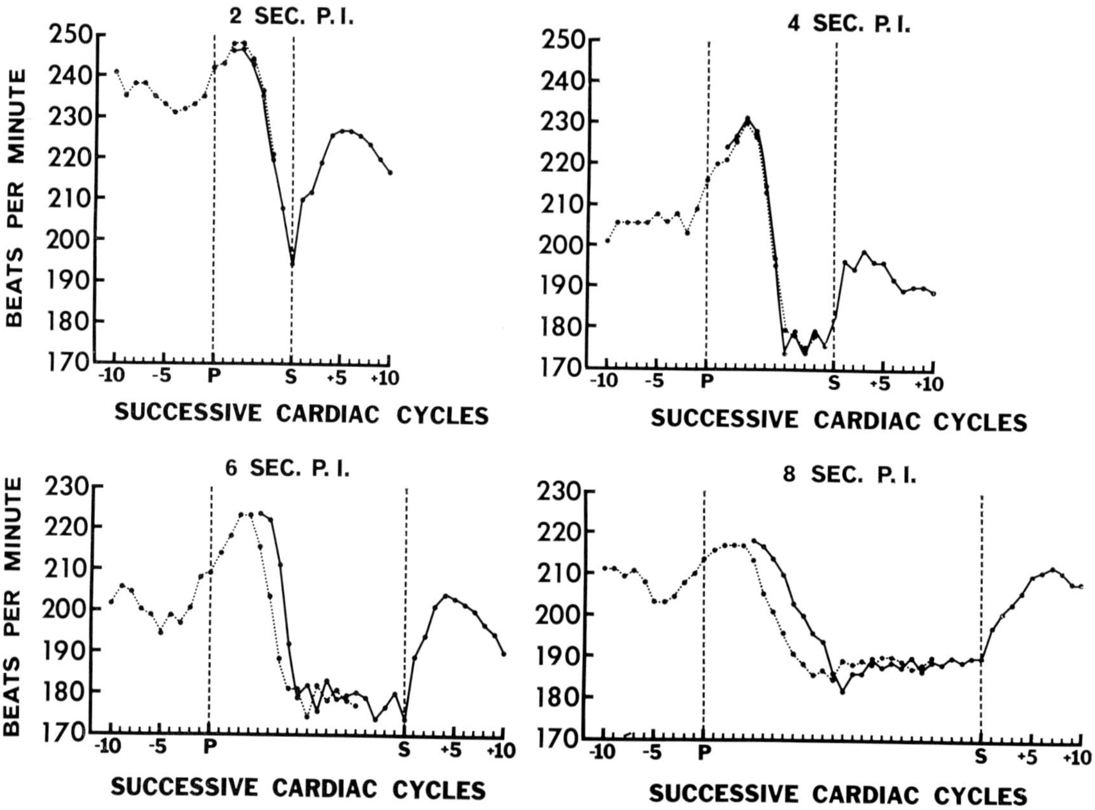

Figure 11–14. Representative median heart rate response curves for a cat being trained progressively to respond in a simple auditory reaction time experiment with longer and longer preparatory intervals. "P" is the moment the cat presses the bar after it is presented. This press initiates timing of the preparatory interval which is terminated by an auditory signal, "S." Each curve is for a single session. The curves are oriented both with respect to "S" (solid line) and with respect to "P" (broken line).

acceleration obviously is disturbing. As a practical matter, it means that the number of animals in an experiment has to be increased and that generalization of the results will be difficult. The theoretical consequences are even more serious. How can we explain the failure to decelerate during reaction-time behavior, where attention to external stimuli is so crucial to the control of behavior? Dr. Galin and I reasoned that perhaps the animals were no longer paying attention to the environment and that their behavior was routine and overly automatic. We desired, therefore, to require more consistent attention from the cats. We eliminated some extra cues in the environment, and we attenuated the imperative signal. The heart rate continued to accelerate in the foreperiod! We then suspected that these cats were timing the foreperiod and were not listening for the tone at all. We tested this by omitting the imperative stimulus entirely, and to our surprise and gratification, we found that these two cats were able to estimate the foreperiod interval well enough to produce a "pseudo-reaction time" when there was no imperative stimulus at all! Since they could rely on internal timing, the task was not requiring them to attend to environmental stimuli. In order to force the cat to attend to the imperative stimulus, we changed to a variable foreperiod program with foreperiods of three, four and five seconds. The response of the less experienced cat immediately converted to deceleration, as is shown in Figure 11–15. On the left, we have plotted the median response curve for the last session on a fixed foreperiod of four seconds. On the right we have plotted the median response curve only for trials with four-second foreperiods, administered within a prearranged haphazard order of presentation of foreperiods of three, four and five seconds. The motor performance, the high heart rate level, the conditions of deprivation of food and water, the reward contingencies—all were the same. Only the requirements for attention were increased. In accordance with our "psychophysiological prescription" we found, in

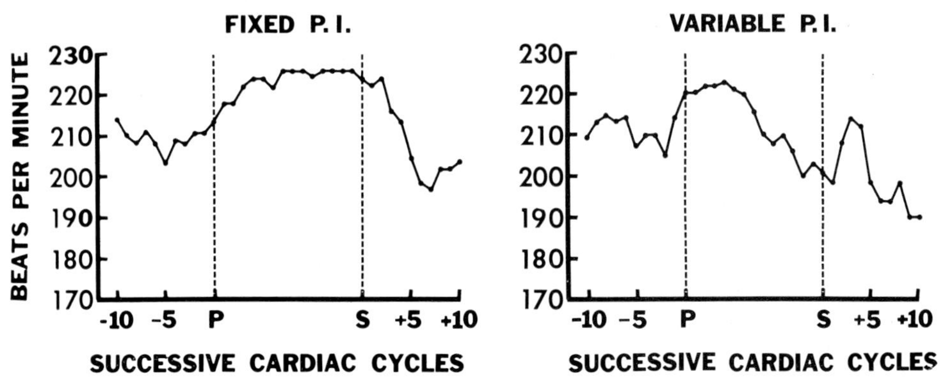

Figure 11–15. Median heart rate curves for a cat who showed only acceleration during the 4-second preparatory interval in a simple auditory reaction time experiment with a fixed 4-second preparatory interval (FIXED P.I.). Upon training on a variable foreperiod schedule, with preparatory intervals of 3, 4 and 5 seconds, the cat showed deceleration during the foreperiod (VARIABLE P.I.). The curve labeled "VARIABLE P.I." is for trials with 4-second preparatory intervals only; trials with 3- and 5-second preparatory intervals were omitted.

this rather notable way, that requiring attention to the external environment did indeed cause cardiac deceleration. Our satisfaction, however, is not complete. The more experienced cat, who had had more than one thousand reaction-time sessions over the course of several years, continued to show only acceleration during the foreperiod.

It is clear that we have a way to go before we can provide an experimental situation in which all or most cats will show deceleration. But it is equally clear that two cats showed the response and did so with great consistency and clarity. With these cats, however, we could not get a clear determination of the relationship of cardiac deceleration to reaction time. Temporal trends, even after prolonged training, still could be seen both in reaction time and heart rate. These trends were cyclic rather than linear, and the variables were not normally distributed. Statistical evaluations of the data, then, are rather complex. Much work remains to be done, but we do have modest encouragement that this experiment can be modified to provide the decisive tests we need.

In the meantime we are left, both in cat and man, with a number of psychophysiological facts that could not have been predicted from our more traditional modes of thinking about autonomic correlates of behavior, but which are congruent with the neurophysiology of the negative feedback loop from the heart to the brain.

REFERENCES

1. Baccelli, G., Guazzi, M., Libretti, A., and Zanchetti, A.: Pressoceptive and chemoceptive aortic reflexes in decorticate and in decerebrate cats. *Amer. J. Physiol., 208:*708, 1965.
2. Bartorelli, C., Bizzi, E., Libretti, A., and Zanchetti, A.: Inhibitory control of sinocarotid pressoceptive afferents on hypothalamic autonomic activity and sham rage behavior. *Arch. Ital. Biol., 98:*308, 1960.
3. Bonvallet, M., and Allen, M. B.: Prolonged spontaneous and evoked reticular activation following discrete bulbar lesions. *Electroenceph. Clin. Neurophysiol., 15:* 969, 1963.
4. Bonvallet, M., Dell, P., and Hugelin, A.: Influence de l'adrénaline sur le contrôle reticulaire des activité's corticale et spinale. *J. Physiol. (Paris), 46:*262, 1954.
5. Dell, P., Bonvallet, M., and Hugelin, A.: Tonus sympathique, adrénaline et contrôle reticulaire de la motricité spinale. *Electroenceph. Clin. Neurophysiol., 6:*599, 1954.
6. Gero, J., and Gerová, M.: The role of parameters of pulsating pressure in the stimulation of intracarotid receptors. *Arch. Int. Pharmacodyn., 140:*35, 1962.
7. Lacey, J. I., Kagan, J., Lacey, B. C., and Moss, H. A.: The visceral level: Situational determinants and behavioral correlates of autonomic response patterns. In Knapp, P. H. (Ed.): *Expression of the Emotions in Man.* New York, International Universities Press, 1963.
8. Nowlin, J. B., Eisdorfer, C., and Thompson, L. W.: Cardiovascular response during reaction time performance. In press.
9. Peterson, L. H.: The mechanical properties of the blood vessels and hypertension. In Cort, J. H., Fencl, V., Hejl, Z., and Jirka, J.: *The Pathogenesis of Essential Hypertension.* Prague, State Medical Publishing House, 1962.
10. Spickler, W. J., and Kezdi, P.: Dynamic response characteristics of the carotid sinus baroceptors. *Amer. J. Physiol., 212:*472, 1967.
11. Walter, W. G., Cooper, R., Aldridge, V. J., McCallum, W. C., and Winter, A. L.: Contingent negative variation: An electric sign of sensorimotor association and expectancy in the human brain. *Nature, 203:*380, 1964.

DISCUSSION

Dr. Lindsley: If the cat immobilizes itself, does it take a stance while it is waiting during the preparatory interval? In other words, the question I'm asking is to what extent does the behavior—that is, action versus inaction, or respiration, as the depth of it increases or decreases—affect heart rate, since we know that movement and things of that kind can affect it.

Dr. Lacey: I do not think that activity on the part of the cat will do anything except to decrease the attentional deceleration. I have never been able to convince myself that these deceleratory responses are driven by respiratory maneuvers on the part of the cat. While some responses may well be based on artifacts of respiration, this is not true for the majority of the decelerations. The mechanism by which the organism gains control of the consistent systematically recurring cardiovascular responses has to be found. I would not have been loathe to find it in the respiratory system which is under obvious voluntary control, but I cannot explain deceleration or hypotension on the basis of respiration. Nor can I explain the bradycardia as a secondary reflex slowing due to hypertension.

Dr. Abrahams: Profound slowing of the heart with a concomitant vasodilatation has been well described and is quite a common cardiovascular phenomenon. Usually, we don't see it because when people faint, their blood pressure is not normally being measured. So it's not surprising that for some strange reason, the organism can self-destruct through its built-in cardiovascular reflexes.

Dr. Lacey: Then why would the cat be responding faster? Why would the organism be in an intensely aggravated circumstance?

Dr. Abrahams: If we come back to the high resting heart rates, I should like to point out that they are quite extraordinary.

Dr. Lacey: What makes you say that they are resting heart rates?

Dr. Abrahams: All right, your control heart rates.

Dr. Lacey: The cat's heart rate is an enormously labile thing, much more labile than I had ever anticipated. I can show you cats at rest whose heart rates are 70 to 80 beats per minute.

Dr. Abrahams: If you try to work with cats in observation chambers, you will find that there are a number of animals in which you cannot provoke active muscle vasodilation, and you find that they don't show it because they've already got it. If you give them atropine, you can bring their resting blood flow right down. There is a population of cats whose cardiovascular responses indicate that the experiment creates a grossly abnormal situation.

Dr. Lacey: Oh, I'm sure it's not a grossly abnormal situation. It is just a situation that you haven't observed. The answer must be that we don't yet understand in detail the mechanisms involved in these responses, as I said before.

Dr. Lindsley: I think I can make a point on that if I understood your question. Some years ago, when we were studying audiogenic seizures in rats and recording heart rate, we turned on a high-pitched tone which often produced seizures. The seizure rats tended to remain immobile; but if a rat had a high heart rate, something around 300 to 400 as opposed to another rat that had a heart rate of around 200, we could predict that the heart rate would go up in the one that had the low rate and would come down, that is do the opposite thing, when the heart rate was high. Is that the kind of question that you are raising?

Dr. Lacey: Yes, I think it is. I can answer the question empirically. I have written quite a bit about the so-called law of initial values, as you may know, Don, and we are not insensitive to the problem in the laboratory. The data were scrutinized to find out whether indeed there was any relationship between the magnitude of the cardiac deceleration and the initial level from which this response started. Those initial levels, incidentally, just wander all over the place, from day to day and from cat to cat. We have had thirteen cats under this regime. Correction for base levels does not modify the basic conclusion that the cat, like man, shows cardiac deceleration in the foreperiod of a reaction-time experiment.

Dr. Abrahams: If there is such a wandering heart rate, how can you not propose a theory in which you say that heart rate is important to the cat? The heart rate is very labile, and yet you are saying that in some way the heart rate has some effect on the levels of attention and other behavioral functions.

Dr. Lacey: Well, that is a good question. A distinction has to be made, and this will lead us along a somewhat different path between phasic responses and the tonic levels of activity. You will notice that I have been describing phasically elicited responses. When my colleagues and I were studying the effects of septal stimulation and posterior hypothalamic stimulation on heart rate in rats, we had to distinguish sharply between the phasic effects of septal stimulation, let us say, and the tonic effects. They were quite distinguishable.

Dr. Gloor: I think that the notion of the feedback loop going out of the brain and back into it again is an extremely fascinating and tempting one. I think that there is one important question that remains to be answered, and that is the possibility that the blood pressure and heart rate changes could co-vary with the reaction times and not really be a part of the loop.

Dr. Lacey: Absolutely.

Dr. Gloor: Have you contemplated doing the following experiment? For instance, stimulating cardiac accelerator nerves in an attempt to see whether in doing so you can improve the performance or impair the performance, or conversely, by stimulating the vagus to see whether the reaction time decreases?

Dr. Lacey: This is why we are conducting experiments both with man and with the cat. In experiments with man, we have no evidence that the visceral afferent feedback pathway that we're talking about is operative. All we have is a suggestive parallel between acute neurophysiology and human psychophysiology. Our program was to find out, first of all, if the cat had the same behavioral responses as the human, then to find out if the cat had the same cardiac responses as the human and then to establish whether cats, like humans, showed faster reactions when their heart rate slowed more. We did indeed find that cats show both current and preceding foreperiod effects on reaction time and that cats show cardiac deceleration. In moving to such a direct test as you propose, Dr. Gloor, we were specifically thinking of thoracic vagal implants for the stimulation, not the reticular formation. The reticular formation was easier to approach for a first look. Now, as I mentioned, this experiment is a partial success and a partial failure. The failure to get an unambiguous correlation in the cat between the reaction-time and cardiovascular responses is a serious one. We must clear this up before resuming stimulation experiments. To date, I repeat, all we have are suggestive parallels.

Dr. MacLean: I was trying to say, John, that with the classical Bechtervian trace-conditioning in the cat, one will get consistently a 15% drop in heart rate. Sound the tone, wait fifteen seconds before applying the shock, and you will get this slowing of the heart rate. This will develop within forty trials, but with four hundred trials, the animal never learns to anticipate and lift the leg. Working with McLennan in 1954, we showed that bilateral propagating hippocampal seizures abolished the slowing of the heart rate. We tried to do these experiments with the monkey in the same experimental situation. The heart rate went up to 190 after the first shock and never came down during the rest of the morning, so we gave up on the monkey.

Dr. Lacey: The use of shock disturbs me.

Dr. MacLean: We have to anticipate a lot of shock in this world!

Dr. Lacey: On no, I don't mean on humane grounds. I am simply looking at it on psychological grounds. We really know very little about the effective parameters of shock in the human work, for example.

Dr. Wolf: John, would you care to speculate on the possibility that intention tremor is connected with cardiovascular phenomena in some fashion—that there may be a relationship with that foreperiod. Do you have any evidence on this in your human experiments?

Dr. Lacey: I know that there are reports that in the early stages of essential hypertension, the labile stage, there are all sorts of interferences with motor performance which disappear, incidentally, when the hypertension becomes stabilized. No, I haven't thought at all about intention tremors, nor can I summon up anything particularly rational to say about it.

Dr. Abrahams: I just wondered if there was anything in the physiological or chemical literature about the long-term experiments with lesions in these areas. Is there any clinical evidence which would relate these two findings?

Dr. Lacey: There is the evidence I quoted, not on lesions but on the labile phase of hypertension.

Dr. Hugelin: In your experiments on men, did you pay attention to the initial values of your parameters?

Dr. Lacey: The so-called law of initial values, as I have said, is not a law at all. If it is a law, there are as many exceptions to it as there are conforming examples. One should always look at the data, however, and if there are strong dependencies of the response upon the level, then one should correct them. I remember in my early work, on the cold-pressor responses, in particular, there were tremendous dependencies there and they had to be taken into account. In the reaction-time experiments, we find only small correlations between initial level and response.

Dr. Dell: I want to make a comment regarding the question that was asked of you. It is possible to make lesions, viable lesions, 1 mm anterior to the obex in the nucleus of the tractus solitarius, and the cat survives very well. Mlle. Bonvallet has such cats, but I don't believe that she has made those particular observations.

Dr. Lacey: Bonvallet's results were as follows: she made bilateral lesions and reported that informal observations revealed no differences between these cats' behavior and the behavior of nonlesioned cats. She put them on the table and found they behaved just the way they should in terms of input stimuli.

Dr. Marczynski: In connection with the very interesting data presented by Dr. Lacey, I would like to mention that the deceleration of the heart rate observed by Dr. Lacey may be interpreted as one of many possible correlates of an active process of Pavlovian internal inhibition. During the last twenty years, a vast electrophysiological and behavioral evidence has accumulated (in the laboratories of Doctors Dell, Hernandez-Peon, Konorski, Clemente, Sterman, Sawyer, Roitbak, Kogan, John, Gluck and Rowland, and others), which shows that peripheral and/or internal arousing stimuli (associated with either innate or learned goal-oriented behavior) or central electrical stimuli delivered to the brain stem reticular activating system, set in motion homeostatic mechanisms which activate neuronal substrates responsible for inhibition and termination of an internal excitatory state. Thus, such things as a monotonous presentation of a sensory stimulus, the withholding of an aversive stimulus, the extinction of a conditional response and the presentation of a negative conditional stimulus that requires inhibition of a certain behavioral response may all unmask or trigger the EEG synchronizing influences associated with active internal inhibitory processes. In an alert and highly motivated subject, the synchronizing influences may suddenly override the internal excitatory and desynchronizing ones and may manifest themselves in a sudden burst of EEG synchronization, changes of the monosynaptic and polysynaptic spinal cord reflexes or in a sudden shift in the tonus of the parasympathetic division of the autonomic nervous system that regulates the heart rate and blood pressure. In cats, trained to press a lever for milk reward, Clemente, Sterman and Wyrwicka (1964) have described dramatic shifts in the EEG patterns. During nonrewarded and prior to the rewarded lever press, a desynchronized EEG pattern was observed, but as soon as the bar press resulted in delivery of reward and the subject had to stop bar pressing in order to consume the reward, a burst of high-voltage slow wave activity of 5 to 8 cps was observed over the parieto-occipital cortex. These bursts of alpha activity, termed "postreinforcement synchronization," has been interpreted as transient but powerful inhibition of the brain stem activating system. Subsequent studies of patterns of cortical evoked potentials, selectively recorded during nonrewarded lever pressing performance or during bursts of postreinforcement synchronization (and the comparison of the latter with those recorded during sleep onset), strongly support the contention (Marczynski *et al.* 1968; 1969; Hackett and Marczynski, 1969). In your cat preparation in which you have observed phasic deceleration of the heart rate, it might be very interesting to see whether there is any correlation between the degree of deceleration and the duration and amplitude of alpha bursts over the parieto-occipital cortex, if the electrode arrangement in your preparation makes such recording possible, for example, over the posterior marginal gyrus where the amplitude of the postreinforcement synchronization is usually very large (up to 200μV), measured peak to peak in epidural recording.

Dr. Lacey: Yes, we have epidural leads implanted in the cats. We have not looked hard at it yet, but that is one of the things that we must analyze.

Dr. Marczynski: It might also be interesting to see whether there is any correlation between the deceleration of the heart rate and the epicortical steady potential shifts, since the latter seem to be an extremely sensitive index of internal excitatory state and inhibitory processes. We have observed dramatic epicortical steady potential shifts in the cat during lever pressing performance for 1 cc of milk rewards.

Dr. Lacey: There were negative shifts?

Dr. Marczynski: Yes, there were very marked sustained negative shifts during nonrewarded and prior to the rewarded bar press, but what is more interesting with regard to your observation is that after the presentation of milk reward, there was always an abrupt positive steady potential shift of 250μV to 400μV associated with alpha bursts over the posterior marginal gyrus, recorded with respect to a distant ectosylvian gyrus or subjacent white matter (the latter electrode arrangement excluded the possibility of the contamination of the epicortical steady potential shift by the strong corneoretinal potential field associated with eye movements). The occurrence of the positive shift after each reward depended on the taste and appropriateness of reward, since it could be abolished simply by the substitution of milk for water. Therefore, we have termed this shift "reward-contingent positive variation" (Marczynski *et al.* 1969). Interestingly enough, the topographical distribution of the "reward-contingent positive variation" was indistinguishable from phasic steady potential shifts observed in the same subject during grooming or sleep onset. Furthermore, this localized bilateral positive shift over the posterior marginal gyri disappeared as soon as delta wave sleep patterns developed, thus suggesting an active process of internal inhibition during the onset of sleep.

Dr. Lacey: You may remember that when Dr. Smythe spoke yesterday, he showed the effect of infused adrenaline on blood pressure and electroencephalographic activity—the EEG behaved just the way it should. Darrow, years and years ago, showed that in stimulating human subjects, the greater the increase in blood pressure and heart rate, the shorter the duration of alpha block.

Chapter 12

Bodily Changes During Arousal, Attention and Emotion

ANDRE HUGELIN

THIS PRESENTATION will deal with the neurophysiological problem of stereotype and nonstereotype in bodily changes during arousal, attention and emotion. First of all, I am going to explain the stereotype and nonstereotype of reticular responses, pass on to review a limbic component of arousal and then discuss results obtained in man.

After the discovery of the activating influence of the reticular formation, it became obvious that reticular discharge simultaneously produces motor modifications, autonomic effects and EEG arousal. I had not intended to give further consideration to this point, and I will simply present two figures both showing an arousal reaction, one obtained from a cat

Note: Preparation of this chapter and the reported research originating in the Department of Physiology, Faculté de Médecine, Saint-Antoine, Paris, has been supported by the Centre National de la Recherche Scientifique (LA-38), by the Institut National de la Santé et de la Recherche Médicale (66–014), by the Délégation Générale a la Recherche Scientifique et Technique (66–00431) and by the Direction des Recherches et Moyens d'Essai (535–68).

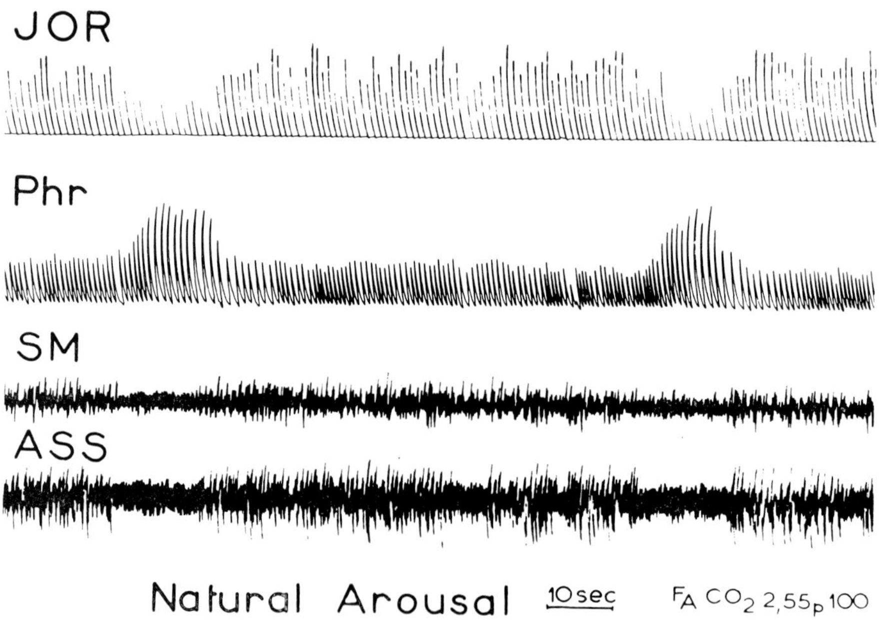

Figure 12–1. Arousal due to natural stimulation in the cat. Encéphale isolé preparation. Explanations in text. (Hugelin and Cohen, unpublished observation.)

and the other from a charming young lady.

The first figure shows the cat's arousal (Fig. 12–1). The upper trace shows a polysynaptic reflex (the jaw opening reflex) produced by stimulation of the lingual nerve; the second trace is the integrated phrenic discharge; and the last two traces are electrocorticographic records from the sensorimotor and associative cortex, respectively. From the resting state, the cat was aroused by series of claps which produced simultaneously EEG desynchronization, an increase in respiratory activity and an inhibition of the jaw opening reflex. These changes are repeatedly induced by electrical stimulation of the reticular formation, and also by natural stimulation that produces arousal and behavioral alertness.

The same kind of effect is observed in man during arousal. In the experiment illustrated in the second figure (Fig. 12–2), the subject was submitted to a vigilance test. The task was to detect, twenty-four times in an hour, a random slight increase in the loudness of a 1000 Hz pure tone. The polygraphic record shows from top to bottom, the cardiotachogram, the pneumotachogram, the capnigram, the spirogram, the electrodermogram and three leads from the EEG. On hearing the change in tone (S of the fifth trace), the subject was instructed to press a key (R on the bottom trace). At the beginning of the record, the subject was drowsy as shown by the disappearance of alpha waves and the appearance of theta waves. On presentation of the signal, the subject awakens, as shown by the reappearance of the alpha waves, and then a complete desynchronization follows. At the same time, an increase in heart rate and respiratory activity is observed, as well as a psy-

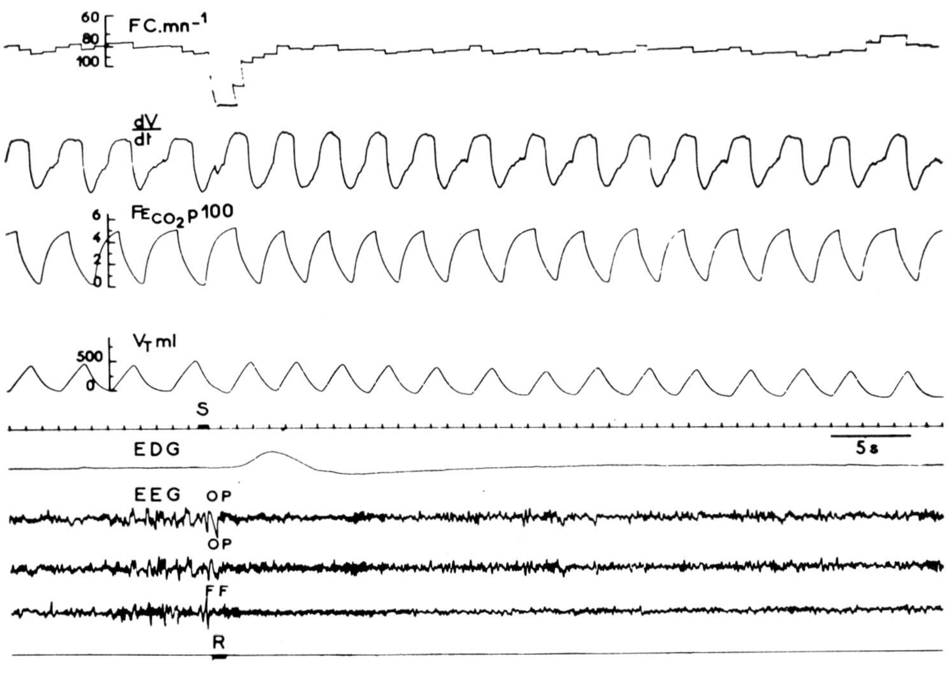

Figure 12–2. Arousal in man during a vigilance test. (Explanation in text.)

chogalvanic response. In this situation also, these multiple changes can be repeatedly induced by attention and alertness.

These two figures show examples of a general activation reaction, the characteristics of which are the simultaneousness and stereotype of the effects. It is perhaps not necessary to add that there is general agreement upon the reticular origin of this response, since it is the same as that observed when the reticular formation is stimulated in lightly anesthetized animals.

AROUSAL IN ANIMALS

In some cases, for example, those reported by Dr. Lacey,[21,22] such stereotype was not observed in man during arousal, attention or emotion. I will show that such variations also occur in animals, even during reticular stimulation, and I would like to propose several neurophysiological explanations of these phenomena: (a) they could be due to differentiation in the reticular efferent discharges resulting from the processing of the information by reticular neurons; (b) they could be the result of changes in the processing of information at the spinal level due to the reticular discharge itself; (c) they could be due to the fact that the effects resulting from the reticular discharge can vary according to the physiological state of the effector; or (d) they could be due to extrareticular mechanisms which are brought into action in these circumstances, the observed effect of which is the summation of reticular and extrareticular effects.

To illustrate the first point (change in

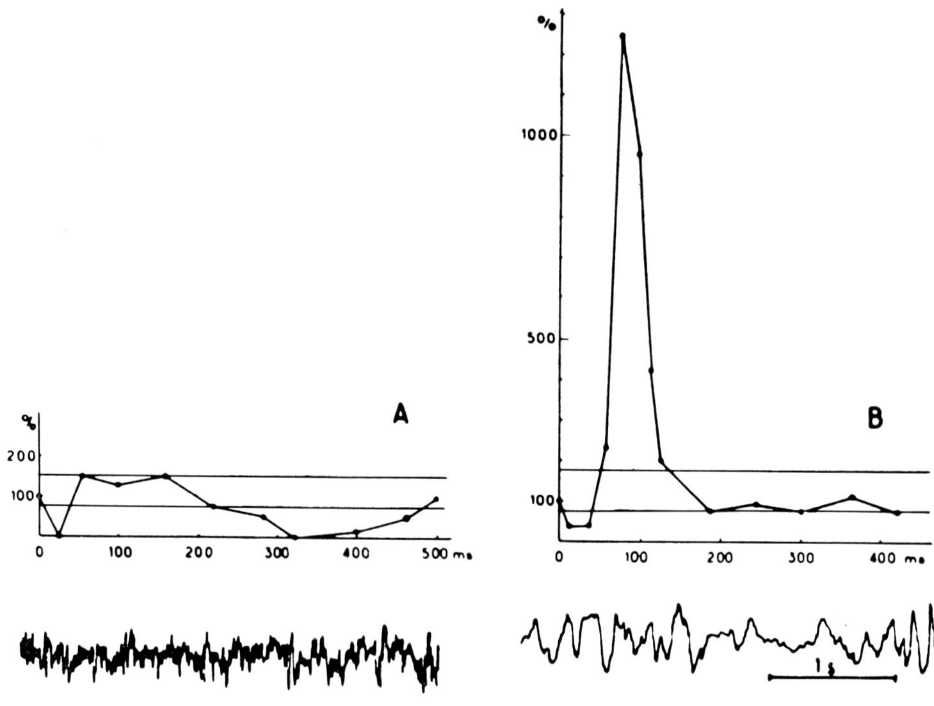

Figure 12–3. Influence of a reticulo-cortico-reticular system activity on monosynaptic reflex facilitation due to repetitive stimulation of the afferent fibers of the ulnar nerve. EEG traces under each curve were recorded before stimulation. (Explanation in text.) (From Hugelin and Bonvallet: *J. Physiol.*, (*Paris*), *50*:951, 1958.)

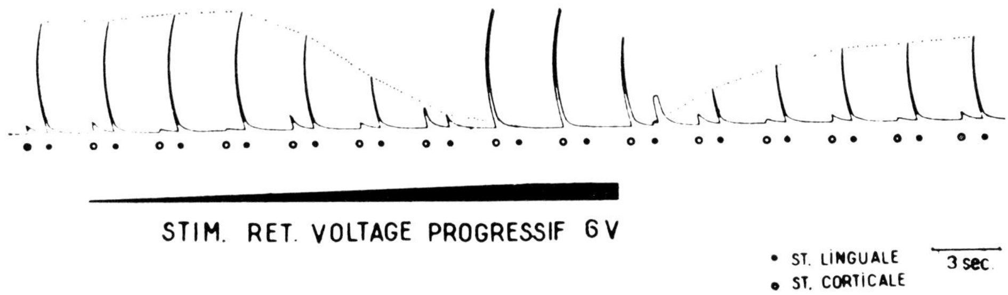

Figure 12–4. Opposite effects of repetitive reticular stimulation on cortico-motor response and on polysynaptic nociceptive reflex using the same final common path. (From Hugelin: *Arch. ital. Biol.*, *99*:244, 1961.)

the processing of information at the reticular level), I will show the influence of a reticulo-cortico-reticular feedback loop on the classical motor facilitation of reticular origin. In Figure 12–3 are shown the facilitation curves of a monosynaptic reflex, the masseteric reflex, to reticular stimulation; on the left, stimulation is given when the animal is excited, while on the right, the same animal is asleep as indicated by the EEG records.

In the first case, no facilitation is observed, while in the latter case, there is a large facilitation. The differences between the two responses are due to the action of the negative feedback loop, which does not

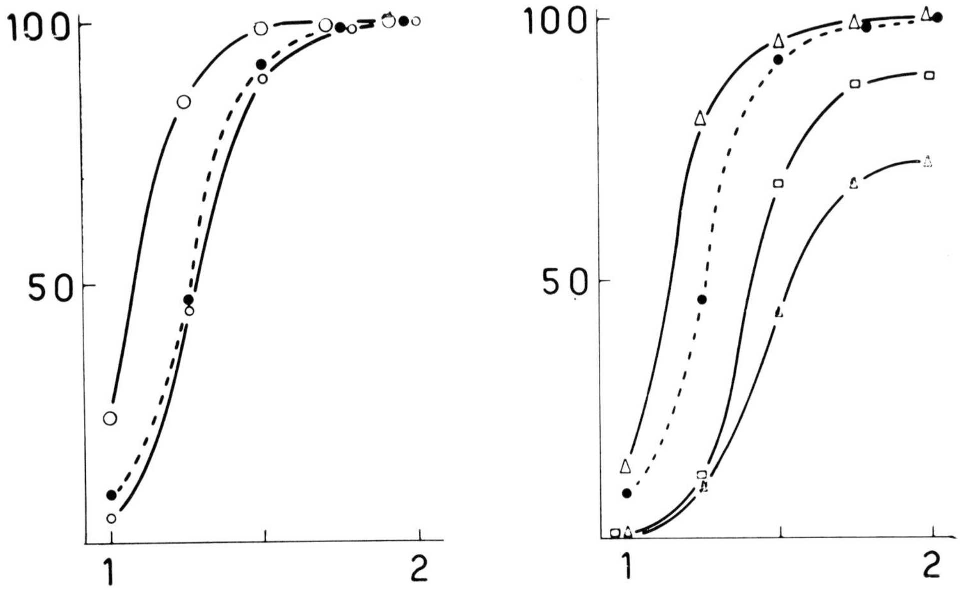

Figure 12–5. Reversal of reticular effect on the monosynaptic masseteric reflex in relation to both reticular stimulation intensity and motoneuron conditioning. Each curve represents the input-output relations of the two neuron arc. (*Left*) Masseteric reflex (•); additional reticular stimulation at 3 volts (o) and 5 volts (O). (*Right*) Conditioning of the two neuron are by supratrigeminal nucleus stimulation (□); additional reticular stimulation at 3 volts (△) and 5 volts (△).

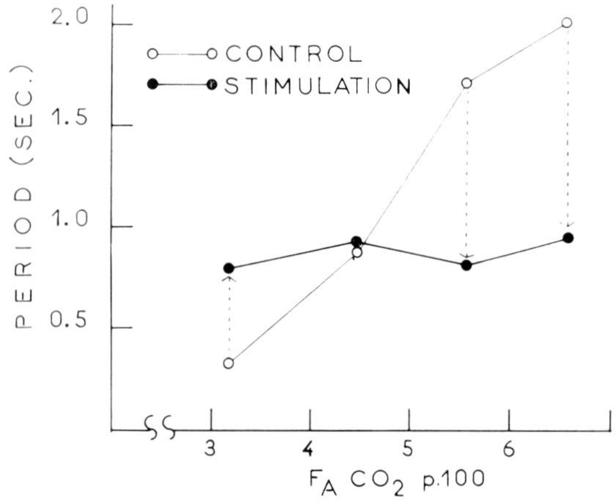

Figure 12–6. Effects of prestimulation state on the respiratory responses to reticular stimulation. (From Hugelin and Cohen, unpublished data.)

come into operation in the second case until reticular stimulation has produced cortical arousal.[17-19] In this case the cortico-reticular feedback system acts as a buffer memory, and the information obtained at the reticular output depends on the information received at the reticular input several seconds before.

I shall illustrate the second point (changes in the processing of information at the spinal level) with an example in which the motor response is facilitated or inhibited by the same reticular stimulation, according to the stimulus producing the reflex. In Figure 12–4, each vertical signal represents a contraction of the digastric muscle in response to alternative stimulation of nociceptive afferents of the lingual nerve (dots) and of the motor cortex (circles). At the beginning of the record in the resting state, the nociceptive reflex amplitude is large while the response to pyramidal stimulation is small. Repetitive reticular stimulation, delivered at a slowly increasing voltage level, produces first a decline in nociceptive response which is then followed by a marked facilitation of the corticomotor response. The decrease in the nociceptive reflex is due to afferent inhibition and the increase in corticomotor response to facilitation of motoneurons both of reticular origin. These changes in opposing directions operate a switch in the activity of the final common path.[16,19] Thus according to the input impinging on the final common path, reticular activation produces either a facilitation or an inhibition of motor activity.

The next figure illustrates the quantitative aspect of the same point. The curves in Figure 12–5 represent the input-output relation of the monosynaptic masseteric reflex in the cat. The curve with the interrupted line represents the animal at rest. Effects of reticular stimulation can be observed in the left part of the figure. A 3-volt repetitive stimulation does not modify the input-output relation, whereas a 5-volt stimulation facilitates the reflex. It can be seen that the input-output relation is nonlinear; thus, effects of reticular stimulation differ according to the magnitude of the afferent volley. Moreover, when the monosynaptic reflex is conditioned by an inhibitory influence due to excitation of the supratrigeminal nucleus, the direction of the effect resulting from reticular stimulation varies according to the current intensity. It can be seen in the right part of Figure 12–5 that a 3-volt reticular stimulation produces an inhibition of the conditioned masseteric reflex, whereas a 5-volt stimulation produces a facilitation. Here, the direction and the magnitude of changes vary as a function of both input level and reticular excitatory state.

The next figure (Fig. 12–6) illustrates the third point (change in the information processing due to altered physiological conditions). It is an example concerning the respiratory center. Experiments were done on an animal with a spinal section at

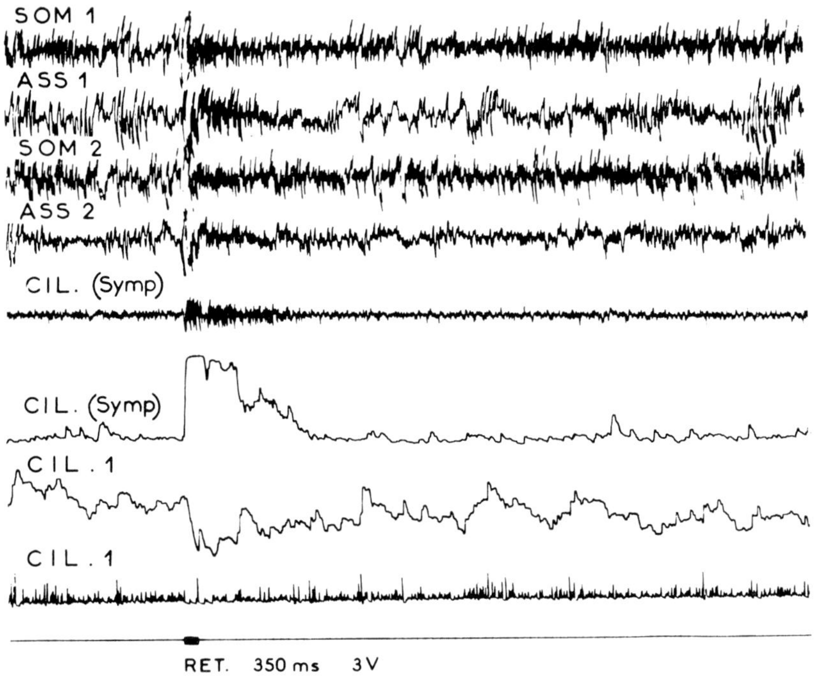

Figure 12–7. Reciprocal effects of brain stem stimulation inducing arousal on the long ciliary nerve (sympathetic) and the short ciliary nerve (parasympathetic). Direct and integrated activity of each nerve are presented. Note the decrease of parasympathetic discharge during arousal. (From Bonvallet and Voloschin: *Electroenceph. Clin. Neurophysiol., 26*:296, 1969.)

the C_1 level, under curare and after vagotomy. Phrenic nerve discharge was recorded in order to measure the respiratory period. Reticular stimulation was carried out at different levels of CO_2. It can be observed that reticular stimulation increases the respiratory period when the control value is small but decreases it when the initial value is large; it should also be noted that during reticular stimulation the absolute value of the respiratory period remains the same, even though the prestimulation state differs markedly. We know that the amplitude and period of respiration are controlled by several neuronal subsystems. It would appear that the activity of each of these subsystems depends on the physiological state and, according to the level of respiratory activity, the reticular discharge will produce an effect of one type or another.[8]

Concerning the fourth point on the nonreticular component of arousal, I would like to present results obtained recently by Miss Bonvallet's group.[6,7,12] The experiments were carried out on the ciliary nerves of the cat, in encéphale isolé preparations. Parasympathetic discharge has been compared with sympathetic and EEG activities during rest and arousal. In Figure 12–7, the vegetative discharges to pupil muscles are recorded on the lower four traces. It was shown that a stereotyped response can always be obtained during arousal produced by a brief stimulation of the mesencephalic reticular formation: the activity of the sympathetic fibers (long ciliary nerve) is always in-

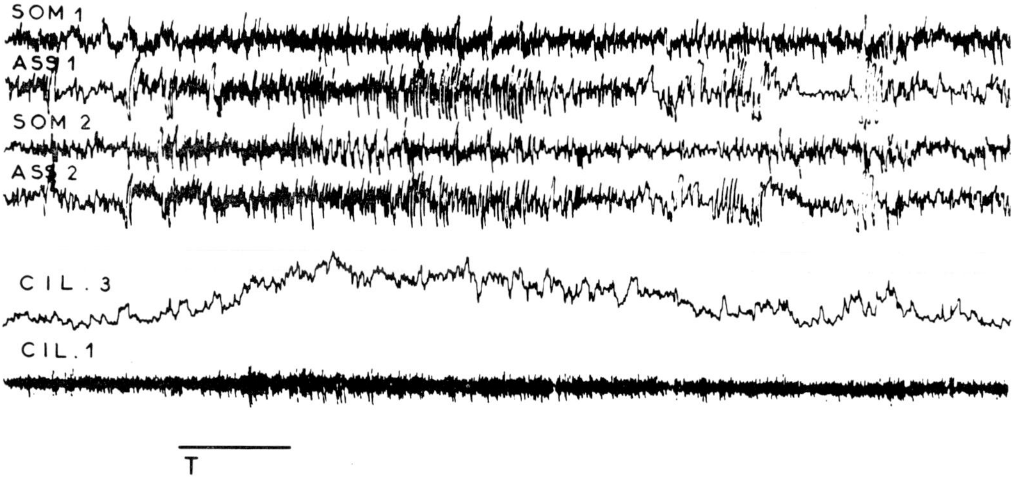

Figure 12–8. Increase in parasympathetic ciliary nerve discharge during arousal. (From Bonvallet and Voloschin: *Electroenceph. Clin. Neurophysiol., 26*:296, 1969.)

creased while an inhibition of parasympathetic discharge (short ciliary nerve) is simultaneously observed. This is a classical example of reciprocal inhibition at the autonomic level. When, however, arousal is brought about by a *natural* stimulation (Fig. 12–8), it often happens that the amplitude of parasympathetic discharges increases in contrast to that obtained by direct reticular stimulation. Observation of short ciliary nerve (SCN) discharges on a cathode-ray oscilloscope showed that an increase in amplitude corresponds to the appearance of large spikes which are known to represent the discharge of fibers to the ciliary muscles (producing accomodation to near vision) while a decrease in amplitude corresponds to the disappearance of the small spikes which are known to represent the discharge of fibers running to the constrictor muscles. The discharge of the latter fibers is tonic at rest and stops during arousal. In the series of experiments that ensued, the large spikes were sifted out by using an electronic gate and they could be analyzed separately. It was thus ascertained that the appearance of large spikes during arousal coincides precisely with a dilatation of the pupil—that is, to an inhibition of pupiloconstrictor neurons.

The next problem was to find the neural structure that receives the afferent messages and is responsible for this effect. Bonvallet and Gary Bobo [6,12] tried to reproduce the effects of natural stimuli by artificial stimulation of the brain. Stimulation of the amygdaloid complex in the region of

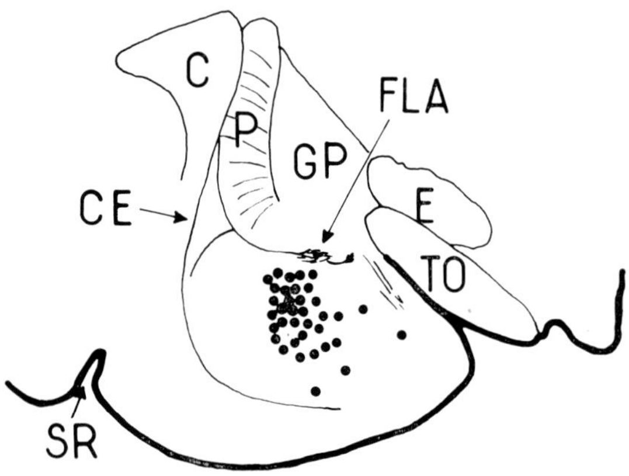

Figure 12–9. Topography of points where stimulation produces the incrementing discharge of parasympathetic fibres to ciliary muscles (accommodation to near vision). (Reprinted by courtesy of Bonvallet and Gary Bobo.)

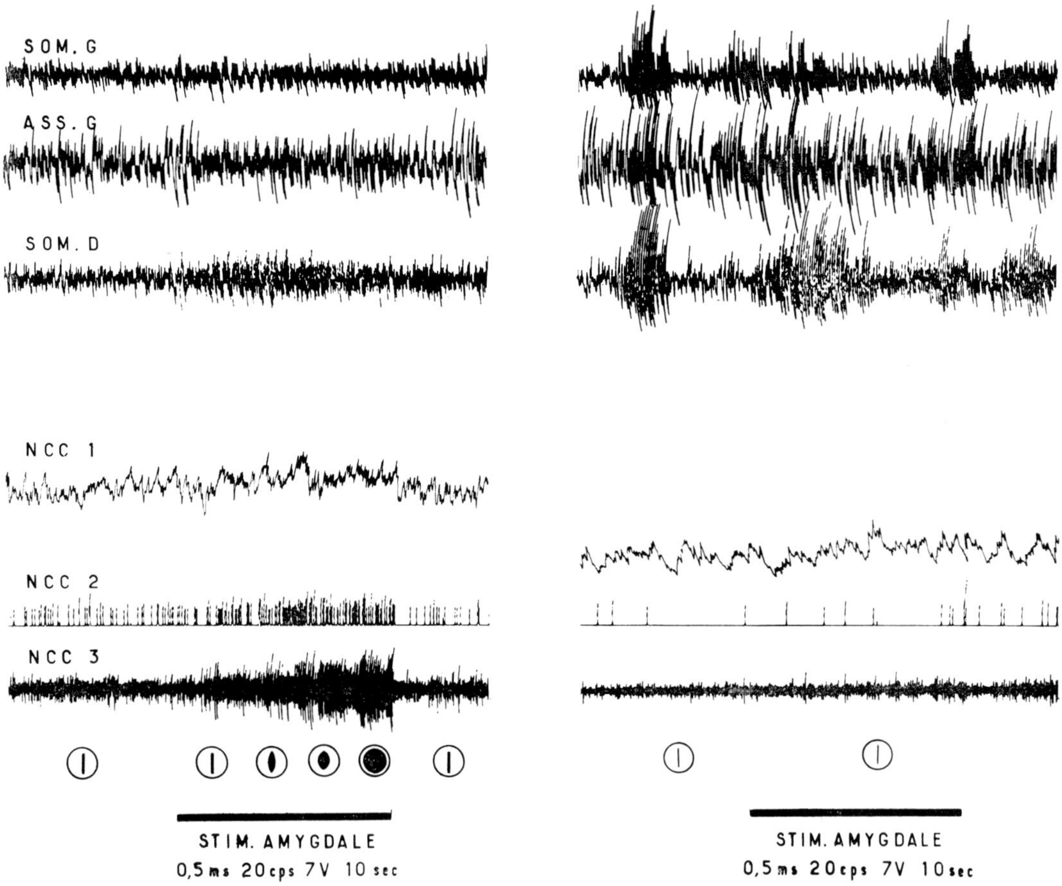

Figure 12–10. Response of fibres to the ciliary muscles according to the level of wakefulness. (Reprinted by courtesy of Bonvallet and Gary Bobo.)

the basal nucleus (or, more precisely, the magnocellular part of this nucleus) produced the same type of response (Fig. 12–9). Similar results were also obtained by stimulation of the afferent pathway to the basal nucleus (stria terminalis). The efferent system is the ventral amygdalofugal pathway (VAF) and its projection to the prerubral field where the ultimate relay to the Edinger-Westphal nucleus has been located. It should be noted that stimulation of the same area has been reported to produce strong affective responses,[10] fear, anger and autonomic effects[24] or defense reactions.[15] A characteristic of this response must be mentioned: repetitive stimulation of the amygdala with small bursts of impulses produced a progressive building up of the ciliary nerve discharge which can be called an "incrementing response."

The most important point, however, is drawn from a comparison of ciliary nerve responses to amygdala stimulation, according to the state of wakefulness as shown by the EEG record in Figure 12–10. During arousal (left record), stimulation easily produces an increase in large spike discharge, while during sleep (right record) no such response can be obtained. Moreover, if amygdala stimulation is started when the EEG record shows a state of drowsiness, the large spikes of the parasympathetic discharge only appear when an arousal reaction has been obtained. Presumably, a summation of both reticular and amygdaloid discharges is necessary before the ciliary neurons can respond. It is probable that during emotion, events similar to these also occur and, in point of fact, an arousal reaction is always associated with changes related to specific behavior.

AROUSAL IN MAN

I now come to the problem of attention in man, and I would like to describe some experiments done by Drs. Gautier, Bathien, Mrs. Bertrand and myself during the past few years. In these experiments, we investigated the effect of experimental conditions on the stereotype of somatic and autonomic responses during attention.

First of all, it must be remembered that the concept of attention covers a large field of psychological mechanisms. The many meanings of this term have recently been reviewed by Berlyne.[5] Briefly, there is general agreement in separating them into at least two behavioral classes concerning the intensive and the selective aspect, respectively. The intensive dimension of attention was first recognized by Duffy[9] and Freeman[11] and was then widely accepted.[14,22] It is generally used as a synonym for "arousal." The intensity of attention or "attentiveness" depends mainly on the flow of information being processed. Into the intensive aspect fall the channel capacity, and the equivocation and variation in the intensity of attention as a function of time.

In our experiments with Dr. Bathien,[4] we decided to investigate the effect of attention tests in which no stimulus selection was required and where the subject had to perform a task within a limited time. We used two types of attention tests called the "letter test" and the "XY plotter test." With the letter test, the letters of the alphabet were arranged at random, and the subject had to find a given sequence of three letters and count the number of times it occurred. For the XY plotter test, the subject was required to draw a circle of 15 cm in diameter by activating the two knobs of an XY plotter. Both tasks had to be performed within four minutes. The time limit insured a high flow rate of information, and both tests called for a large amount of equivocation.

The first problem was to ascertain that this type of attention test produced the same changes in man as does a reticular stimulation that, in the cat, induces a very characteristic pattern of effects on spinal reflexes. It was decided to explore human reflexes in a search for the same changes during these tests. Figure 12–11 shows records of five different reflexes from two muscles in the leg (soleus and biceps). From top to bottom are seen (a) the H reflex, (b) the soleus tendinous reflex, (c) the biceps tendinous reflex, (d) the biceps polysynaptic reflex to stimulation of group II flexor reflex afferents and (e) the biceps polysynaptic reflex to stimulation of group III flexor reflex afferents. Each trace is the average of fifty successive reflexes. On each pair, the upper trace is recorded during rest and the lower trace during the letter test. It can be observed that attention facilitates all reflexes except the nociceptive response. A statistical analysis has shown that the results are highly significant. In addition, using a battery of six different tests and a scaling

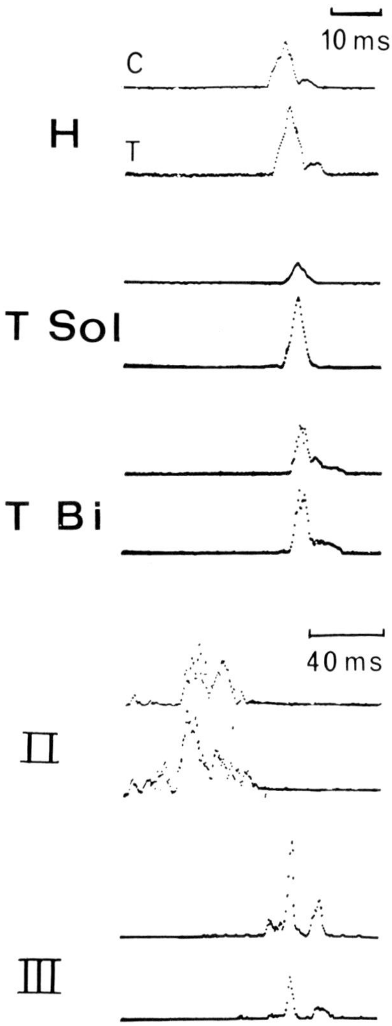

Figure 12–11. Variation in five reflex responses during attention. Each trace is the average of the negative phase of fifty consecutive responses. *Abbreviations:* C (control), T (test), H (H reflex), T sol (soleus tendon reflex), T bi (biceps tendon reflex), II (the polysynaptic reflex of the biceps to stimulation of group II afferents) and III (the nociceptive polysynaptic reflex of the biceps in response to stimulation of group III afferent fibers). (From Bathien and Hugelin: *Electroenceph. Clin. Neurophysiol.,* 26:640, 1969.)

technic, Dr. Bathien [1] concluded that tendinous reflexes (gamma motoneurons) were the most easily modified by attention, then came the polysynaptic reflexes (interneurons) and the H reflex (alpha motoneurons) had the least sensitive motor response. It should be noted that these results are exactly the same as those already dealt with in the first section of this chapter. Thus, there exists a striking likeness between what is observed during attentiveness in man and what is seen during reticular stimulation in the cat.

The second problem was to verify the stereotype of somatic, cortical, respiratory

	t_E	PE	EKG	Pente	Refl.	EDG	Tonus
AH_1	+	+	+	+	+	·	+
ST_1	+	+	+	+	+	·	+
CM_2	+	+	+	+	+	+	–
FC_1	+	+	+	+	+	·	+
AH_2	+	+	+	–	+	+	–
RC_2	+	+	–	+	+	+	–
ST_2	+	+	+	–	+	+	–
MS_1	+	+	+	+	–	·	–
CM_1	+	+	+	+	–	·	–
MS_2	+	+	–	+	–	–	–
NG_1	+	+	+	–	–	·	–
RC_1	+	+	–	–	–	·	–

Figure 12–12. Effect of attentiveness on somatic and autonomic activities. + indicates results significant at the level $P < 0.5$; – indicates nonsignificant results and absence of measurement. Note that the threshold of significant responses is reached in a set order. (From Bathien *et al.,* in preparation.)

	t_e (s)			pente ($ml.s^{-1}$)			V_T (ml BTPS)			t_i (s)			$\frac{t_i}{t_e}$		
	C	T	Δp100	C	T	Δp100	C	T	Δp100	C	T	Δp100	C	T	Δp100
ST_1	3,04	2,24	-26	227	253	+11	534	293	-45	2,35	1,16	-51	0,721	0,533	-26
	73	101	.001	72	95	.001	74	99	.001	74	99	.001	73	99	.001
CM_2	2,59	1,92	-26	286	386	+35	515	464	-10	1,80	1,20	-33	0,700	0,625	-11
	59	111	.001	61	114	.001	61	114	.001	61	114	.001	59	111	.05
AH_1	2,71	2,04	-25	256	307	+20	472	376	-20	1,84	1,22	-24	0,591	0,601	+2
	71	134	.001	76	134	.001	77	134	.001	77	134	.001	71	134	NS
RC_2	2,89	2,37	-18	277	296	+7	423	389	-8	1,53	1,32	-14	0,533	0,565	+6
	118	75	.001	123	75	.001	123	75	.001	123	75	.01	118	75	NS
MS_2	2,41	2,21	-8	269	284	+6	402	387	-4	1,50	1,36	-10	0,623	0,616	-1
	67	80	.001	65	77	.001	65	77	.001	65	77	NS	65	77	NS
FC_1	3,68	2,61	-29	259	327	+26	556	510	-8	2,14	1,56	-27	0,582	0,598	+3
	50	72	.001	51	69	.001	51	71	.01	51	71	NS	50	71	NS
MS_1	2,83	1,96	-30	319	358	+12	470	458	-3	1,47	1,28	-13	0,522	0,659	+26
	84	111	.001	87	111	.001	87	115	NS	87	115	.01	84	111	.02
CM_1	2,84	1,95	-31	307	411	+34	510	510	0	1,66	1,24	-25	0,693	0,638	-8
	70	53	.001	66	69	.001	69	69	NS	69	69	.01	69	53	NS
ST_2	2,09	1,37	-34	245	250	+2	389	276	-29	1,59	1,10	-31	0,755	0,815	+8
	87	154	.001	85	148	NS	85	150	.001	85	.150	.02	85	150	NS
AH_2	2,60	2,26	-13	206	212	+3	327	318	-3	1,59	1,50	-6	0,610	0,663	+9
	86	114	.001	82	100	.05	82	100	NS	82	100	NS	82	100	.01
RC_1	2,43	2,07	-15	290	299	+3	350	330	-6	1,20	1,10	-8	0,497	0,532	+7
	75	102	.001	80	101	NS	81	102	.05	81	102	.05	75	102	NS
NG_1	2,10	1,90	-10	277	282	+2	413	415	0	1,49	1,47	-1	0,707	0,770	+9
	83	84	.001	88	83	NS	88	85	NS	88	85	NS	83	84	NS

Figure 12–13. Effects of attentiveness of five respiratory parameters. *Abbreviations:* te (expiratory duration), pente (mean slope), V_T (tidal volume) and t_i (inspiration duration). The mean values are indicated in each case during control (C) and test (T) as well as △ p. 100 (in large characters) and their level of significance. (From Bathien *et al.*, in preparation.)

and autonomic responses during attentiveness. We performed a series of experiments on seven subjects using the letter test [2] and the XY plotter test.[1] We measured (a) the expiratory duration, (b) the peak-to-peak amplitude of an averaged somesthesic evoked potential, (c) the cardiac period, (d) the mean slope of the spirogram during inspiration, (e) the surface of a polysynaptic reflex discharge, (f) the mean value of the electrodermal activity and (g) the mean value of the quadriceps integrated electromyographic record. Differences were observed according to the subject and to the type of test. As shown in Figure 12–12, however, there exists a relative stereotype in the pattern of responses. In this table, crosses represent significant changes at the level P ≤ .05. It can be seen that positive results were obtained for the expiratory duration and the evoked potential in all cases, but muscle tone was changed in only three. The organization of the table offers the opportunity to observe a stereotype in the pattern of responses. This shows that for all subjects, changes in the parameters at the threshold level take place in a set order. In the acute cat, an identical sequence is observed during reticular stimulation.[8] The same phenomenon can be observed for several respiratory parameters. In Figure 12–13, the black line indicates the limit of results significant at the P < 0.001 level, the mean variations being indicated for each subject and for each parameter. It can be seen that according to the subjects, the extent of change is very variable for a given parameter and a given test, but for the same subject and the same parameter, the magnitude of changes varies with the test in an unpredictable way; however, the sequence in which the different thresholds are reached can always be predicted. It is likely that the internal organization of respiratory centers (and the interplay of feedback systems) is responsible for the large variation in the effects obtained.

Recently, Dr. Gautier[13] investigated the effects of arousing stimuli on respiration. He observed that stimuli such as brief tones, light flashes or tactile excitations when given during expiration produced either a lengthening or a shortening of this phase. It was then observed that the direction of the effect depended on the initial value of the respiratory period. With a high breathing rate, expiratory duration was increased, while in subjects with a

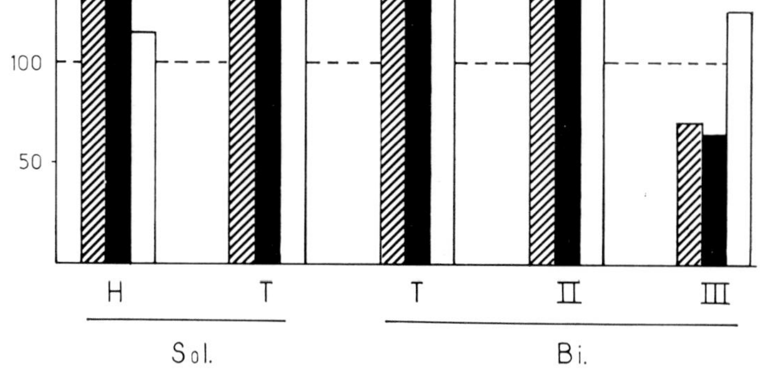

Figure 12–14. Comparison of the effects obtained on five reflex responses during the letter test (LET) and the XY plotter test (XY) and from the Jendrassik manoeuvre (JK). Abbreviations as in Figure 12–10. (From Bathien and Hugelin: *Electroenceph. Clin. Neurophysiol., 26*:604, 1969.)

low respiratory frequency, it was decreased. This observation is again very similar to that given in the first part of the chapter.

These results should be compared with those obtained in experiments where other kinds of attention have been investigated. Briefly, effects of somatic, respiratory and autonomic activities differed when dimensions other than that of intensity were explored. In Figure 12–14, for example, motor effects during the XY plotter test and the letter test are compared with those obtained during the Jendrassik test. In this latter test, the subject strongly clenches his fist and keeps it clenched for three minutes. This test is accompanied by a marked cortical arousal, but it can be seen that the intensity and/or direction of reflex changes is markedly different from that observed during the attention test.

Recently, Dr. Bathien observed the same phenomenon with selective visual attention (selection by location) which produced changes in spinal reflexes that were significantly different from those observed during the letter test and the XY plotter test.

The most likely neurophysiological explanation of the differences between attentiveness and selective attention effects is that during selection of information neural events, specific to this type of behavior, take place together with reticular discharge. According to this hypothesis, the intensive component of attention (attentiveness) coincides with a pure reticular stereotyped response, whereas other mechanisms are simultaneously brought into action in the case of selective attention.

AROUSAL AND EMOTION

During the last few years, we had the opportunity to analyze physiological changes in seven subjects during psychoanalytical investigations.[3] For each of these subjects, the appearance of an asthmatic disorder was clearly related to the development of a psychological conflict. Several records were obtained for each subject during a period of a few months up to more than a year. The H reflex, the muscle tone, EKG and the electrodermal activity were recorded, as well as the interview itself. Preliminary observations under these experimental conditions indicated very complex phenomena. The results obtained with five asthmatic subjects, using the letter test and the XY plotter test before and after psychotherapeutic interviews, were compared with those obtained with five normal subjects under the same experimental conditions. Results from normal subjects did not differ from those already obtained. On the other hand, asthmatic subjects showed a different pattern of response. On the left side of Figure 12–15 are shown results from the five normal and the five asthmatic subjects during the letter test. It can be seen that with normal subjects no change in muscle tone was observed and that the EKG frequency and the GSR were increased in three cases. For the five asthmatic subjects, muscle tone and heart rate were increased in two cases, whereas the GSR was increased in three cases and decreased in one. The fact that this change in the pattern of response was not directly related to the psychotherapeutic interview itself is demonstrated by the fact that it was still observed during special recording sessions for which the schedules did not include psychological investigations. The most

Letter Test	Ss	EKG	EDG	MTone
Normal Ss	C	+	+	0
	A	+	+	0
	S	+	+	0
	M	0	0	0
	R	0	0	0
Asthmatic Ss	F	+	+	+
	G	0	+	+
	H	0	+	+
	D	0	0	+
	B	+	−	+

Interview	Ss	EKG	EDG	MTone
Illness	F	+	+	+
	G	0	+	0
	H	0	+	+
	D	0	+	+
	B	+	0	−
Trigger	F	−	−	±
	G	0	+	+
	H	+	+	+
	D	0	+	+
	B	+	+	−

Figure 12–15. Changes in heart rate (EKG), electrodermogram (EDG) and muscle tone during attention test and during a psychotherapeutic interview. Changes significant at the level $P < 0.5$ are indicated by + for an increase and − for a decrease; O; non-significant changes. (Explanation in text.)

likely hypothesis is that this shift in the pattern of responses is due to changes in experimental conditions related either to anxiety or to a disturbance of the respiratory function.

In order to compare results of attentiveness tests with those of psychoanalytical sessions, the psychotherapist was instructed to manage the interview in such a way that each topic of conversation was maintained during periods of at least four minutes. Analysis of physiological changes were done on data recorded during sequences of 192 seconds.

Under these conditions, it has been observed that physiological changes have a much larger magnitude than those occurring in normal subjects during an ordinary conversation. Even when psychotherapy had been going on for several months, the simple sight of the psychoanalyst and an exchange of trivial remarks induced significant changes in almost all the parameters under study.

The use of scaling techniques, however, showed that certain topics produced significant variations in physiological parameters relative to both the average for the whole interview and the mean value for the previous topic discussed. These were either related to psychological conflict or could even be considered as the *primum movens* of the illness. These can be called stressful subjects of conversations and are divided into conflict-related and trigger topics.

During psychotherapeutic interviews, significant changes in a given parameter could occur in opposite directions according to the topic of the conversation. For example, with one subject, conversation concerning his mother or his wife (provoking resentment and aggressiveness) caused a decrease in heart rate, whereas when a conversation about his father (provoking fear and culpability) was begun, the opposite effect was observed. These observations are in agreement with those reported several years ago by Lacey.[21,22] If we now consider the pattern of physiological change induced by a conflict-related or a trigger topic, it can be seen that there exists a predictable pattern of responses which varies with the topic. For example, this phenomenon was repeatedly observed with one subject where asthma began at the same time as an increase in professional responsibility. Conversation about work produced a very large increase in cardiac frequency, muscle tone, the H reflex and the GSR, whereas the possibility of a change in his employment produced a sudden and marked drop in muscle tone and GSR but, on the other hand, a large increase in the H reflex and the heart rate. From the physiological point of view, it can be concluded that in the first case the sympathetic system, as well as alpha and gamma motoneurons, were facilitated and the parasympathetic cardiac system inhibited. In the second case, however, gamma motoneurons and the sympathetic system were inhibited and the alpha motoneurons were facilitated.

When all the physiological responses observed during psychotherapeutic sessions are now compared with those obtained during the attention test, it can be seen that for a given subject, the pattern of responses differs widely. For example, in Figure 12–15, responses to the attention test are different from those obtained during the interview where the topic discussed was either his own illness (B) or the trigger topic (B, F). For subject B, responses were different in every case. On the other hand, for three subjects (G, H, D), the pattern of the response, to attention tests and illness and trigger topics, probably did not differ other than in their intensity. Since EEG arousal was always observed during the entire psychoanalytical interview, it can be presumed that during emotion a variety of extrareticular mechanisms comes into play at the same time as reticular mechanisms. This leads us to conclude that these physiological changes which occur during mental activity, such as selective attention or emotion, never seem to be as simple as those observed during tests investigating the intensive dimension of attention.

SUMMARY

1. In animals, nonstereotyped somatic and autonomic responses to reticular stimulation, which are sometimes observed, can be explained by changes in experimental conditions. The nonstereotype of behavioral arousal, however, could be due to association of reticular mechanisms with extrareticular mechanisms such as those of the limbic system.

2. In man, attention tests exploring the intensive dimension of brain information processing (attentiveness) produced the

same kinds of somatic and autonomic effects as direct stimulation of the reticular formation in animals.

3. It is confirmed that in man the somatic and autonomic effects of selective attention and emotion may differ from those of attentiveness, and it is suggested that the observed differences are due to additional extrareticular mechanisms.

REFERENCES

1. Bathien, N.: Effets de tests d'attention de niveaux différents sur les réflexes spinaux de l'Homme. *J. Physiol. (Paris), 61* (suppl 1): 209, 1969.
2. Bathien, N., Bertrand, F., Gautier, H., Hugelin, A., and Vincent, J.: Sensibilité comparée de tests sensitifs, moteurs, végétatifs et respiratoires au cours de l'attention. *J. Physiol. (Paris), 59:*342, 1967.
3. Bathien, N., Bertrand, F., Hugelin, A., and Kourilsky, R.: Détection physiologique du conflit-clé au cours de séances d'investigation psychologique chez des asthmatiques. *Rev. Méd. psychosom. Psychol. méd., 2:*147, 1971.
4. Bathien, N., and Hugelin, A.: Réflexes monosynaptiques et polysynaptiques de l'homme au cours de l'attention. *Electroenceph. Clin. Neurophysiol., 26:*604, 1969.
5. Berlyne, D. E.: *Attention as a problem in behavior theory.* In D. Mostofsky (Ed.): *Attention.* New York, Appleton-Century-Crofts, 1971.
6. Bonvallet, M., and Gary Bobo, E.: Décharges des nerfs parasympathiques oculaires déclenchées à partir des corps striés, du pallidum et de l'amygdale. *J. Physiol. (Paris), 61* (suppl 1): 228, 1969.
7. Bonvallet, M., and Voloschin, L.: Niveaux d'activation et variations des décharges toniques de deux systèmes de fibres parasympathiques oculaires. *Electroenceph. Clin. Neurophysiol., 26:*296, 1969.
8. Cohen, M. I., and Hugelin, A.: Suprapontine reticular control of intrinsic respiratory mechanisms. *Arch. Ital. Biol., 103:*317, 1965.
9. Duffy, E.: *Activation and Behavior.* New York, John Wiley & Sons, 1962.
10. Fernandez de Molina, A., and Hunsperger, R. W.: Central representation of affective reactions in forebrain and brainstem: electrical stimulation of amygdala, stria terminalis and adjacent structures. *J. Physiol. (London), 145:*251, 1959.
11. Freeman, G. L.: *The Energetics of Human Behavior.* Ithaca, Cornell University Press, 1948.
12. Gary Bobo, E., and Bonvallet, M.: Résponses incrémentales associées du noyau d'Edinger-Westphal, du cortex et du tronc cérébral à des stimulations de l'amygdale. *J. Physiol. (Paris), 61* (suppl 1): 295, 1969.
13. Gautier, H.: Effets respiratoires de stimulations sensorielles chez l'Homme. *J. Physiol. (Paris), 60:*360, 1968.
14. Hebb, D. O.: Drives and the CNS (conceptual nervous system). *Psychol. Rev., 62:*243, 1955.
15. Hilton, S. M., and Zbrozyna, A. W.: Amygdaloid region for defence reactions and its efferent pathway to the brain stem. *J. Physiol. (London), 165:*160, 1963.
16. Hugelin, A.: Intégrations motrices et vigilance chez l'Encéphale isolé. II. Contrôle réticulaire des voies finales communes d'ouverture et de fermeture de la gueule. *Arch. Ital. Biol., 99:*244, 1961.
17. Hugelin, A., and Bonvallet, M.: Tonus cortical et contrôle de la facilitation motrice d'origine réticulaire. *J. Physiol. (Paris), 49:*1171, 1957.
18. Hugelin, A., and Bonvallet, M.: Etude expérimentale des interrelations réticulo-corticales. Proposition d'une théorie de l'asservissement réticulaire à un système diffus cortical. *J. Physiol. (Paris), 49:*1201, 1957.
19. Hugelin, A., and Bonvallet, M.: Effets moteurs et corticaux d'origine réticulaire au cours des stimulations somesthésiques. Rôle des interactions cortico-réticulaires dans le déterminisme du réveil. *J. Physiol. (Paris), 50:*951, 1958.

20. Hugelin, A., and Dumont, S.: Intégrations motrices et vigilance chez l'Encéphale isolé. I. Inhibition réticulaire du réflexe d'ouverture de la gueule. *Arch. Ital. Biol., 99:*219, 1961.

21. Lacey, J. I., Kagan, J., Lacey, B. C., and Moss, H. A.: The visceral level: situational determinants and behavioral correlates of autonomic response patterns. In P. H. Knapp (Ed.): *Expression of the Emotions in Man.* New York, International University Press, 1963, pp. 161.

22. Lacey, J. I.: Somatic response patterning and stress: some revisions of activation theory. In Appley, M. H., and Trumbull, R. (Eds.): *Psychological Stress.* New York, Appleton-Century-Crofts, 1967. pp. 14.

23. Malmo, R. B.: Activation: A neuropsychological dimension. *Psychol. Rev., 66:*367, 1959.

24. Ursin, A., and Kaada, B. R.: Functional localization within the amygdaloid complex in the cat. *Electroenceph. Clin. Neurophysiol., 12:*1, 1960.

DISCUSSION

Dr. Hall: I would like to comment on the first figure that you showed regarding stimulation of the amygdala. It appears that the arousal effect is localized primarily in the large-celled part of the basal nucleus.

Dr. Hugelin: It is the large-celled part, the magnocellular region.

Dr. Hall: Yes. However one or two of the dots indicating an arousal response may be within the small-celled part of the nucleus. As well, stimulation produced a positive response in the stria terminalis, which is more directly related to the parvocellular than the magnocellular part. In considering the anatomical pathways underlying these responses, one could postulate that axon collaterals in the junctional region of the two parts of the basal nucleus are involved. Stimulation of collaterals of the large-celled part might activate cells of the small-celled part which send their axons into the stria terminalis. One might also suggest that afferents coursing via the stria terminals to the parvocellular region are involved in the production of the arousal response.

Dr. Hugelin: I cannot answer that because I have not done the experiments myself, but I can say that in the amygdala the effects are very restricted. The entire amygdala was explored, and it was not possible to get effects from all parts that were stimulated.

Dr. Sigg: Did your stimulations in the amygdala set up any after-discharges?

Dr. Hugelin: No.

Dr. Sigg: Or any spread into the mesencephalic reticular formation?

Dr. Hugelin. I don't think so.

Dr. Hall: One other interesting point is that the large-celled part of the basal nucleus is stained by the acetylcholinesterase method. I wonder if this is significant in terms of your findings.

Dr. Gloor: In relation to your suggestion and also to the observations of Miss Bonvallet that stimulation of the stria terminalis produces this response, I wonder whether you're not dealing with the same system that Hilton and Zbrozyna were dealing with when they elicited the defense reaction by amygdaloid stimulation. The graded stimulation response that you get in this series is essentially like the behavior of the defense reaction. In which case, I would imagine that the stria would be the afferent limb. I thought that they had shown quite clearly that this response is afferent—is elicited by the afferent limb—and that the clustering of points in the magnocellular part would favor the suggestion that this is VAF outflow and not stria outflow, although there are a few points that are more medial.

Dr. Hugelin: The stimulation parameters indicate that they are very similar to those described by Hilton and Zbrozyna when they produce the defense reaction and its vascular component. It is likely that the discharge in the fibers running to the ciliary muscle is also a component of the defense reaction, allowing accommodation to near vision when an animal attacks.

Dr. Wolf: Would either Dr. Hugelin or Dr. Lacey care to comment on an observation in two patients who had frequent and fairly regular premature ventricular contractions? We gave each of these individuals mathematical problems to solve. When the individuals were distracted and confused by the problem and unable to concentrate, the frequency of the premature ventricular contractions increased; however, when the problem was grasped, concentrated on and correctly solved, the premature ventricular contractions during the period of computation dropped out altogether in one individual and decreased substantially in the other.

Dr. Lacey: Neither Dr. Hugelin nor I are surprised by the fact that different behavioral circumstances produce different physiological responses. In the light of describing general principles, however, I can't begin to conceive of the mechanisms by which premature ventricular contractions would be made to disappear. I don't know, Stewart, do you?

Dr. Wolf: No.

Dr. Hockman: I'd like to comment on the disappearance of the ventricular premature contractions. There are many regions within the forebrain midbrain limbic circuit which, when stimulated electrically, will give rise to ventricular premature contractions. In seeking mechanisms to explain these phenomena, it is reasonable to assume that inputs to these regions produced by different behaviors could, either by inhibiting or facilitating autonomic reflexes, dramatically alter both cardiac rate and rhythm.

Dr. Andy: Have you observed any pupillary constrictions, or has Dr. Bonvallet observed pupillary constrictions from stimulation of the amygdala?

Dr. Hugelin: I'm not sure, but I don't think so.

Dr. Sigg: We have done a number of studies on pupillary dilatation and constriction. As a matter of fact, we measured short ciliary nerve activity and from nowhere except the direct light-reflex pathway, of course, could we elicit pupillary constriction in the unanesthetized animal.

Dr. Andy: Have you stimulated in the anterior cingulate area?

Dr. Sigg: In the unanesthetized animal, we stimulated the cingulate cortex but observed no constriction.

Dr. Andy: I have observed constriction from the anterior cingulate occasionally in patients, but that's the only place, and I feel that this is almost happenstance because I don't know of any work confirming it.

Dr. Lacey: I would like to make one point related to something that Walle Nauta brought up. Dr. Hugelin described two kinds of data, with both of which you know I agree. The individual differences in response patterns in common behavioral circumstances are possibly due to constitutional differences, and if there are differences in activity of peripheral organs, this goes along systematically with different kinds of behavioral responses. Of course, the big problem is to specify what the differences are in these behaviors. The problem of diffuseness of somatic reactivity makes this very different.

SESSION VI

Chairman: Ebbe Curtis Hoff

Chapter 13

Pharmacological Aspects of Limbic Function

KEITH F. KILLAM, JR.

A PHARMACOLOGIST'S approach to the study of the limbic system varies somewhat from that of the anatomist, physiologist, psychologist or clinician. The focus is at two levels: (a) the description of brain structure(s) and function(s) affected by a drug and (b) the evaluation of features of the spectrum of physiological or behavioral changes induced by a drug to select those alterations in function essential to the action of the drug on the organism—that is, a study of the spectrum of drug influence versus the mechanism of action of the drug. For example, the intravenous administration of a drug which produces anesthesia may at the same time increase recovery times of neuronal populations measured from reticular formation, thalamic nuclei and hippocampus. The subsequent task is to uncover whether the "anesthetic state" induced by the depressant agent is dependent upon the entire spectrum of alterations or is related to one or a combination. Part of the strategy by which this question is approached should include studies of dose/response relationships, the use of chemical analogs which may share some but not all of the properties of the anesthetic, a comparison of the new drug with conventional anesthetics and finally the study of drugs that either partially or totally reverse the action of the experimental drug. Unfortunately no agent is entirely specific so the pharmacological approach is always fraught with imponderable variables, few of which can be absolutely controlled.

Drug effects on the limbic system are studied by methods similar to those commonly used for other structures: the assessment of variables related to state and the assessment of transient variables.

In the former, the spontaneous rhythms and characteristic responses from the various parts of the limbic system are evaluated under differing behavioral states. Examples are the theta activity from the hippocampus during arousal and REM sleep and the origin and progression of spontaneous seizure activity. While the data tend more to be descriptive and less precisely quantifiable than from the other type of study, they are closely related to the behavioral variable, and it is generation of behavior which is the *raison d'etre* of the nervous system.

The assessment of transient variables implies interference by the experimenter usually in the form of evoking responses in the nervous system by any of a variety of techniques. While these techniques may precisely categorize the biophysical status of neurons, they have not in the classical studies included aspects related to informational content of stimuli. More recently, as conditioning techniques have come into use, the behavioral components have been added. Such correlates would seem crucial to current evaluations of limbic activity and the importance of drug effects thereon. For example, the pathways transferring information regarding a conditioning stimulus to structures generating behavior have been shown to include the hippocampus at a definite point in the learning curve before correct responding at a high rate is stabilized. This finding in avoidance conditioning[1] fits with earlier evidence about the periods at which rhinencephalic lesions prevent full development of conditioned responses.[2]

The pharmacology of synapses and synaptic transmission is a fundamental part of drug action in any neuronal population. At least three factors must be taken into consideration: (a) the integrity of metabolic systems maintaining membrane characteristics and generating, as byproducts, substances with powerful influences on synaptic junctions; (b) the characterization of such modulator substances influencing synaptic zones; and (c) the physical and chemical factors related to classical transmitter substances. All three factors have differing time constants and subsystems which, in my view, make the central nervous system essentially different from the peripheral nervous system and will in time force rethinking of the current models of brain function.

It is within the framework just outlined that certain aspects of the pharmacology of the limbic system will be discussed.

Alterations of the cholinergic substratum of the brain by the administration of anticholinesterases produces theta rhythms as the dominant pattern from the hippocampus with asynchrony from other limbic structures such as the amygdala.[3] The pattern is indistinguishable from the theta rhythms seen during neocortical arousal or REM sleep. But while in the nondrugged state the rhythm will appear and disappear as the behavior of the subject varies along the sleep-wakefulness continuum, such plasticity of rhythms is lost following the administration of anticholinesterases. The obverse is seen with the administration of anticholinergic drugs such as atropine and scopolamine. Theta rhythms of the hippocampus are abolished. Pseudosynchrony appears on the neocortex[4] with desynchronized patterns in other limbic structures. But as was seen after the anticholinesterases, the rhythms become stereotyped or independent of fluctuations within the behavioral sleep-wakefulness continuum. The effects of these two classes of drugs have been considered as examples of ways to separate EEG changes from spontaneous behavior. On one hand, the anticholinesterases produce rhythms consonant with the arousal state even during behavioral fluctuations involving lack of attention and sleep. On the other hand, the anticholinergic drugs produce changes bearing a resemblance to spindle or slow-wave sleep, yet the subjects are attentive and responsive to the environment. If one examines conditioned behavior and attendant conditioned brain waves following either class of drugs, the subjects are unable to perform previously learned responses. The conditioned brain wave indicators are also disrupted. Thus, despite earlier gross observations that an animal's general comportment is intact under such compounds, learned behavioral patterns are disrupted in proportion to the alterations in limbic and neocortical brain rhythms.

For example, following atropine administration conditioned approach behavior dependent upon form or light flux discrimination was blocked.[5-7] Conditioned avoidance performance after atropine was also abolished.[8] Peripheral factors are not involved in that neither topical application of atropine nor parenteral administration of atropine methyl nitrate, which does not pass the blood brain barrier, altered the conditional behavior. Similarly, following the administration of physostigmine both approach behavior (light-flux discrimination controlled) [7] and conditioned avoidance behavior are blocked.[9]

Data from studies employing iontophoretically applied acetylcholine (ACh) indicate a great disparity in sensitivity between cells in the hippocampus and those of the neocortex.[10,11] Most cells from the hippocampus are sensitive to ACh and respond with increased firing. In the neocortex the responsive cells are patchy in distribution and may exhibit either an increase or decrease in firing. It could be inferred, therefore, that the function of the limbic system, or more specifically the hippocampus, is more dependent upon cholinergic transmission than that of the neocortex owing to the more systematic organization of cholinoceptivity. The behavioral data that either hyperactivity via anticholinesterase administration or hypoactivity via anticholinergic therapy interrupts learned behavior suggests a further hypothesis relating to the fundamental impact of this system on limbic functions. With either manipulation of cholinergic transmission, the brain wave patterns become stereotyped and the critical factor may thus be neither inhibition nor facilitation but the loss of plasticity of the nervous systems. Such plasticity can be conceived of as necessary for all but a basal level of behavioral responsiveness.

The role of catecholamines or the adrenergic system is less clear. The administration of drugs inhibiting the catabolic enzymes mono-amine oxidase or o-methyl transferase have been found to have little effect on spontaneous or evoked rhythms of the limbic system or neocortex provided the specific drug had no sympathomimetic activity in addition to that of enzymatic blockade. The lack of effect of enzymatic blockade may most logically be explained by the finding that adrenergic transmission is terminated primarily by rebinding of the transmitter to subcellular specialized particles.[12] Data from iontophoretic application of norepinephrine(NE) indicate more similarity between the neocortex and hippocampus than that seen after ACh application and thus less specificity of the adrenergic system to the rhinencephalon.[10,11] The distribution of receptive cells was shown to be diffuse and when sensitivity was found the response was usually a decrease in firing. To my knowledge the monumental task of assessing iontophoretic sensitivity in relation to storage of biogenic amines in the same preparation has not been attempted.

Studies with reserpine, a tranquilizer known to deplete the storage of adrenergic transmitters, shed some interesting light on the pharmacology of the limbic system. In some animals spontaneous seizures occurred following reserpine beginning in some instances in the amygdaloid complex and in others in the hippocampus.[13] While these findings cannot explain the full spectrum of activity of reserpine, a side effect often seen in patients involving decreasing seizure thresholds and surfacing of subclinical epileptic states is more easily understood. Following reserpine, especially chronic administration, there appears a stabilized hypersynchronous rhythm in the hippocampus not exactly at theta frequencies. Conditioned behaviors of a wide variety are blocked with attendant changes of conditioned EEG indicators.[1,14] Attempts to reverse the effects of reserpine with a precursor of NE, DOPA, are of interest. When a conditioned avoidance response was employed, the effects of reserpine could be completely reversed by DOPA with corresponding increases in brain levels of DOPamine.[15] However, when the behavioral paradigm was an approach response there appeared to be a separation between the reversal of the spontaneous behavior changes versus the alterations in conditioned response.[16] In our laboratories in twelve animals the marked generalized depressions and other autonomic signs of reserpinization were completely reversed by DOPA for one to three hours. However, in only two of the twelve was a milk-reinforced behavior returned to control responding levels. Computer analysis of the EEG indicators confirmed both states. In the same animals, a sympathomimetic amine, amphetamine, reversed the effects on both the spontaneous and conditioned behavior. This is of particular interest in that from studies on the peripheral autonomic systems, the mechanism of action of amphetamine is postulated as being dependent upon intact stores of NE. The drug is thought to prevent the rebinding of NE as the sympathetic system tonically fires. The behavioral and EEG data suggest that some other alternative must be operative in the central nervous system including the possibility of amphetamine acting as a false transmitter.

Tranquilizing agents of other chemical classes than reserpine have much less obvious effects on the limbic system. Chlorpromazine was originally thought to act as a central adrenergic blocking agent because of its powerful peripheral alpha adrenergic-blocking properties. However, more potent analogs of chlorpromazine, trifluperazine and perphenazine are devoid of adrenergic-blocking activity while having enhanced potency in inhibiting a variety of conditional behaviors.[1,17] Implication of altered limbic system activity as one aspect of chlorpromazine action depends upon the appearance of epileptoid activity at doses five to ten times that needed for effects on conditional behavior.[18] Further, chlorpromazine has a variable effect on seizures elicited by stimulation of the hippocampus or amygdaloid complex.[19] Like reserpine, chronic treatment with chlorpromazine increases the likelihood of seizures in the epileptic but the high doses needed in the studies mentioned above do not support the view that the limbic system is the focus of this action.

A similar pattern is seen with the butyrophenones. Haloperidol will produce spontaneous seizure activity involving the limbic system at six to eight times the dose required to block a conditioned arousal response.[20]

The benzodiazepines exhibit another spectrum. Chlordiazepoxide, diazepam and nitrazepam were introduced originally as minor tranquilizers and central muscle relaxants.[21,22] They were found to have, in addition, a wide spectrum of anticonvulsant activity including blockade of seizures elicited by stimulation of the amygdala or hippocampus.[23,24]

Other minor tranquilizers such as meprobamate also alter thresholds at which electrical stimulation causes limbic seizures and shorten the duration of afterdischarge.[25] This property is shared generally with barbiturates, including those not considered to be anticonvulsants. For example, at doses of pentobarbital showing selective depression of brain stem reticular formation, the threshold for eliciting limbic seizures is markedly elevated.[26] These findings may be interpreted as either a dual and similar susceptibility of the reticular formation and the limbic system or the interdependence of the two systems for the propagation of limbic seizures.

This effect of barbiturates serves as an

example of the importance of correlated studies of a number of compounds before assigning to any one central effect an important role in the mechanism of a drug's action. Rhinencephalic seizure repression, while characteristic of barbiturate action at anesthetic doses and below, is not related to the origin of the state of anesthesia per se since ether administration tends to elicit rather than suppress seizure responses in hippocampus [27] while diazepam or chlordiazepoxide suppress hippocampal seizures but are not anesthetic agents.

The phenothiazines,[19] the butyrophenones [20] and the benzodiazepines [22] share the property of blocking the EEG arousal of the limbic system at doses leaving the neocortical systems virtually intact. However, as in the case of electrically induced limbic seizures, the mechanisms coupling somatic integrative systems to the limbic system may be the site of action rather than the limbic system per se.

Abnormal hypersynchrony in the limbic system induced by LSD-25 [28] and phencyclidine [29] has been taken as an indicator of the mechanism for the hallucinogenic properties of these drugs. However, the degradation of conditional behavior after these drugs is not totally dependent upon the appearance of such activity.[5,30]

As mentioned earlier, hypersynchrony of the hippocampus is a consistent, excellent correlate of the appearance of REM sleep. In attempting to evaluate the effects of drugs on sleep cycles, a number of other indicators of various sleep stages become less reliable. For example, drugs with central muscle relaxant properties will alter the appearance of rapid eye movements and concomitant decrease in somatic muscle tone. At such times the external manifestations of REM sleep are difficult to assess. However, periods with spike transients from the lateral geniculate corresponding with hippocampal theta activity are observable. Thus, despite the loss of peripheral correlates, central REM states may be identified.

Studies comparing barbiturates, tranquilizers and sedative antihistamines indicate that alterations of sleep cycles are paralleled with alterations of the limbic system indicators.[32] Thus, the limbic system is intimately involved in and interlocked with the somatic integrative systems in the regulation of sleep cycles, but the site of interference of such regulation by the various agents can not be assigned to either system from such data.

As an overview and in an attempt to unify these findings, one should examine the generalizations as to the function of the limbic system and consider the actions of various drugs in that perspective. On the "sensory side," the sensation of olfaction has an exceptional amount of cognitive and experiential overlay. Novel odors or those out of context evoke personalized rather than generalized ideation and behavior. With respect to integrative mechanisms, autonomic activity, the learning process or sexual behavior, the emphasis of limbic function is on modulation. If one contrasts these properties of the limbic sytsem with those of the central reticular core, striking conceptual differences emerge. The reticular formation receives direct information concerning enteroceptive and exteroceptive fields. Modulation of this information at first is in relation to classical reflex activity. Further, primitive overall regulation of sleep cycles and wakefulness parameters tonically regulates the total capability of the entire nervous system. The rhinencephalon receives directly only from the olfactory system; it gathers the distillate of other modified activity. In simple conceptual terms, the somatic systems including the reticular formation may be thought to determine the capability and action of the organism, the limbic system to define the flavor or appropriateness of actions. Stereotyped behavior occurs with loss, malfunction or hyperstability of the limbic system. If this hypothesis is correct, then we have barely scratched the surface of the pharmacology of the limbic system. More complex and better controlled experiments need be designed to address directly the parameters related to limbic functions, especially those related to the plasticity of response in functional systems of the brain. Furthermore, some systematization of a massive base of controlled empirical data is required from which may emerge more rewarding theoretical hypotheses.

REFERENCES

1. John, E. R., and Killam, K. F.: *J. Pharmacol. Exp. Ther., 125:*252, 1959.
2. Hunt, H. F., and Diamond, I. T.: *Proc. Int. Cong. Psychol., 22:*163, 1957.
3. Funderburk, W. H., and Case, J.: *Electroenceph. Clin. Neurophysiol., 3:*213, 1951.
4. Wikler, A.: *Proc. Soc. Exp. Biol. Med., 79:*261, 1952.
5. Lindsley, D. F., Carpenter, R. S., Killam, E. K., and Killam, K. F.: *Electroenceph. Clin. Neurophysiol., 24:*497, 1968.
6. Seiden, L. S., and Killam, K. F.: Unpublished data.
7. Matsuzaki, M., and Killam, K. F.: Unpublished data.
8. Rougel, A., Verdeaux, J., and Gogan, P.: *Int. J. Neuropharmacol., 4:*265, 1965.
9. Pfeiffer, C. C., and Jenney, E. H.: *Ann. N.Y. Acad. Sci., 66:*753, 1957.
10. Salmoiraghi, G. C., and Stefanis, C. N.: *Arch. Ital. Biol., 103:*705, 1965.
11. Krnjević, K., and Phillis, J. W.: *J. Physiol. (London), 166:*328, 1963.
12. Hertting, G., Axelrod, J., and Whitly, L. G.: *J. Pharmacol. Exp. Ther., 134:*146, 1961.
13. Killam, E. K., and Killam, K. F.: In Fields, W. S. (Ed.): *Brain Mechanisms and Drug Action.* Springfield, Charles C Thomas, 1957.
14. Brady, J. V.: *Science, 123:*1033, 1956.
15. Seiden, L. S., and Carlsson, A.: *Psychopharmacologia (Berlin), 5:*178, 1964.
16. Killam, K. F., Killam, E. K., and Seiden, L. S.: *Jap. J. Neurochem., 4 (Suppl. 4)*, 1965.
17. Cook, L., and Weidley, E.,: *Ann. N.Y. Acad. Sci., 66:*740, 1957.
18. Preston, J. B.: *J. Pharmacol. Exp. Ther., 118:*100, 1956.
19. Killam, E. K., and Killam, K. F.: *Proc. As. Res. Nerv. Ment. Dis., 37:*245, 1959.
20. Monti, J. M., Hance, A. J., and Killam, K. F.: *Fed. Proc., 25:*229, 1966.
21. Zbinden, G., and Randall, L. O.: *Advances Pharmacol. 5:*213, 1967.
22. Randall, L. O., and Schallek, W.: *Psychopharmacology: A Review of Progress, PHS Public 1836:*153, 1957–1967.
23. Requin, S., Lanoir, J., Plas, R., and Naquet, R.: *Soc. Biol. (Paris), 157:*2015, 1963.
24. Stark, L. G.: Ph.D. Dissertation, A neuropharmacological comparison of three models of epilepsy including the baboon, *Papio papio.* Stanford University.
25. Gangloff, H.: *J. Pharmacol. Exp. Ther., 126:* 30, 1959.
26. Killam, E. K., Killam, K. F., and Shaw, T.: *Ann. N.Y. Acad. Sci., 66:*784, 1957.
27. Naquet, R., and King, E. E.: Unpublished data.
28. Adey, W. R., Bell, F. R., and Dennis, B. J.: *Neurology (Minneap.), 12:*591, 1962.
29. Adey, W. R., and Dunlop, C. W.: *J. Pharmacol. Exp. Ther., 130:*418, 1960.
30. Gehrmann, J. E.: Ph.D. Dissertation, A neuropharmacological and behavioral study of phencyclidine and two of its congeners. Stanford University.
31. Domino, E. F.: *Int. Rev. Neurobiol., 6:*303, 1964.
32. Prinz, P. N.: Ph.D. Dissertation, Pharmacological alterations of patterns of sleep and wakefulness in the cat. Stanford University.

DISCUSSION

Dr. Hoffer: Dr. Killam just mentioned that there is some evidence to indicate that amphetamines may play a direct rather than just a releasing role in the central nervous system. If I may, I would like to present some evidence supporting this view. If you apply norepinephrine iontophoretically to a Purkinje cell in the intact rat, you get a prompt inhibition. You can see a similar inhibition when you apply amphetamine or tyramine, both of which are considered to work by releasing norepinephrine. If you now pretreat the rat with 6-hydroxydopamine, there is a complete destruction of norepinephrine containing nerve terminals and elimination of all biochemically detectable norepinephrine in the cerebellum. In such a treated rat, tyramine, amphetamine as well as norepinephrine will again produce a very prompt inhibition of Purkinje cells, so in this case both tyramine and amphetamine appear to be working directly.

Dr. Killam: Do you believe that this is a false transmitter type of action?

Dr. Hoffer: No, we believe that amphetamine and tyramine possess direct postsynaptic sympathomimetic activity.

Dr. Hornykiewicz: Have you tried serotonin on the cerebellar cells? I wonder what serotonin would do, since there are hypotheses linking the effects of amphetamine on a "tryptamine receptor." Do you think that the effects of amphetamine might be explained by an action on such a "tryptamine receptor" in the central nervous system as has been claimed several times by Vane and others?

Dr. Hoffer: We have tested serotonin and find an admixture of both excitatory and inhibitory effects. The evidence we have suggests that serotonin effects may be induced.

Dr. Killam: I might say that we have been unsuccessful to reverse reserpine depression with serotonin (5-HT) in our behavioral experiments. Serotonin was administered both centrally and peripherally with and without monamine oxidase inhibitors.

Dr. Hornykiewicz: This would argue against "tryptamine receptors" being involved.

Dr. Jasper: I would like to make one comment and ask one question. Firstly, regarding your statement about the effects of anticholinesterases, atropine and scopolamine on learning. In certain types of learning situations where we are using a tactile discrimination task in the monkey, we came to quite a different conclusion than you mentioned. Light does of scopolamine, sufficient to allow the animal to continue performing the task, have never interfered with the percentage of accuracy of discrimination in the learned task, but they will always prevent or retard the acquisition of learning if given during the learning process. These seem to be quite different results than those which you were reporting. We repeatedly tried to show the effects of well-learned tasks, and in some cases, performance seemed to be improved due to an increase in percentage of correct responses under scopolamine, partly due to the diminution in number of chance key presses—the number of responses decreases and the percentage of accuracy increases with scopolamine. The second comment was the question about the reversal of action by the administration of DOPA, and you commented on the relations if you increase DOPamine. Of course, DOPA is a precursor of noradrenaline, and if you also find a large increase in noradrenaline, this could be a better explanation for your results than DOPamine.

Dr. Killam: In answering Dr. Jasper's first question, the data reported referred to drug effects on trained behavior and at successive stages in training. Since there is variability of sensitivity of all animals, each was examined over a reasonable dose spread. In general, the degree of behavioral deficit was directly proportional to the amount of cortical hypersynchrony induced by the drugs. Generally, scopolamine was ten times more active than atropine. Further, the more complex the task, the more sensitive the behavior to drug disruption. For example, when an animal is asked to select lighted versus darkened panels—a simple light-dark discrimination—one needs to administer enough drug to cause persistent and continuos hypersynchrony. On the other hand, if the same animal with further training is required to discriminate among three geometric figures, at the first sign of drug-induced neocortical hypersynchrony, a behavioral deficit will be apparent.

Dr. Lacey: Is this also true of atropine?

Dr. Killam: Yes, this is also true of atropine, and it is directly related to the amount of hypersynchrony that appears, or the pseudohypersynchrony. We have some other interesting findings from our laboratories which we believe are almost specific to a species of rat.

The data from our laboratories on acquisition changes are curious. The experiments were designed to demonstrate the "amnesic effect" of scopolamine. The specific paradigm is as follows: The animals were subjected to intensive shock and subsequently tested for retention of shock experience. Specifically, rats were given inescapable shock periodically every five seconds for fifteen minutes. Four weeks later they were trained on a continuous reinforcement schedule for food pellets. Once stabilized, each lever press produced a foot shock at one-tenth of the original shock level and, of course, a food pellet. Scopolamine was administered only during the period of inescapable intense shock. Appropriate paired controls were run throughout the procedure. The dosage of scopolamine was sufficient to produce behavioral depression. We, therefore, expected some degree of amnesia in these animals for the initial shock phase. However, the animals receiving intensive shock plus scopolamine were hypersensitive to minute shock rather than being less sensitive. The response was so severe that the animals stopped eating in their home cages and required forced feeding for survival. Subsequent retraining and retesting elicited the same pattern. Unfortunately, the phenomena appear to be strain and/or species specific.

With respect to the comment about DOPA and DOPamine, from V. Carlsson and Seiden's experiments, the degree of reversibility was proportional to brain and heart levels of DOPamine and not to DOPA or norepinephrine. There are those who believe that the central modulator is DOPamine rather than epinephrine or serotonin. The latter products would be simply as by-products. Certainly the provocative findings with DOPA in the treatment of parkinsonism must cause reevaluation of central neurohumoral transmission.

Dr. Ling: Do you not think that DOPamine may be postulated as the neural transmitter and that norepinephrine is the by-product of this effect?

Dr. Killam: Let me be a bit more provocative. Over the years we have become more convinced that the peripheral model, the model of sympathetic and parasympathetic divisions of the autonomic nervous system, either does not apply or is inappropriate for the central nervous system. Further, if we are to relate protein synthesis to memory, then in some way synaptic function must be linked to the metabolism of the cell. I realize that this is a very large jump but as far as I know, no such linkage has been proposed for excitable cells. If one considers studies using microiontophoretic techniques, the sensitivity of specific membranes to drugs and the response latency can be described. The so-called classical transmitters such as acetylcholine, norepinephrine, epinephrine, DOPA and DOPamine are several orders of magnitude less effective and with longer latencies as compared with glutamic acid, glycine or gamma aminobutyric acid (GABA). These three substances are under metabolic control and can figuratively make the cells dance as their supplies to membranes are turned on and off.

Glutamic acid happens to be in a very critical place with respect to the whole metabolic cycle, and we know that in the central nervous system it is the only place in the body where there is the so-called GABA shunt. This particular step in the enzymatic pathway also accounts for the largest production of high-energy phosphates within the whole sequence of the TCA system. Glycine is probably the most uniformly used amino acid within the central nervous system involved in transaminations and with the building of brain proteins and gangliosides. It is quite possible that we should then be able to come up with some statement on what makes a neuron more hyperexcitable than supportive elements. This could be specifically related to instabilities reflecting these kinds of pools of substances that are being generated by neuronal metabolism. However, such a system would inevitably oscillate. Thus, there is needed some system that performs a role of smoothing function. It is this role that I see for our classical transmitters, such as acetylcholine, norepinephrine and 5-HT. This formulation is in addition to the kind of depolarization that is related to the conduction of impulses over the boutons. Further, some of the findings in protein synthesis may be brought into this formulation. Consider the proposition that when a cell fires the ion imbalances established are enough to scramble the foregoing metabolic sequences, particularly partially formed structures on the ribosomes. Thus, when Hyden describes base-paired differences, the changes reflect past history of temporal sequences of biochemical interruptions and/or cell firing. I would hope that you would find the formulation stimulating if nonclassical.

Dr. Abrahams: I would like to make a point since we are dealing with cholinergic drugs. Some years ago, we did enzyme histochemistry to show that acetylcholine occurs in the brain stem, and it became apparent immediately that there are large quantities of pseudocholinesterase in neuronal and non-neuronal areas. The medial aspects of the ependyma is very rich. One finds all kinds of glial cells in the hippocampus very rich in cholinesterase, and we have no idea what these enzymes are doing there, but presumably if the enzyme inhibitor is in the brain, these are inhibited, and we can base our interpretations solely on the neuronal model that we have.

Dr. Snider: This is a very complex field, and I would like to bring up the point about blocking agents. To cite a specific example, if seizure activity is induced in the hippocampus, and this is quite easy to do, electrical stimulation of the cerebellum can stop the seizure activity promptly.

This is easy to demonstrate with an animal under Flaxedil, but hard to demonstrate with an animal under d-tubocurarine. You get it through the first time and stop the seizures, and then this thing won't work the second time. Here is an example of blocking agents that do not act in the same way insofar as the cerebellohippocampal systems are concerned. Embarassingly small amounts of Nembutal will block this effect. I note that you left the barbiturates out of your discussions. Would you like to make any additional comments?

Dr. Killam: I only mentioned barbiturates in passing. In our hands, the cerebellum, the reticular formation, the hippocampus and the amygdala are equally sensitive to the barbiturates. In studies with Drs. Brazier and Adey, cerebellar unit activity promptly disappears after 3 to 4 mg/kg of pentobarbital or thiopental. Recovery takes forty-five minutes to one hour. The same range of effects may be seen in the reticular formation. At that time, it is possible to evoke limited activity, but in general the background tone dies away. Most anesthetics share this property except for ether. Ether in small doses elicits seizure-like activity in the hippocampus and amygdala, first described by R. Naquet in his thesis in 1951. Concomitant with this activity there is profuse salivation. This coupling of amygdaloid seizure-like activity and salivation can be demonstrated without the classical buccal, mucosal stimulation usually invoked to explain salivation following ether.

Dr. Gloor: Electroencephalographic seizure activity?

Dr. Killam: Yes.

Dr. Hornykiewicz: I am particularly interested in your findings with reserpine and DOPA on different types of conditioned behavior. You mentioned that the decrease in locomotor activity could be easily restored with DOPA, but you couldn't restore milk-reinforced behavior with DOPA. On the other hand, it has been shown that the conditioned avoidance response which is also interrupted after reserpine can also be restored with DOPA. To my mind, this shows that in the conditioned avoidance response, different regions might be involved than in the milk-reinforced behavior. The conditioned avoidance response might involve the striatal region, at least insofar as locomotor activity is concerned, whereas the milk-reinforced behavior might involve regions for which DOPamine does not have any physiological function, so you cannot restore the disrupted behavior with DOPA. I was wondering if you didn't possibly try serotonin in these experiments and if it could not have had an effect on the disrupted milk-reinforced behavior.

Dr. Killam: In the particular experiment reported here, we have not assessed the effects of serotonin. We did, however, assess one of the other aspects that you did mention with respect to DOPA. In some of our twelve animals, we established a double-conditioning situation. Animals were, of course, trained to the milk reinforcement with the particular flicker stimulus configuration. Some were also trained in a separate chamber to perform a conditioned-avoidance response in a classical shuttle box to the same frequency or flicker stimulation. In those particular animals, DOPA completely reversed the depression of the conditioned-avoidance response while having little or no effect on the conditioned-approach response reinforced by milk.

Some time ago in the mid-fifties when Dr. John and I worked together, we tested the effects of serotonin on the reversal of reserpine effect, and we were unable to reverse the reserpine depression with either peripheral administration of serotonin or the administration of serotonin by an intraventricular cannula.

Dr. Hornykiewicz: Are you referring now to the avoidance response or the reinforcement?

Dr. Killam: Neither the spontaneous depression nor the conditioned avoidance response depressed with reserpine could be changed by serotonin. DOPA, on the other hand, would completely reverse the so-called pharmacological side effects of reserpine irrespective of whether or not the conditioned behavior was altered. Further, when the animals are offered milk, they will take the milk even if they will not perform the conditioned behavior.

Dr. Hornykiewicz: I would also like to make a remark on Dr. Jasper's suggestion that noradrenaline might also be involved in the DOPA effect. Experiments with threo-3,4-dihydroxyphenylserine, threo-DOPS, which yields noradrenaline without the intermediate formation of DOPamine seem to show that in spite of an increase in brain noradrenaline, there is no anti-reserpine action; so it seems that noradrenaline is not really responsible for the DOPA effect in question. I have a rather unorthodox opinion on the conditioned avoidance response and the antireserpine effects in this situation. It seems to me that part of this conditioned response involves locomotor activity, and of course, reserpine causes rigidity and a kind of hypokinesia which is probably of striatal origin. Under these conditions, the avoidance response is blocked by reserpine not because of some actions on, I don't know what brain function, but just because the animal doesn't have the initiative to move and can't move because of muscle rigidity. DOPA reverses the rigidity and the hypokinesia.

Dr. Killam: In the cat at the doses we used (70μg/kg IM), there is hypokinesia but no rigidity. Further, the animals will exhibit escape behavior. Now, we have evidence that learning can go on while the avoidance paradigm is blocked.

The evidence is as follows: When the cat is trained to multiple cues only one of which is reinforced in the avoidance paradigm, it will generalize its behavior to several of the cues. Under the influence of reserpine, negative reinforcement is only paired with the appropriate cue. After the effects of reserpine have worn off, the animal no longer generalizes to the other cues but generates avoidance behavior only to the appropriate cue.

Dr. Hornykiewicz: It shows that learning is a separate process, and performance as such is another one.

Dr. MacLean: When do they come out of the reserpine? What doses do you give?

Dr. Killam: The dosage that we used was 70μg/kg.

Dr. Hornykiewicz: IV?

Dr. Killam: Intraperitoneally or intramuscularly, either one.

Dr. MacLean: This wouldn't be comparable to Brodie's doses which would deplete the brain of serotonin pretty well?

Dr. Killam: We did not have any direct measurement of catecholamines, but our animals were depressed for ninety-six hours or more. If one studies blood pressure effects in the cat over this period, the true sympatholytic activity of reserpine is evident. From Brodie's data, the cat takes much longer than any other animal to replete its stores of biogenic amines. However, there is something curious about the cat in conditioned-avoidance behavior and the reserpine effect. Again from data gathered with Roy John, we observed that it took about five days for the cats to recover from 70μg/kg of reserpine. At that time they will hop into the recording chamber as is their custom; however, their response to latencies, instead of being crisp and around five to seven seconds, will drift to around cutoff time, requiring negative reinforcement. When the cats are reinforced, they completely go to pieces, and all the so-called pharmacological side effects of reserpine return—bradycardia, meiosis, diarrhea and depression. Whether this is another manifestation of conditioned behavior we do not know. The phenomenon was repeatable in every animal we used! Thus, after presumably the stores of biogenic amines have been resynthesized, one can reinstate a pharmacological response in the absence of the drug by applying the negative reinforcement.

Dr. Marczynski: I have very much enjoyed your penetrating analysis of pharmacological approaches to the problems of CNS function. I would like to mention only that reserpine is probably the worst drug to study the physiological role of catecholamines in the central nervous system because of its unselective depleting action on both catecholamines and serotonin and also because of its peculiar and poorly understood action on central and peripheral cholinergic systems. In contrast to more selective monoamine depletors and inhibitors of their synthesis, reserpine significantly increases acetylcholine levels in most brain structures and in peripheral organs such as the heart and gastrointestinal tract. This effect does not seem to be caused simply by an overall depression of the central nervous system. Little is known about the mechanism of this action of reserpine. It appears that the well-known increase in the tonus of the parasympathetic division of the autonomic nervous system observed after reserpine administration results from both central and peripheral action of this drug on cholinergic and/or cholinoceptive neuronal substrates.

Dr. Snider: What would you substitute for it—for the use of reserpine?

Dr. Marczynski: Alpha-methyl-para-tyrosine would be much more selective in its action, since it blocks the synthesis of catecholamines by inhibiting the enzyme tyrosine hydroxylase which catalyzes the conversion of tyrosine to DOPA. In addition, this drug does not seem to influence significantly the levels and synthesis of serotonin.

Dr. Killam: As you know, alpha-methyl-tyrosine has markedly less effects on behavior. Dr. Marczynski has rightfully pointed out lack of specificity or control one has when one uses reserpine. In addition to the changes he has mentioned, there is also a tremendous amount of fluid loss, with attendant ion changes. Still to be explained is the rather controversial work of Dr. H. Zaimais wherein digitalis normalized the reserpine heart more effectively than norepinephrine. Some of this may be related to water and ion loss.

One can control for the water loss by using tetrabenazine. The peripheral effects can be controlled by using judicious doses of syrosingopine. Recently, however, the use of parachlorophenylalanine is in vogue.

Dr. Ling: This acts primarily on serotonin.

Dr. Killam: Yes. There is some curious information about this drug that should be brought to light. If one wishes to administer it in any sizeable dose, one must give it by mouth, and there is very good evidence that it exerts toxic effects on the lining of the stomach. A number of statements concerning the maintenance of REM sleep activity following this substance could be related to this irritant effect on the gut and intraperitoneal cavity. These are variables that are in need of control.

Dr. Smyth: I have two questions. Firstly, does the effect of phenylephrine differ in any way from that of other adrenergic agents on REM sleep cycles? Secondly, the relatively new agent methaqualone is said to be a nonbarbiturate hypnotic which induces sleep without REM sleep deprivation and without a withdrawal overshoot of REM sleep. It is alleged to do this, and if this is so, is there anything known about its peculiarities of action?

Dr. Killam: Phenylephrine is a sympathomimetic agent used to elevate blood pressure in emergency situations, for example, in the operating room. As far as I know, its mechanism of action is similar to that of tyramine. It may be a false transmitter. With respect to its effect on sleep cycles. I know of no data that would indicate that it would modify sleep cycles.

I am sorry that I am not familiar with the pharmacology of methaqualone.

Dr. Ling: Methaqualone is a quinazolinone derivative that depresses the central nervous system and produces sedation. It has a weak antihistaminic effect and is also a local anesthetic in experimental animals. The CNS depression produced by methaqualone is potentiated by other central nervous system depressants, particularly the barbiturates, phenothiazines and butyrophenones. There is no firm data to indicate that this compound does not interfere with REM sleep.

Dr. Snyder: You will probably welcome a change of pace, Keith. I see several clinicians in the audience, and the other drug problem that might be of considerable interest is the anti-epileptic drug called Dilantin ®. As you know, in Dilantin toxicity, a very prominent cerebellar sign appears. An easy way to destroy Purkinje cells is to step up the dose of Dilantin, and yet there are few if any changes in the other cerebellar cells. We have even looked in the hippocampus but have seen no changes and certainly nothing comparable to the Purkinje cell destruction. Do you know of any work where a rather critical study has been done on the pharmacology of Dilantin in reference to any part of the limbic system?

Dr. Killam: We have some interesting data with Dilantin. As you are all aware, the drug must be given chronically to exhibit consistent anticonvulsive properties. We have been able to abolish conditioned-approach behavior for up to six weeks following three to five days of Dilantin at nontoxic doses. The tagged conditional neuroelectric activity from brain stem and central areas was disturbed at this time.

We have also studied Dilantin in the *Papio papio*. It is not effective under acute administration and will alter the photomyoclonic syndrome only with massive chronic doses.

Dr. Hoff: Would you care to comment on the newer exploration in the use of Dilantin —the psychiatric use of Dilantin?

Dr. Killam: Dilantin is also a very good anti-arrhythmic agent. I am, however, not convinced of the data indicating that Dilantin may be a replacement for chlorpromazine or some other tranquilizer. You are all aware of the terrific overlay between subclinical epileptic states and misdiagnosis with respect to psychiatric problems. I cannot help but feel that this is part of what is being uncovered when one reports tranquilizing effects with Dilantin.

Dr. Andy: During a septal or hippocampal discharge, the conditioned avoidance response may be altered, and as the seizure progresses the response is further impaired. We have tried amphetamine to see if this would not decrease the amount of impairment. These drugs made the animal alert but instead of improving the conditioned avoidance response, they impaired it a little more.

Dr. Killam: Again, some of the old findings of Roy John may bear upon the point raised by Dr. Andy. Dr. John was interested in changing slightly the ratios of potassium, magnesium and sodium in the cerebrospinal fluid. Under some circumstances, unilateral motor convulsive discharges were observed. To control for simple motor discharge, Dr. John administered physostigmine, again producing a unilateral convulsion. If the animal in question has been trained to make a conditioned-avoidance response, then his ability to perform during the time of the unilateral convulsion depends upon what the seizuregenic substance or perturbation was originally. If the unilateral seizure is caused by the administration of physostigmine intraventricularly, the animal will perform adequately. If, however, it is secondary to upsetting the potassium and magnesium ratios in the cerebrospinal fluid, the animal just cannot perform and sits there and takes the shock. Thus, the appearance of unilateral seizures is not necessarily debilitating or as disorganizing as we heretofore suspected.

Dr. Andy: May I ask another question related to anesthesia? If one wants to perform an acute experiment with these drugs, one gets into trouble from the point of view of general anesthesia. What do you do?

Dr. Killam: The question has come up, but we still do acute experiments with agents such as curare, and I am constantly hearing the comment, "We will be happy to publish your data if you will assure us that the animal is under no pain." As far as I'm concerned, that question and the response are important, but the question is impertinent. As a scientist, one has at one's command a number of monitors which indicate whether or not one's preparation is reliable. If the preparation is swinging back and forth as a result of pain, then one is a poor scientist and has no business being in the game. From this standpoint, I think that there are a number of ways in which the problem can be attacked. There are times when one must use specialized preparations; however, I believe that the restrictions imposed by a number of national and international journals is tragic. I don't know how to alter this state of affairs, but there are times when you have to do specified types of experiments. One study which I did was to attempt to study the mechanism of action of morphine. To study the action of morphine implies that one must elicit some sort of painful response, and it must be in a controlled manner to prevent debilitation of the organism. It is ridiculous to ask if one can guarantee that the animal was not in pain when one is studying pain!

Dr. Hockman: I wanted to ask you about the experiment in which the conditional response was blocked for a period of six weeks following the chronic administration of Dilantin. What conditional procedure did you use?

Dr. Killam: We have a chamber one wall of which contains a panel onto which we project symbols, and the animal touches it to receive milk or Metrecal.® There is background lighting so that the illumination ratio can be varied, and everything is pre-programmed.

Dr. Hockman: I should like to make a comment in view of some of the results that you reported on activity from forebrain structures with Dilantin, because there still exists some controversy regarding the site of action of this compound. As you know, some investigators have discussed the action of this drug on the myocardium by drawing an analogy between the area surrounding a myocardial infarction and the boundary region around a cerebral post-traumatic lesion. What is your opinion of this?

Dr. Killam: To my way of thinking, most anticonvulsant agents have not been very well studied with respect to both general pharmacology and the nervous system. You can define things concerning the regulation of foci and the like, but the basic problems concern conduction through a number of structures. As you know, it has often been said that one of the reasons that you use phenobarbital in centrencephalic epilepsy is that the drug blocks the central midline structures involved. You know that phenobarbital just does not change conduction in the reticular formation. It is one of the few barbituates that doesn't. As far as I'm concerned, this hypothesis just does not hold. Some investigators use the model of some of the spinal reflexes and extrapolate that to the epileptic process. I'm not sure, because as far as I am concerned, part of epilepsy is the ictal period, but the other part is the aperiodic nature and other things that control, in the epileptic, the appearance and the nonappearance of those states which will allow a focus to fire. We are not beginning to touch this with the antiepileptic drugs which we have today.

Dr. Hockman: When you mentioned that Dilantin was a good anti-arrhythmic agent, I remembered that Dr. Mauck and I showed, a few years ago, that this drug also abolishes centrally induced ventricular arrhythmias in both cats and dogs.

Chapter 14

Closing Comments

Dr. Ebbe Curtis Hoff: The idea of chapter 14 is not to have a summary of what we have done, because this symposium in itself has been a summarizing and critical evaluation. We thought that we would ask Jack French, Stewart Wolf and Paul Yakovlev briefly to do one or both of two things: either to say a few words about where our field should go, what are the profitable directions ahead or to ask one or two questions to make sure that we draw together what has been said. In that order, I have asked Jack, Stewart and Paul to do this.

I

John D. French

I think it was a wise decision not to attempt to summarize this splendid meeting. So much essential information has been presented which is of a summary nature itself that it would be anticlimactic to attempt such an additional summation. My own contribution, if it may be called that, will be to call attention to what I am taking away from this conference, in terms of my own interests. I am a physician, and I suppose it is logical for us to attempt to apply information a little more than those among you who are primarily basic scientists. To me, the great carry-home item from this meeting will be a better awareness of what all this means to medicine, and it means a lot. I have been interested for a long time in the gastrointestinal tract and more recently in the cardiovascular system as it is influenced by the central nervous system. I think that the great failing of medicine in the past is that it has not recognized that most of the visceral ailments to which man is subject are dependent on the nervous system, either as the primary cause or as a contributory cause. I am perfectly sure, for example, that 75 percent of man's disorders are going to get worse now that man is being herded in ever larger numbers into cities and subjected to invasion of privacy, environmental pollution and other stresses to which he must be exposed in an urban setting. We are going to have to expect, therefore, that the elements of stress which normally manifest themselves through the anatomical pathways that Walle told us about and the physiological mechanisms that Pierre and Orlando and others described are going to be evermore a part of the practice of medicine, and any solutions to these problems are going to come from a better understanding of these mechanisms.

Perhaps it is relevant to mention just a few of these. Cardiac arrest is a very common tragedy which occurs in the operating room and at the dinner table, and this is quite understandable to me in terms of the neural mechanisms which were discussed here. Stewart will probably talk about this more.

Mental hospitals are full of patients with temporal lobe seizures or limbic system discharges. In patients with implanted electrodes being studied for temporal lobe epilepsy, my colleagues have seen that depths of the brain, such as the amygdala and perhaps the hippocampus, may exhibit a veritable storm of electrical activity while the rest of the brain is little disturbed. This seizure activity may be undetectable on the cortex or in other regions of the brain. Some of these patients exhibit unusual behavior at the time. Others show nothing at all in terms of behavioral abnormalities in spite of this discharging pattern in regions in which we have been particularly interested here. Some patients with schizophrenia show firing patterns in the septal region about which Orlando spoke. We have a lot to look forward to, therefore, in terms of finding medical handles vitally important in correcting such malfunction in the limbic and related systems. The searching investigation you discussed here provide a springboard to a better understanding of these mechanisms.

I can offer one more illustration of an important contribution that material presented at this conference can make to society and that is in its application to man's intense preoccupation with some of the remarkable new environments to which he is subjecting himself. First, in space, our NASA program has been planned largely on the basis that man will be his own experimental subject in assessing his ability to accommodate to exposures to space environments. The animal program which has been planned has been trivial in terms of the total manned effort. To me, this disregard of animal studies is wrong because most of the important information required cannot be obtained on man alone. It is not possible to apply internal sensors in astronauts to find out the autonomic consequences to cardiovascular function of a column of blood which weighs nothing in outer space. I cannot imagine that in outer space, a full but weightless stomach will produce the same satiety that it does on earth or that a full bladder which does not compress the pelvic floor will have a normal effect. I am impressed by the fact that under 1 g these visceral afferents are constantly bombarding the brain with physiological controls which will not be available in outer space, and I cannot imagine that the brain which was designed to work under circumstances in which gravity plays an important part will permit it to function in the same way that it does on earth. I think, therefore, we are in for trouble. I think that man's internal milieu must have a lot of support for these extended excursions, support which must be developed through such studies as those described here and not exclusively by clinical observation.

The same comments can be made in connection with our invasion of the depths of the sea. Man is going down to the sea in suits, not ships, to live there for periods of three months to a year. It is too difficult to send him down in one day and bring him back on the same day; yet these mechanisms that have been talked about at this symposium are all going to be sharply distorted in the underwater environment. Since we are going to be spending billions of dollars on these two enterprises, the problem of economics must be added to those of public health, medicine, environmental physiology and science.

Much attention will be paid to the subject of this conference in the decade to come, hence it is very timely that information summarized and discussed at this symposium shall be available to the new era of medicine, space and the sea.

II

Stewart Wolf

Among important things emphasized at this conference was the need to disentangle ourselves from the toils of conventional categorical thinking. Dr. Yakovlev referred to the way one's nervous system is set by the prevailing attitudes of the establishment. We have learned that one long-established dogma, the distinction between visceral and general behavior, is highly artificial. The responses of smooth muscles and glands depend on the same enteroceptive and exteroceptive networks as do the responses of the skeletal muscles. Moreover, the circuits that integrate the information and formulate somatic and visceral responses reverberate among the same forebrain and midbrain structures. Finally, the discrete, patterned and purposeful responses often involve both visceral and somatic structures working together.

The misleading conceptual separation of the autonomic from the somatic nervous system may have been due in part to the extraordinary intrinsic capability of the viscera not only to function but to some extent to adapt. Such visceral virtuosity diverted the attention of physiologists from the study of the hierarchy of regulatory mechanisms in the central nervous system.

Social behavior, like the behavior of organs, is modified by neural events in the limbic system. Moreover, life experiences contribute to the programming of visceral as well as social responses, and I suppose that this is the basic trend of psychosomatic medicine. Lucretius is quoted as saying, "I am a part of all that I have seen." That may be true, but for our purposes today it would be more appropriate to say, "All that I have seen is a part of me."

Perhaps there is a therapeutic implication here. In something like a setting of operant conditioning the reinforcement, instead of the promise of candy, may be the hope that things are going to get better.

In the ultimate regulation of the person and his various bodily equipment, inhibitory modulation appears to be important to the structures innervated by autonomic nerves as it does to those innervated by somatic nerves. It is evident that blocking of synaptic transmission may occur at almost any site from sensory nerve to various levels of the neuraxis concerned with perception, interpretation and response. The importance of epitome has been emphasized. When it was pointed out that in 1891 most of the nuclei had been seen and identified in the limbic structures, but that understanding had to await interpretation, I was reminded of Charles

Richet who got the Nobel Prize in 1913 for discovering anaphylaxis. Actually, he did not discover anaphylaxis. It had been known for a long time that one might die from a second injection of something, but Richet epitomized or interpreted the phenomenon. What has gone on at this meeting is certainly, in a way, a step toward the same goal. The comment Dr. Hockman made after I mentioned our experiment in which ventricular premature contractions were suppressed during mental concentration is particularly relevant here. He invoked the possibility of forebrain inhibition of autonomic reflexes. I was reminded that we have other indirect evidence of inhibitory damping of autonomic reflexes. In experiments in which we attempted to manipulate the amplitude of sinus arrhythmia, we found that the range of heart rate variation was greatly reduced during intense mental concentration and increased during anxiety or mental confusion. The inhibitory effect would suggest a principle of economy in a busy brain. With the human computer hard at work, any excess input, either exteroceptive or interoceptive, may be regarded as noise and therefore shut out. The tendency to shut out irrelevant information is illustrated by some experiments of a colleague of mine, Dr. Robert A. Schneider. He has been studying adaptation to smell with a very accurately quantified odor delivery system. Odors at threshold are turned off very quickly. When the quantity of the same odor is raised slightly, it is extinguished even more quickly, and so on, until finally the odor is turned off so quickly that it is hardly smelled at all. Schneider found adaptation impaired in the presence of anxiety.

It would appear from all this that the integrative process in which the limbic system shares is a matter of algebra where past experience, state of attentiveness, motivation, mood and preoccupations become letters in the formula that determines behavioral response.

III

Paul I. Yakovlev

A PROPOSED DEFINITION OF THE LIMBIC SYSTEM

First I want to briefly pay tribute to James W. Papez. There are still many of us who have known and remember him personally. A dedicated and humble man, he built himself a lasting monument, unbeknownst to himself as it were. Papez' concept of the limbic system, as it is known at present, was not a hypothesis. It was a statement of an empirical generalization, highly original and personal to him.

A hypothesis, to be a scientifically relevant one, is constructed always in terms of some accepted notion of what is true. It is proposed in the framework of a prevailing theory of reality and is tested by experiment. Should the experiment contradict the hypothesis, a new hypothesis is then formulated in different terms, yet always in the framework of some accepted theory of reality. Should the statement conform to the prevailing theory of what is true, it is then no more than a banality. However, should the empirical generalization contradict the theory, it is then either a delusion or a discovery!

Papez' generalization was a discovery. In his now classic article [40] of 1937, he humbly proposed, and at some calculated risk, that "emotions" have an anatomical "mechanism," and he marshaled evidence for the location of the mechanism in the brain. This empirical generalization contradicted the notion widely accepted in his time, that experience so exquisitely "mental," as are "emotions," are a preserve of psychology and that a generalization proposing an anatomical mechanism was a delusion.

For a whole decade, Papez' article remained unnoticed. It was Paul MacLean [33-36] who brought the significance of Papez' idea to the attention of clinicians and physiologists. Since then, Papez' empirical generalization has become itself a theory of the limbic system. It provided the framework for scientific hypotheses and for important discoveries of new facts of anatomy and physiology of the brain. This symposium attests to the fruition of an inspired idea.

To summarize the information received during these three days requires more thought than is possible ex promptu. One naturally tends to fit new facts and ideas into the framework of one's own experience and conception of the limbic system. Some delusions tend to creep into any generalization. My generalization cannot be free of them. At some risk, therefore, I would like to outline the framework.

The objective of this discussion is to outline a concept of the organization of the body as a biological action system, of the brain as the hub of this system and of behavior as bodily movements within and outside the system. I will propose a tectogenetic definition of the limbus of the hemisphere and of the limbic system in the framework of this concept. For the sake of candor as much as for the sake of brevity, I will dispense with discussion of the literature and will cite the sources by reference only.

1. The Symmetries of the Body and of the Brain

One is often admonished to envisage the organism "as a whole." Yet it is difficult to study the organism as if it were—in Lorenz'[32] humorous expression—some kind of "holistic jelly"! The empirical representation of a living organism is inherently tripartite.[66] It has a "body" and occupies a finite, structured and symmetrical space, distinct from the nonfinite, wide open and dyssymmetrical space, outside the closed space occupied by the body. It has texture, external form and species-specific internal symmetries. It consists of three systems of organs: the visceral organs within the body hollow, the somatic organs of the body wall and the brain, a hollow viscus within the head, leading the body and, in a sense, leading also the world about the body.[11]

The three systems of organs differentiate in an orderly topological sequence, each from its own germinal layer in the wall of the blastocyst: the entoderm, the mesoderm, and the neuro-ectoderm (Fig. 14–1,A).[1,15,28] These three germinal layers of the blastocyst are recapitulated in the corresponding topological sequence by the matrix, the mantle and the marginal layers of the wall of the neural tube (Fig. 14–1,B).[22]

Each system of organs arises in its own cephalocaudal axis in the median ventrodorsal plane of the bilateral symmetry of the vertebrate body.[42] These three axes are the primitive gut or *visceral* axis, the

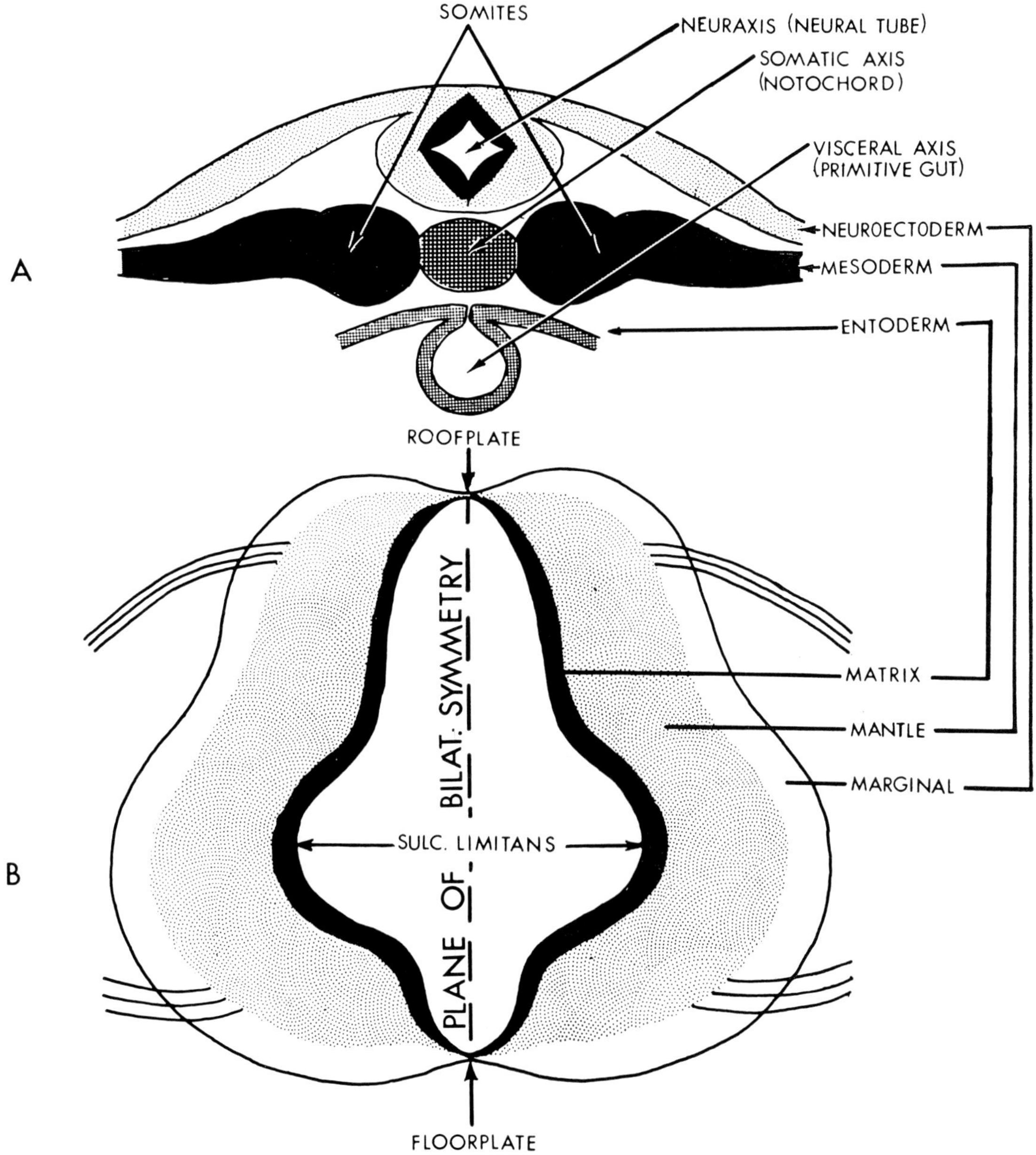

Figure 14–1. (*A*) Three germinal layers of von Baer [1] in the wall of the blastocyst represented schematically in cross section at right angle to the plane of bilateral symmetry and to the three cardinal axes of cephalocaudal polarization of the vertebrate body. (*B*) Recapitulation of the three germinal layers of von Baer in the wall of the neural tube by the three zones of His.[22]

notochord or *somatic* axis, and the neural tube or *neuraxis proper*, represented by the metameric brain stem and spinal cord.

The organization of the three systems of organs may be defined in terms of the topological symmetries [53] of three orders: (a) the *ablateral* or azygous symmetry, such as that of a cylinder which has an

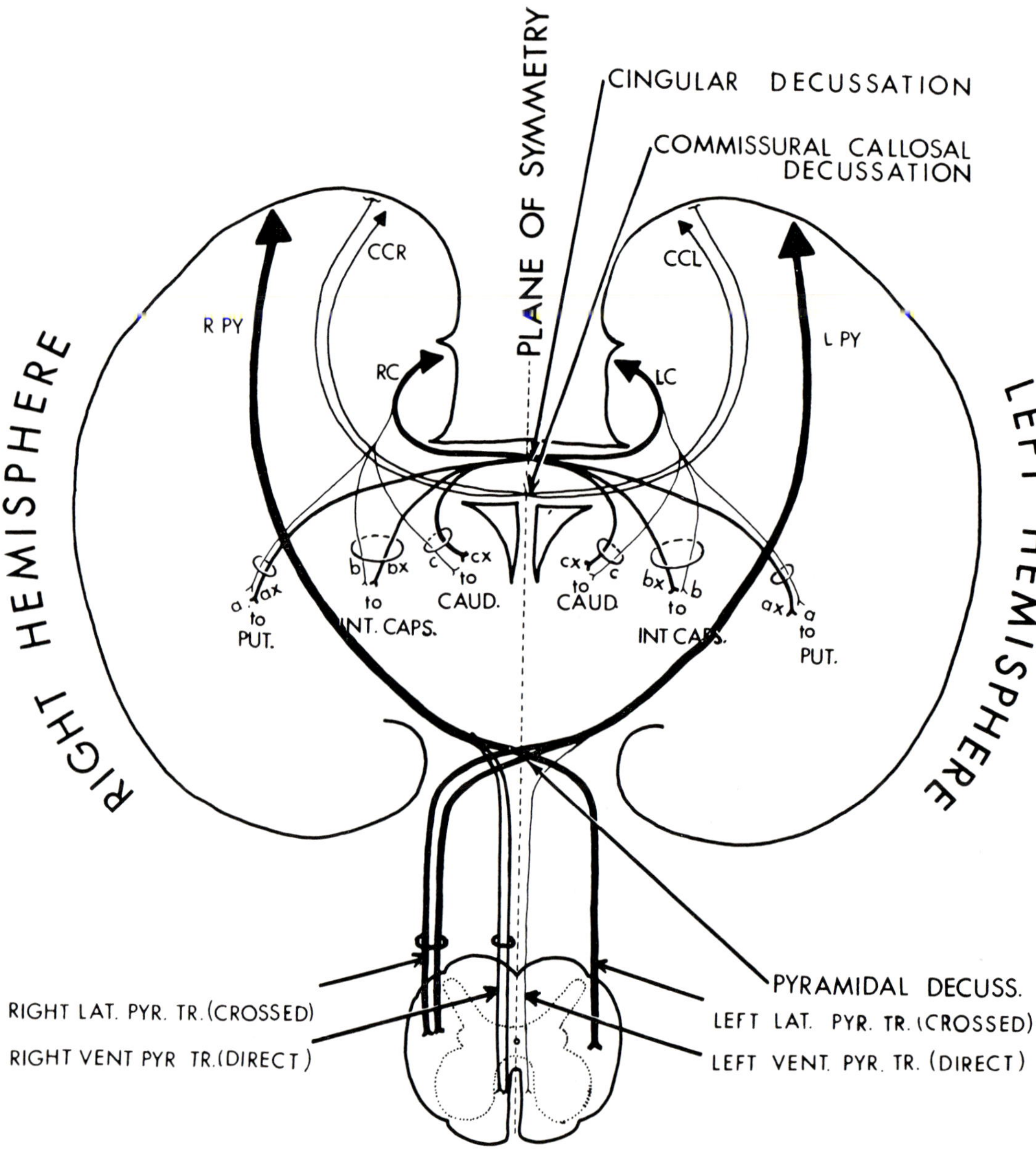

Figure 14–2. Schematic representation of the principle of the double spiral (helicoid) symmetry [53] of the "commissures" and of the "decussations" of the long corticofugal fiber systems from the *limbic* and from the *supralimbic* divisions of the hemispheres proper. *Abbreviations:* CCL and CCR—commissural (callosal) fibers from the *supralimbic* divisions of the hemispheres crossing the "geometric" median plane in the corpus callosum ("commissural" decussations). LC and RC—cingular projection fibers from the left and from the right *limbic* divisions of the hemispheres and their collaterals: *a, b, c* to the ipsilateral caudatum, internal capsule and putamen; *ax, bx* and *cx* to contralateral caudatum, internal capsule and putamen ("transcallosal" cingular decussations). LPY and RPY—pyramidal (corticospinal) fibers from the *special heterotypical* ("motor") areas of the left and of the right *supralimbic* divisions of the hemispheres to the neuraxis proper. Note that each hemisphere projects corticospinal fibers to *both* sides of the spinal cord with an assymmetrical torque skewed preferentially to the right side. In the case of man, this is a statistical constant in approximately 80 percent of adult individuals. (See further, section 6 and Figure 14–14A and B.)

axis but no plane of symmetry of its own; (b) the *bilateral* symmetry, such as that of enantiomorphic crystals—that is, one which has the axis and the plane; and (c) the *spiral* symmetry of a double helix, lateralized with a torque turned on its axis two ways, clockwise and counter-clockwise, such as the symmetry of the double-threaded shaft of a power drill.

In these terms, the visceral organs, arising from the entoderm in the axis of primitive gut, are azygous, *ablateral* organs. The somatic organs of the body wall, arising from the mesoderm of the paired somites in the axis of the notochord, are *bilateral* organs (skeletal musculature); and the central nervous system, arising in the axis of the neural tube, presents symmetries which in the case of the *neuraxis proper* (the brain stem and the spinal cord) is an outspoken bilateral symmetry of the neuromeres, which reflects and duplicates the bilateral symmetry of the somatomeres of the body wall. However, in the case of the *forebrain*, the symmetry, presented by the commissures and decussations of major fiber systems of the forebrain, is conspicuously that of a double helix turned on the cephalocaudal axis clockwise and counterclockwise (Fig. 14–2).

The forebrain is the hub of the three cardinal cephalocaudal axes of the vertebrate body: the visceral and somatic axes and the neuraxis. I shall outline briefly the morphogenesis of the forebrain, and I will attempt to correlate the three orders of symmetries in the structure and functions of the three systems of organs.

2. Morphogenesis of the Forebrain

The morphogenesis of the forebrain is radically different from that of the neuraxis proper.[2,10,27,30] The latter, developing in the caudal part of the neural tube is coextensive with the notochord (Figs. 14–3, A and B). It has a floor plate, a roof plate and bilaterally symmetrical, *aboriginally paired,* basal and alar plates. Accordingly, the brain stem and spinal cord, developing in this "epichordal" part of the neural tube, present the *aboriginal* bilateral symmetry. In contrast, the forebrain which arises in the "praechordal" part of the neural tube overlying the foregut (stomadeum), has no floor plate, and its roof plate extends cephalad over the thalamus only to the conventional border between the latter and the endbrain. (Figs. 14–3, A, and 14–4C). Accordingly, the bilateral symmetry of the forebrain is of a radically different order than that of the neuraxis proper. The forebrain arises in the median head process in the *visceral* axis from a median, *originally ablateral* prosencephalic brain vesicle. (Fig. 14–4A and B). The paired hemispheres, corpora striata and thalami assume only later a *secondary,* purely "positional," symmetry in relation to the bilateral osmic, optic and statoacoustic sensory placodes of the head process. The septal area and the primitive hippocampus from which the hemispheres expand bilaterad (Fig. 14–4,C) remain median, ablateral structures (Fig. 14–5).[57,65]

The forebrain, the hollow viscus in the head, is divisible on morphological grounds into three zones: the median, nonpaired (azygous) zone *between* the hemispheres and the paired *limbic* and the *supralimbic* zones, bilaterad in each hemisphere (Fig. 14–6).[65] The hemispheres proper are defined by the cortical plate (neocortex, isocortex) which covers each hemisphere and has sharp, clearly definable borders with the median zone. The median zone *has no cortical plate.*

The median zone, or telencephalon "impar" (Fig. 14–5),[23] comprises the olfactory

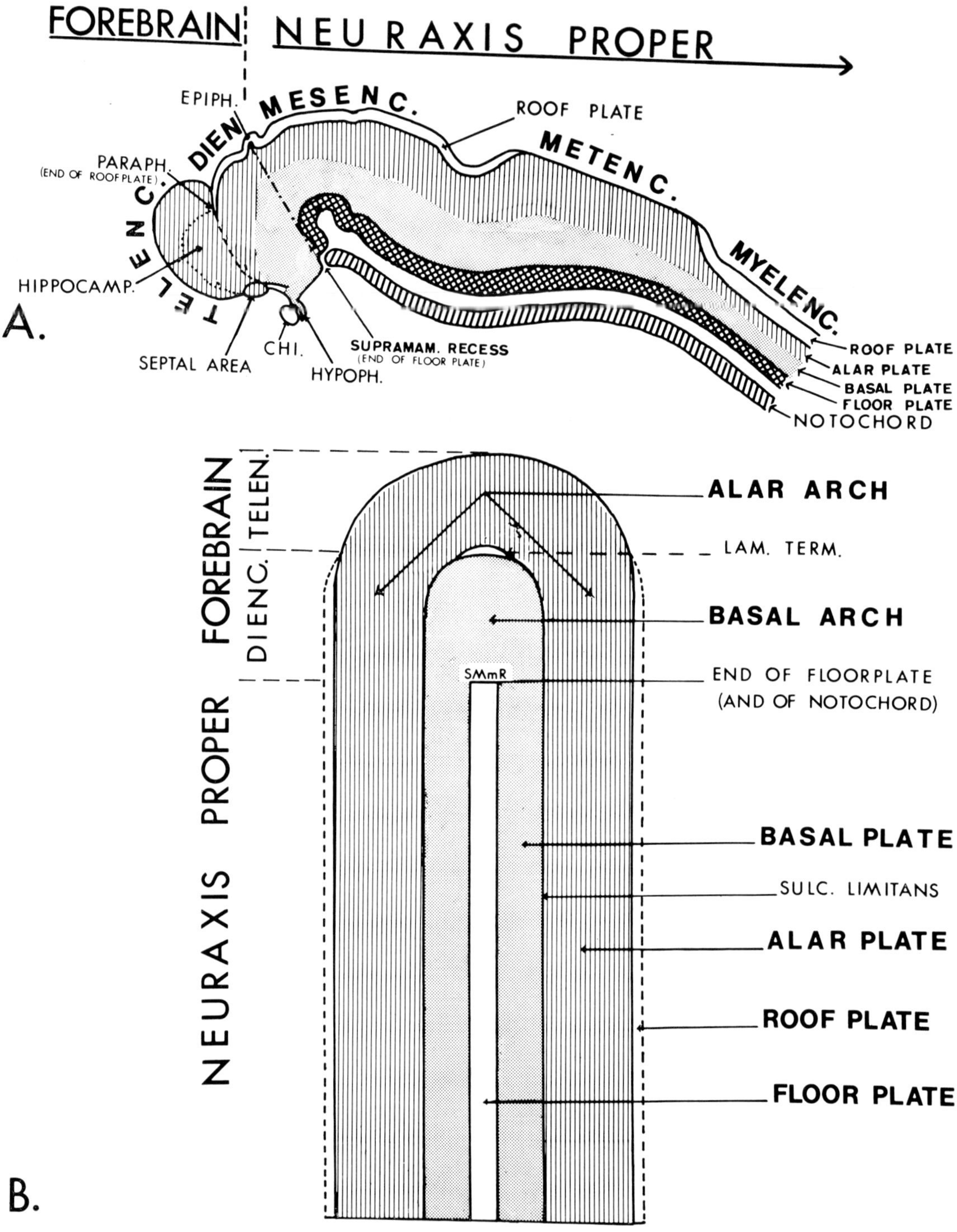

Figure 14–3. (*A*) Neural tube (the forebrain and the neuraxis proper) is represented in sagittal (median ventrodorsal) plane (redrawn and modified from Kingsbury[27]). The neuraxis proper is coextensive with the notochord. The forebrain is at nearly a right angle to the neuraxis due to the mesencephalic flexure. The floor plate (cross-hatching) ends at about the level of the supramammillary recess (SMmR in B). The basal plate (fine stipple) extends to about the level of the chiasmatic ridge. (Chi) and lamina terminalis. The alar plates (vertical lines) join in a continuous alar arch (see B) dorsal →

lobes, the septal area (Figs. 14–7, A and B) and the hippocampus which includes the paired Ammon's horns.[65] The Ammon's horns bracket the thalamus bilaterad.[64] The hippocampus differs radically in its origin, development and structure from the hemisphere proper. [13,14,43] The *limbic* zone in the *borders* of each hemisphere (hence, "limbic") comprises the corpora striata and white matter of the *centrum semiovale* (Fig. 14–8, see Note 1). The massive *supralimbic* zone of the paired hemispheres covers (opercularizes) the limbic zones and is separated everywhere from the telencephalon impar by the intervening limbic zones (Fig. 14–6) and so represents the telencephalon "totopar." [65] This latter zone of each hemisphere comprises the conventional "lobes" of the hemispheres (Figs. 14–7, A and B) and consists of the intricately folded cortical plate (mantle, pallium) (see Note 2) and white matter of the *corona radiata* (Fig. 14–8) (see Note 3).

Each of these three zones, the median or *"impar,"* the limbic or *"semipar,"* and the supralimbic or *"totopar"* zones (Fig. 14–6) [65] are clearly distinguishable one from the other on definitive morphogenetic and on cyto- and myelo-architectonic criteria.

The limbic division of the hemisphere is, on morphological grounds, a cerebral "lobe" in its own right. (Figs. 14–7, A and B). The corpora striata which represent the core of the limbic lobes of the hemispheres proper (Fig. 14–12A and B) are continuous with the septal area and with the basal gray matter of the olfactory lobes of the telencephalon impar. The limbic lobes represent the incompletely paired telencephalon "semipar." [65] The cingular and parahippocampal gyri (Fig. 14–7,A) represent together the dorsomedial and posterior "limbus" of the "epihippocampal" part of each hemisphere (Fig. 14–9, A and B) (see Note 4). This border is coextensive with the hippocampus ("archicortex").[13] The uncus (Fig. 14–7,A), the insula (Fig. 14–7,B) and the orbital border of the hemisphere (Figs. 14–7, A and B; 14–9, A and B) represent together the ventrolateral and anterior "limbus" of the "epistriatal" part of each hemisphere (see Note 5). This border is coextensive with the olfactory lobe (paleocortex).[13] The para-olfactory lobule of Broca (Fig. 14–7,A), adjacent to the septal area, and the uncus of the parahippocampal gyrus, adjacent to the Ammon's horn (Fig. 14–7,A), represent the zones of junction of the ventrolateral (epistriatal) with the dorsomedial (epihippocampal) sectors of the annular limbic lobe of each hemisphere; the striatum is comparable to the "signet" of this limbic ring.

The cortical plate (neocortex) of each hemisphere develops in the phylogeny of mammals *between* the olfactory lobe (paleocortex) and the hippocampus (archicortex) (Fig. 14–5). The deep layers (V and VI) of the cortical plate in the

to lamina terminalis (LAM. TERM. in B). (*B*) Neural tube is represented as if it were opened through the roof plate and spread bilaterad in one plane. Note the rostral extent of the floor plate (overlying the notochord) which defines the extent of the "epichordal" part of the neural tube or the neuraxis proper. Rostral to the floor plate, the paired basal and alar plates form in the forebrain two concentric arches demarcated by the sulcus limitans. Sulcus limitans between the basal and alar plates terminates at about the level of the telodiencephalic junction. The hypothalamus arises from the basal arch of the forebrain tube. The dorsal thalamus and the *entire* telencephalon arise from the alar arch.

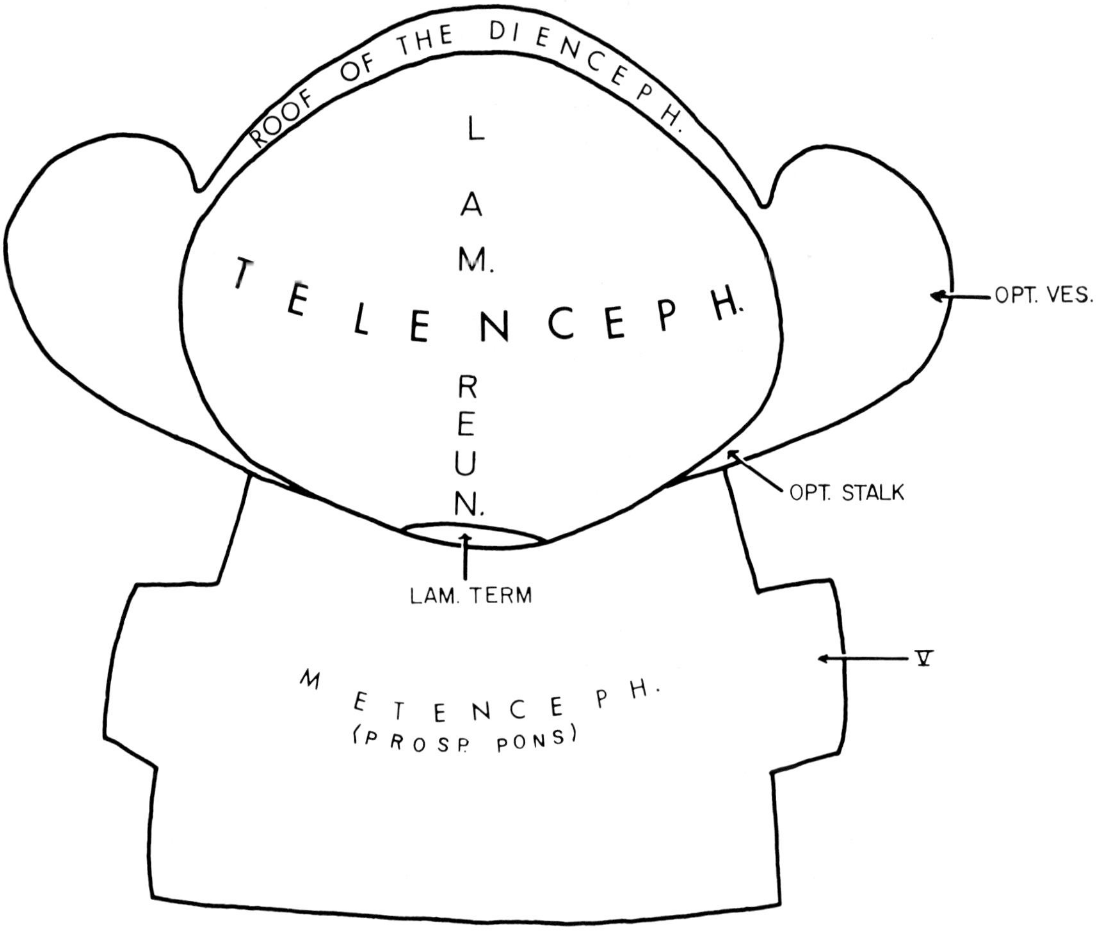

Figure 14–4A. The anterior and slightly dorsal aspect of the forebrain of a 3.5 mm human embryo redrawn and somewhat modified from Hochstetter's atlas [23] to show that at this early stage the telencephalic vesicle is a median, spherical outpocketing of the alar arch of the prosencephalon, between the paired optic vesicles, rostral to the roof of the diencephalon, and dorsal to the lamina terminalis (LAM. TERM.). The lamina reuniens (LAM. REUN.) corresponds topologically to the median region of the telencephalic holosphere. The relative positions of the prospective septal ventrad area and of the hippocampus dorsad in the lamina reuniens, and of the paired corpora striata and cerebral hemispheres bilaterad from it, can be indicated approximately. All these formations exist at this stage only *in potentiam*.

borders of the hemispheres proper blend, on the one hand with the gray matter of the olfactory lobe in the banks of the *sulcus rhinalis* (Fig. 14–10,A) and on the other hand with the hippocampal plate of the subiculum (Fig. 14–10, B and C).[13,14,43] However, the superficial layers II, III, IV of the cortical plate attenuate along these boundaries in a sharp, clinoid border and disappear over the olfactory lobe and over the hippocampus (Figs. 14–10, A, B, C and D).[13,14] This clinoid border of the superficial layers of the *isocortex* (neocortex) provides a clear cytoarchitectonic boundary with the telencephalon impar and defines the *limbus* ("limes isocor-

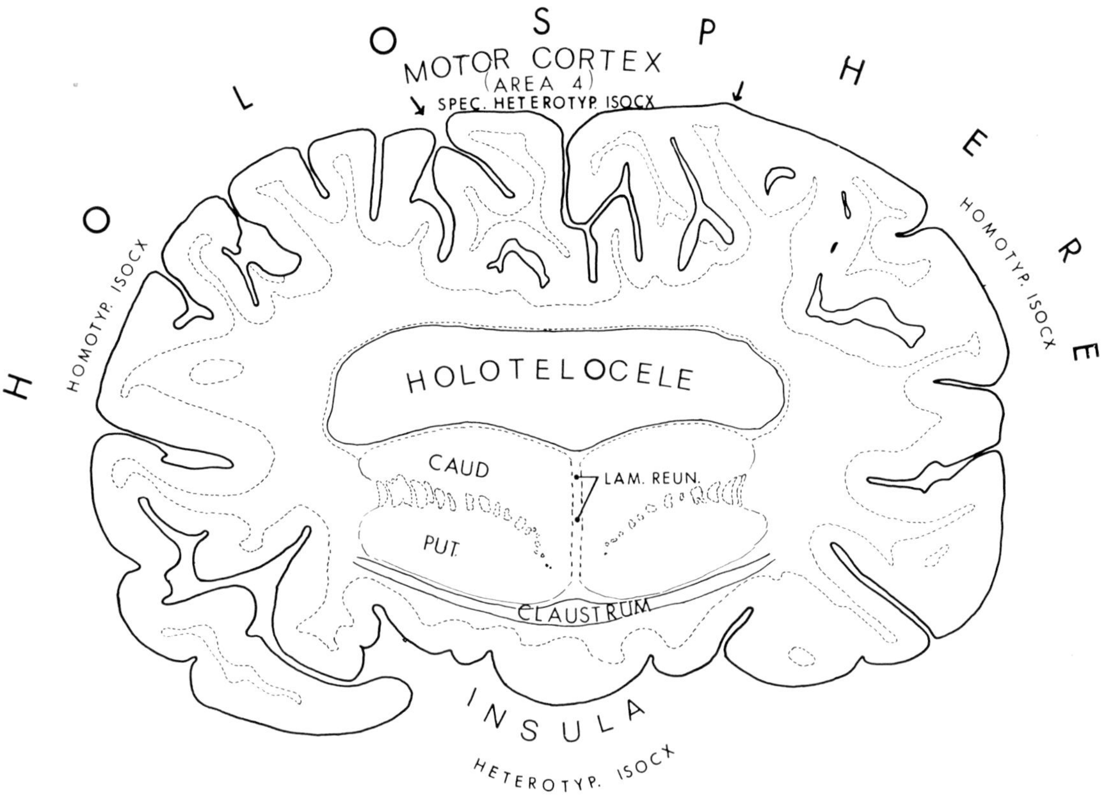

Figure 14–4B. Outline of the transwerse section of the malformed end-brain of an otherwise well-formed 3-year-old arrhinencephalic boy in whom the paired hemispheres proper failed to cleave from the primary median (nonpaired) telencephalic holosphere (see Fig. 14–4A) and a *holotelencephaly* resulted. Such malformations are common and are convincing morphogenetic evidence of the fundamental *ablaterality* and of a merely positional bilateral symmetry of the paired hemispheres. (For details on this type of malformations, see reference 57.)

ticalis")[13] of the hemisphere proper (see Note 6).

The neocortex covering the limbic division of each hemisphere is a *heterotypical* cortex (Figs. 14–7, A and B).[12] It intervenes between and is transitional from the telencephalon impar or "entocortex" (see Note 7) to the cortex covering the phyletically more recent supralimbic (totopar) division of each hemisphere. The limbic cortex, or "mesocortex" (see Note 7), differs in structure from the *special* heterotypical[12] cortex of the specific *projection* areas (kinesthetic, somesthetic, acoustic and visual) of the supralimbic division and from the *homotypical*[12] cortex ("ectocortex")[55] (see Note 7) of the nonspecific *"association"* areas surrounding the projection areas of this division of each hemisphere (Fig. 14–7).

It is significant that the areas of the special heterotypical cortex (projection areas) are continuous in a gradual architectonic transition with the heterotypical cortex of the limbic division. On the contrary, they are demarcated by sharp architectonic boundaries from the homotypical "association" areas bordering on them in

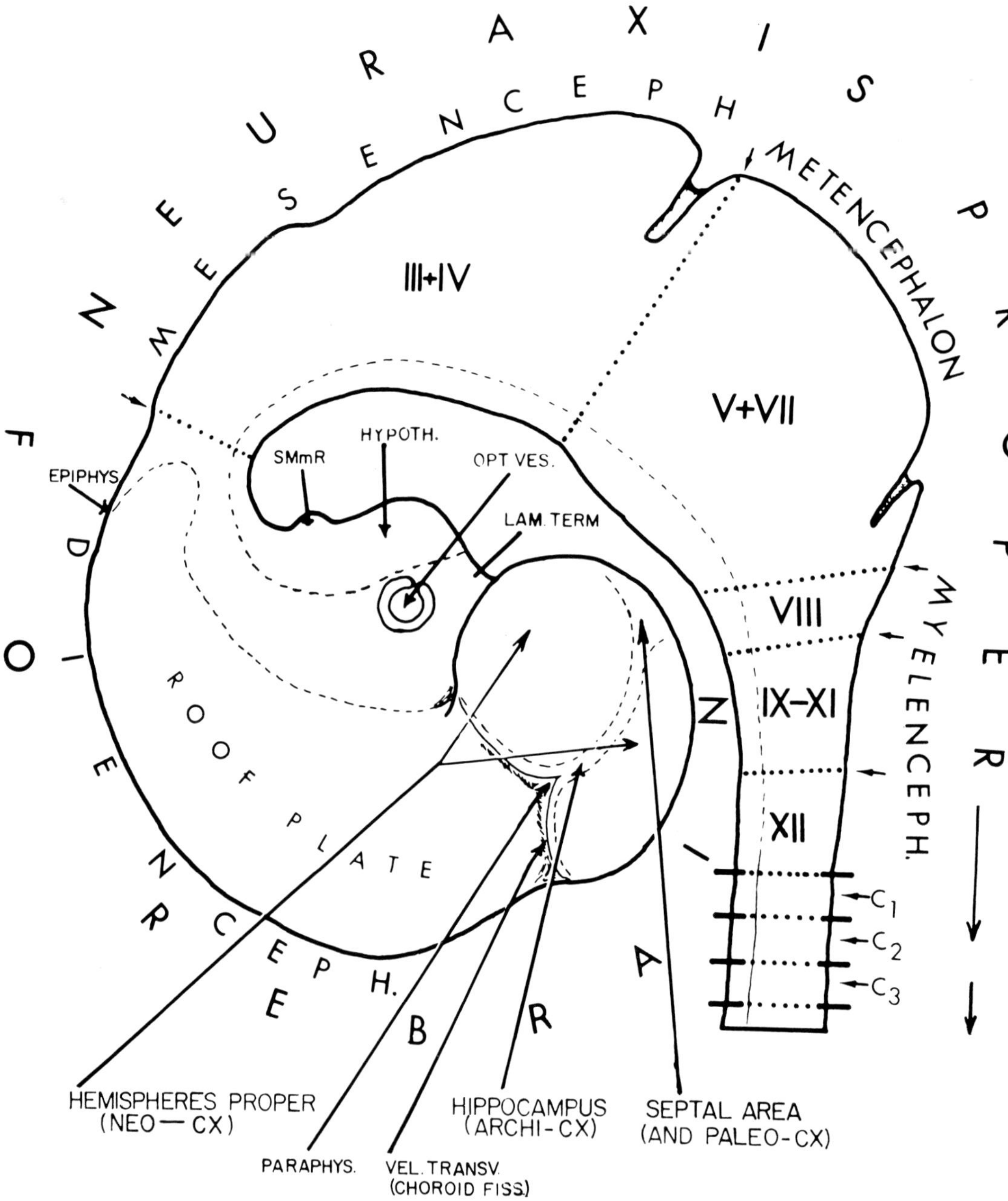

Figure 14–4C. The forebrain and the metameric neuraxis proper (highly schematic) of an embryo of 7 to 10 mm, to show the early stage of cleavage of the paired hemispheres proper ("neocortex" and striatum), bilaterad from the lamina reuniens (see at A LAM. REUN.), which represents the prospective *septal area* and *olfactory* cortex ("paleo-cortex") and the prospective *hippocampus* ("archicortex").

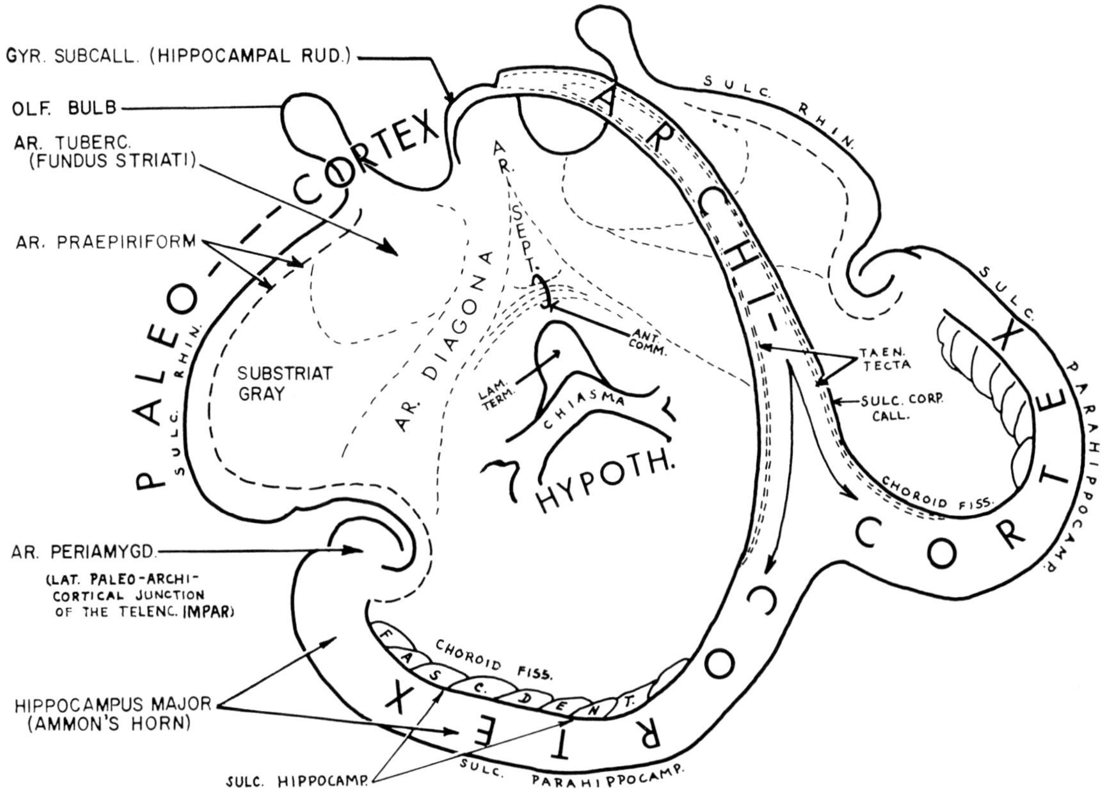

Figure 14–5. Outline of the olfactory lobes ("paleocortex") and septal area and of the hippocampus ("archicortex"), the latter bifurcated into paired Ammon's horns with their dentate gyri to show the topographic relationships (primordial continuity) between the olfactory and the hippocampal formations of the median telencephalic zone ("rhinencephalon" of old nomenclature) as they would be visualized if the hemispheres proper, corpora striata and thalami bilaterad, between these "ancient" (Gr. *paleos*) and "old" (Gr. *archeos*) formations, were "not visible." (From author's pencil sketch used by Mr. Obaya to illustrate Figure 3 of Jacobs, Morgane and McFarland's publication [26]).

the supralimbic divisions.[12,14,43] This is in accord with the other phylogenetic and ontogenetic evidence [43,45,46,57] that the areas of special heterotypical cortex are phyletic elaborations of the limbic heterotypical cortex and are shifted bilaterad, away from the hippocampus, as the neocortex expands in mammals from the telencephalon *impar* (hippocampus and olfactory lobe) of all vertebrates and forms the supralimbic, *totopar* division of the paired hemispheres in primates (Figs. 14–6 and 14–11).

The homotypical association areas, surrounding the specific projection areas, become specially developed in anthropoid apes and man. These areas may be regarded as the elaborations of the neocortex, "supplemental" to the special heterotypical projection areas which are present in all mammals. In man the areas of homotypical cortex are asymmetrical and exhibit the widest *individual* variations in structure, topography and surface extent in the two hemispheres.[27] The nonsymmetries of the paired *hemi*spheres proper

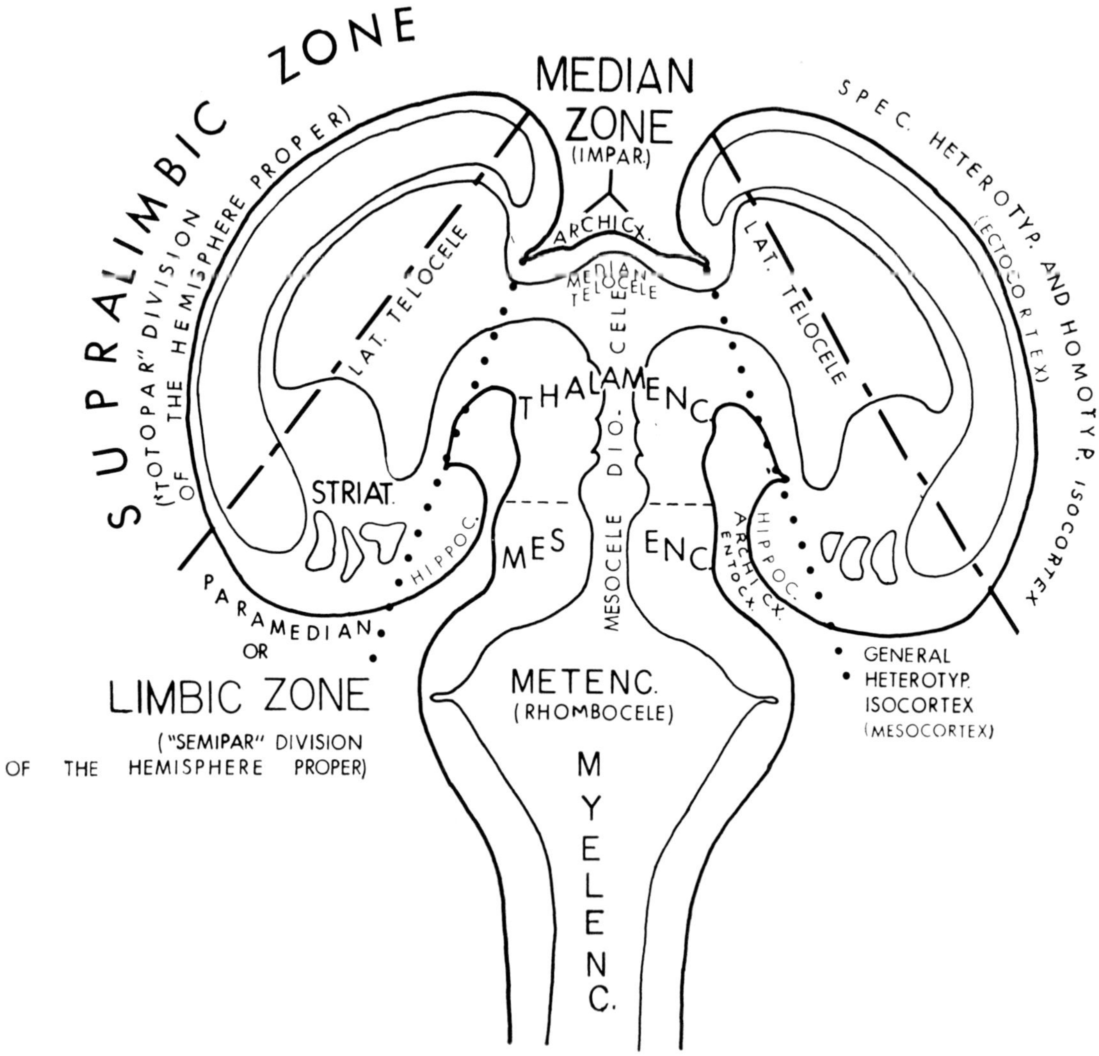

Figure 14–6. Schematic representation of the forebrain and of the cephalic part of the neuraxis proper in the latero-lateral plane to show the topological disposition and topographic sequence of the three cardinal tectogenetic and architectonic zones of the endbrain (from within out): the median telencephalon "impar" between the hemispheres proper, the partially paired ("semipar") *limbic* divisions of the two hemispheres and the completely paired ("totopar") *supralimbic* divisions of the hemispheres proper, bilaterad from the median telencephalon "impar."

is a strong evidence that they arise from the primordial nonpaired *holosphere* (see Note 8) (Figs. 14–4A, 4B and 4C) and each follows its own program of evolution, development and function.[56,65] They assume *secondarily* the positional symmetry of the two *hemi*spheres as a result of the bilateral (paired) but *nonsymmetrical* evaginations from the azygous telencephalon impar (Fig. 14–6). The praechordal forebrain, developing in the axis of the foregut and stomadeum, presents (even as the other visceral organs arising in the axis of the primitive gut) no plane of the *aboriginal* morphogenetic symmetry comparable to that of the neuraxis proper.[65] It is an *ablateral,* hollow viscus.

In the framework of this definition of the forebrain, I will define the morphological and functional symmetries of the three divisions of the forebrain and of the three systems of organs.

3. The Three Neuropils of the Forebrain

Three neuropils differentiate in the wall of the embryonal forebrain in an orderly temporal sequence from within outward [56,66] (Figs. 14–12, A and B): (a) the deep, *reticulate,* periventricular neuropil develops in the zone corresponding to the former embryonal matrix in relation to the entoderm and visceral organs; (b) the intermediate, *nucleated* neuropil develops in the zone of the former mantle layer in relation to the mesoderm and somatic organs of the body wall; and (c) the superficial, *stratilaminate* neuropil, or cortical plate (palium) (see Note 2), develops in the zone of transition between the mantle and the marginal layers, in relation to the bilateral sensory organs of the head region, skin and muscles.

Each neuropil of the forebrain has its own *telencephalic* division.[55,58,65,66] The deep, reticulate neuropil is continuous without architectonic demarcation with the septal area of the telencephalon impar. This division of the endbrain may be regarded as the headmost extension of the "reticular formation" in the core of the forebrain and brain stem. Similarly, the intermediate, nucleated neuropil is continuous with the limbic division of each hemisphere represented by the superficial, stratilaminate neuropil (*mesocortex*) in the borders of the hemispheres and by the striatum (Fig. 14–12,A). In primates, this heterotypical cortex of the limbic division of each hemisphere extends in a gradient of architectonic transition (see above) into the special heterotypical *projection* areas and *homotypical* association areas of the supralimbic (totopar) division of the paired hemispheres.[12,14,43,46,58,65]

The great development of superficial neuropil and of the corona radiata of the supralimbic divisions of the cerebral hemispheres, relative to the development in length and mass of the neuraxis proper, distinguishes the human brain from the brain of the other mammals (see Note 9).[16,17] These differences increase with the complexity and range of changes effected by the individual organism in the "biosphere" (see Note 10).[16,49-51]

The three neuropils, first described by C. Judson Herrick [18] in the forebrain of the amphibia, are clearly recognizable in sections of the normal human brain. (Fig. 14–12) [55,65] Each neuropil presents a characteristic pattern of connectivity of the neurons within it, with the neurons of the other two neuropils, and with the neuraxis proper. These patterns of connectivity reflect in their development and spatial organization the topological symmetries of the respective systems of organs (see further, section 5). I will attempt to show that the functions of these three systems of organs, arising respectively in the visceral and somatic axes and in the neuraxis proper, present corresponding "stereodynamic" symmetries.

4. Symmetries of the Forebrain and of the Organs of Innervation

There are manifest symmetries in the topological organization of the three systems of organs and of the three neuropils and in the functional—that is, dynamic organization of their activities.

It is meaningful that the entoderm faces the cavity of the blastocyst; the mesoderm,

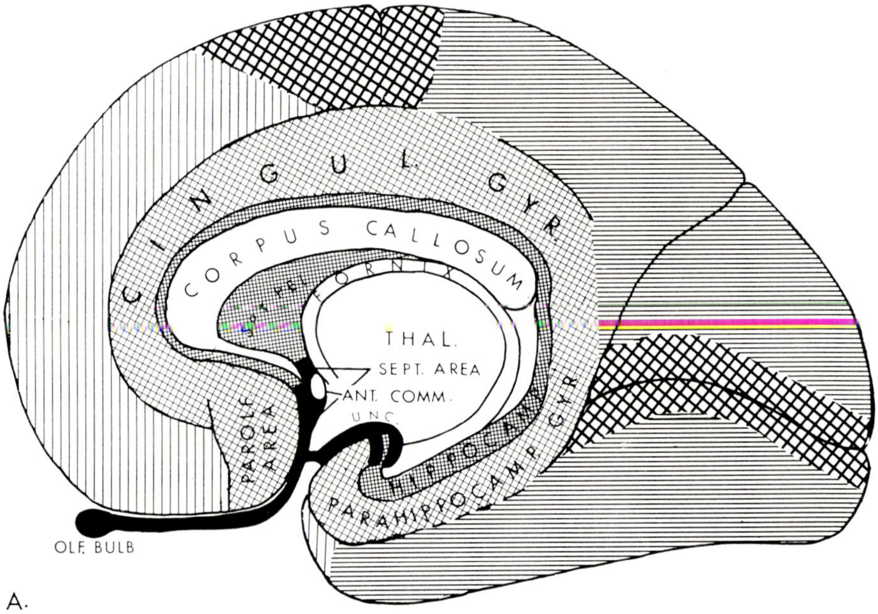

A.

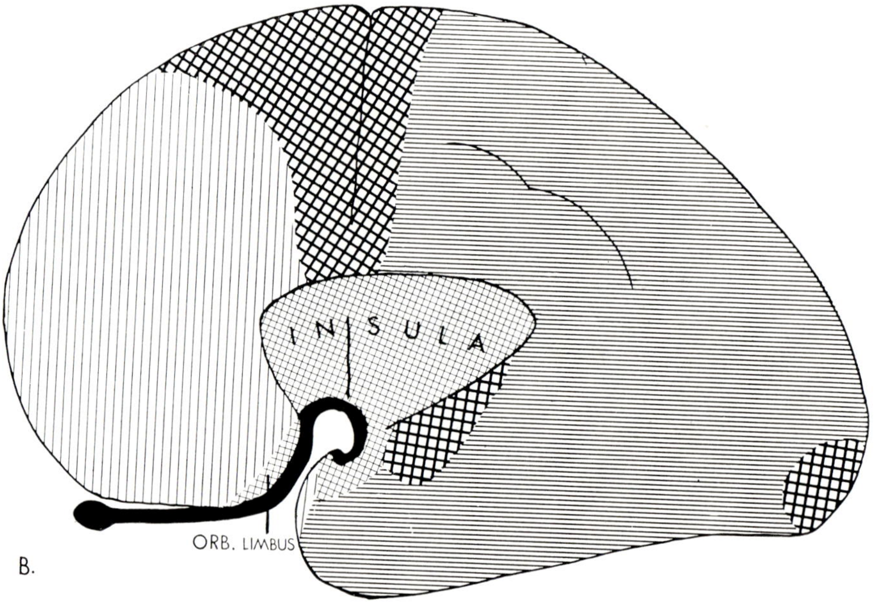

B.

Figure 14–7. Concentric disposition of the cardinal tectogenetic and architectonic zones of the endbrain, as seen on the medial (*A*) and on the lateral (*B*) aspects (highly schematized) of the cerebral hemispheres. *Symbols: Solid black*—olfactory lobe ("paelocortex"). *Closely cross-hatched*—hippocampus ("archicortex"). *Loosely cross-hatched,* in (A)—the parolfactory area and the cingular and parahippocampal gyri (with the uncus) represent the *dorsomedial* and posterior *limbus* of the hemisphere (general heterotypical isocortex or "mesocortex"); in (B)—the insula, continuous with the uncus posteriomedially and with the orbital limbus and parolfactory area anteriomedially, represents the *ventro*lateral (or baso*lateral*) and anterior limbus of the hemisphere. *Coarse cross-hatched* areas indicate the areas of the *special* heterotypical praecentral and postcentral (kinesthetic and somesthetic), calcarine (visual) and

→

interposed between the entoderm and neuro-ectoderm, faces both these layers; and the neuro-ectoderm faces the cavity of the amniotic sac. In an obvious topological relation to this spatial organization of the three germinal layers in the wall of the blastocyst, the activities of the visceral organs, facing the internal environment, are polarized "inwards," as it were, and are autonomous, *interocipient* and *interofacient* activities of cells, tissues and organs, relatively independent of the forebrain. In contrast, the activities of the somatic organs of the body wall (the skeletal musculature) "face" two ways: towards the *finite* internal and towards the *nonfinite* external fractions of the environment. Accordingly, the activities of the skeletal musculature of the body wall are "double-ended," as it were—that is, both *proprio*cipient and *extero*cipient and *proprio*facient and *extero*facient—and are governed wholly by the brain. However, the activities of the superficial neuropil of the paired hemispheres, developing in relation to the special receptors ("distance" receptors) of the head region and to the general exteroceptors and proprioceptors of the skin and muscles, are polarized mainly "outwards" towards the external environment.

The neuraxis proper (brain stem and spinal cord) intercalated as it is between the afferent and the efferent root cells, is interposed between the ablateral visceral and the bilateral somatic organs and the forebrain. It represents a cephalocaudal series of the "metameric brains"—the neuromeres, one for each somatomere. It is reared in the evolution of the vertebrates as a collection of the internuncial (central) neurons upon the afferent or private paths from the recipient surfaces (periphery) of the body and the "final common" path to the muscle, "as on two pillars." [47] On these grounds, the epichordal neuraxis may be regarded as the penultimate path common to all three neuropils of the forebrain. In this sense, the forebrain is the "hub" of all three systems of organs.

It is significant that the activities of the ablateral visceral organs, developing in the axis of the primitive gut, are ablateral *peristaltic* (see Note 11) movements. Accordingly, the activities of the telencephalon impar and of the deep neuropil in the core of the forebrain, monitored via autonomic and endocrine systems to the visceral organs, are *ablateral* ("diffuse") activities unrelated to the laterality of the position of the "target organs" within the body. In contrast to the molility of visceral organs, the activities of the bilateral somatic organs of the body wall (skeletal musculature), developing from the paired somites in the axis of the notochord, are bilateral, *diastaltic* (see Note 12) movements.

The somatic apparatus of the body is comparable to a system of symmetrical levers. Each somatomere is represented by a pair of symmetrical, mirror-image antimeres. The movements of each antimere are duplicates of each other (Fig. 14–13,A). This mechanical symmetry of movements may be called *stereokinetic* and is demonstrable even on a cadaver. The aboriginal bilateral symmetry of the neuro-

superior temporal (acoustic) cortex. All these areas are continuous in a gentle gradient of architectonic transition with the limbic (general heterotypical) cortex (mesocortex) bordering on the hippocampus and in an abrupt gradient with the homotypical *supralimbic* cortex anterior to the plane of the sulcus of Rolando (*vertically* lined areas) and posterior to that plane (*horizontally* lined areas) on the medial (in A) and the lateral (in B) aspects of the hemisphere proper.

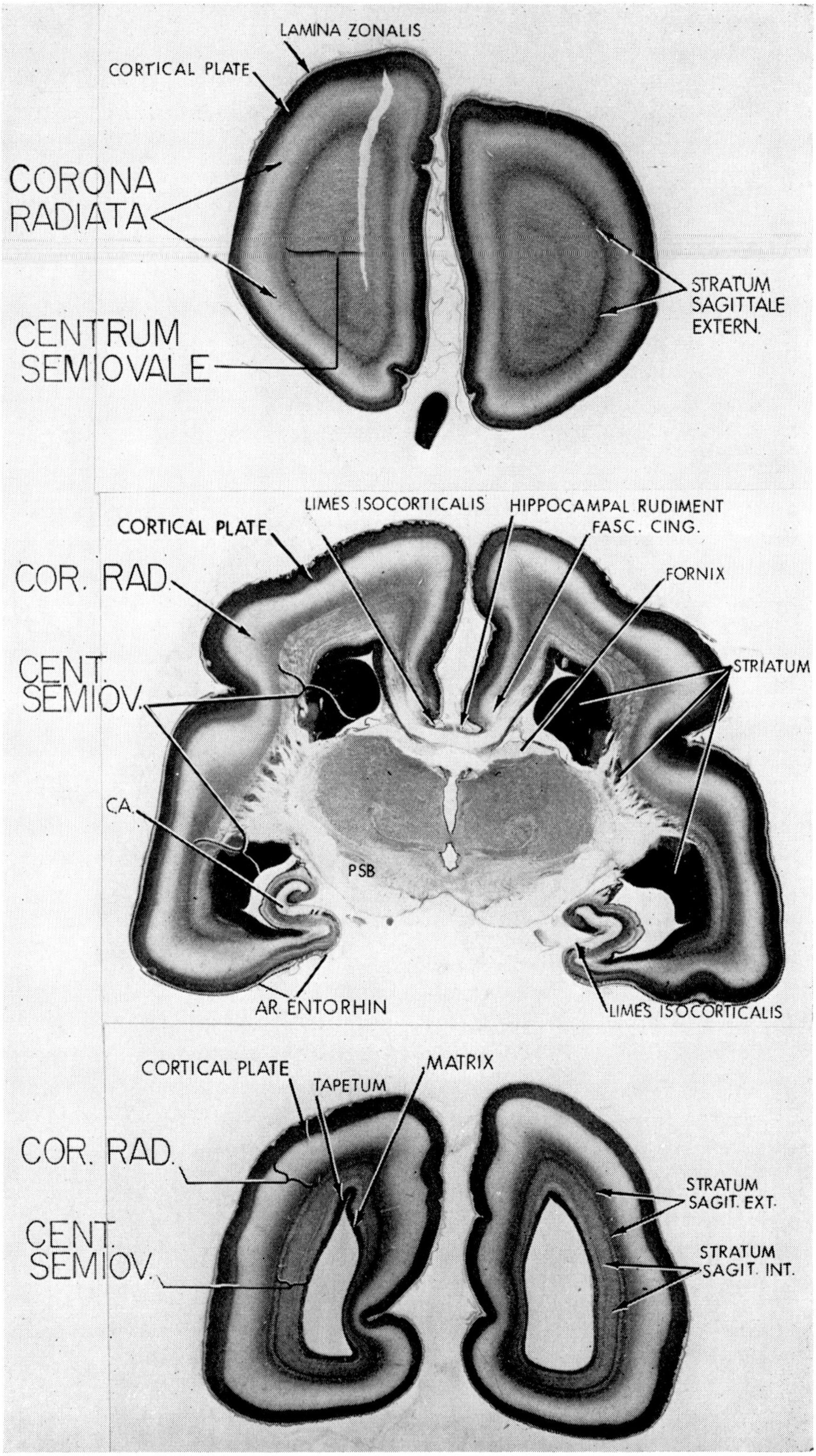
LAMINA ZONALIS
CORTICAL PLATE
CORONA RADIATA
CENTRUM SEMIOVALE
STRATUM SAGITTALE EXTERN.
LIMES ISOCORTICALIS
HIPPOCAMPAL RUDIMENT
FASC. CING.
CORTICAL PLATE
COR. RAD.
FORNIX
CENT. SEMIOV.
STRIATUM
CA.
PSB
AR. ENTORHIN
LIMES ISOCORTICALIS
CORTICAL PLATE
MATRIX
TAPETUM
COR. RAD.
STRATUM SAGIT. EXT.
CENT. SEMIOV.
STRATUM SAGIT. INT.

meres of the epichordal brain stem and spinal cord (the neuraxis) reflects this aboriginal antimeric symmetry of the somatomeres of themetameric body wall and extremities of vertebrates. Each half-neuromere innervates the muscular levers (effectors) on the corresponding (same) side of the plane of somatic symmetry of the body. The entire catalog of possible motor configurations of the body "is built into" the metameric neuraxis proper.

The "reflex figures" of these configurations (Fig. 14–13,B) are reproducible by stimulation of definite loci of the body surface in a "bulbospinal" (decerebrate) or in a "spinal" preparation.[47] However, such experimental preparation is an action system *closed* within itself. The "reflex figures" elicited by the appropriate stimuli in such a preparation are fragments of a machinery which permits us to explain the principles governing the organization of movements of the *open* action systems—the intact organim.[4,5]

In the intact animal and man (Fig. 14–13B), the activities of the cerebral hemispheres, monitored via the neuraxis, exhibit symmetries of a radically different order than the activities of the neuraxis proper shorn of the forebrain. This point of my argument calls for a careful statement which I propose in topological terms as follows:

The functions of the two hemispheres, paired in a *secondary* ("positional")[42] symmetry, are *ablateral* in the sense that each hemisphere governs the motility of the somatic apparatus of the body wall as a *unit,* without reference to the laterality of position of somatic organs on one or the other side of the plane of bilateral symmetry (see Note 13). This is evident from the empirical fact that any motor configuration is reproducible by an intact animal or man in a mirror-image duplicate of its stereokinetic antimere on the other side of this plane. The duplicate motor configurations on the two sides of the plane of bilateral symmetry of the intact vertebrate body (organism) may be said to be equipotential or *isodynamic.* Such are the movements upholding the body in equipoise on the somatic axis in erect stance and locomotion, even in the absence of gravity, and the ordinary movements of respiration, vocalization, mimicry, gesticulation and of articulation of vocal sounds, as vocalized gestures, be they barking, braying or human speech. These are stereotyped, generally rhythmical—that is repetitive movements called variously "instinctive," "automatic," "involuntary" and "emotional" movements—although such terms evade the issue of definition of this order of motility which, in Hughlings Jackson's terms,[25] "marks time and does no work" (see further, section 5).

Yet an apparent conundrum arises in

←

Figure 14–8. The centrum semiovale and the corona radiata represent two distinct layers of the wall of the hemisphere proper. The boundary between the two layers are obscured in the brain of an adult, but are sharp in the brain of fetuses between the 4th and 7th months of gestation. (*Top*) The level anterior to anterior horns of the lateral ventricles. (*Middle*) The level of the thalamus and posterior border of corpora striata. (*Bottom*) The level of the posterior horns of the lateral ventricles (forebrain of a fetus of 5 months). The centrum semiovale of each hemisphere comprises the lateral ventricle, corpus striatum, the lenticulo-caudate sector of the internal capsule and the thalamic radiations which capsulate the centrum semiovale and demarcate the latter from the corona radiata. The centrum semiovale is the *core of the limbic division* of the hemisphere proper. The corona radiata is the white matter of the *supralimbic* division of the hemisphere overlying the limbic division.

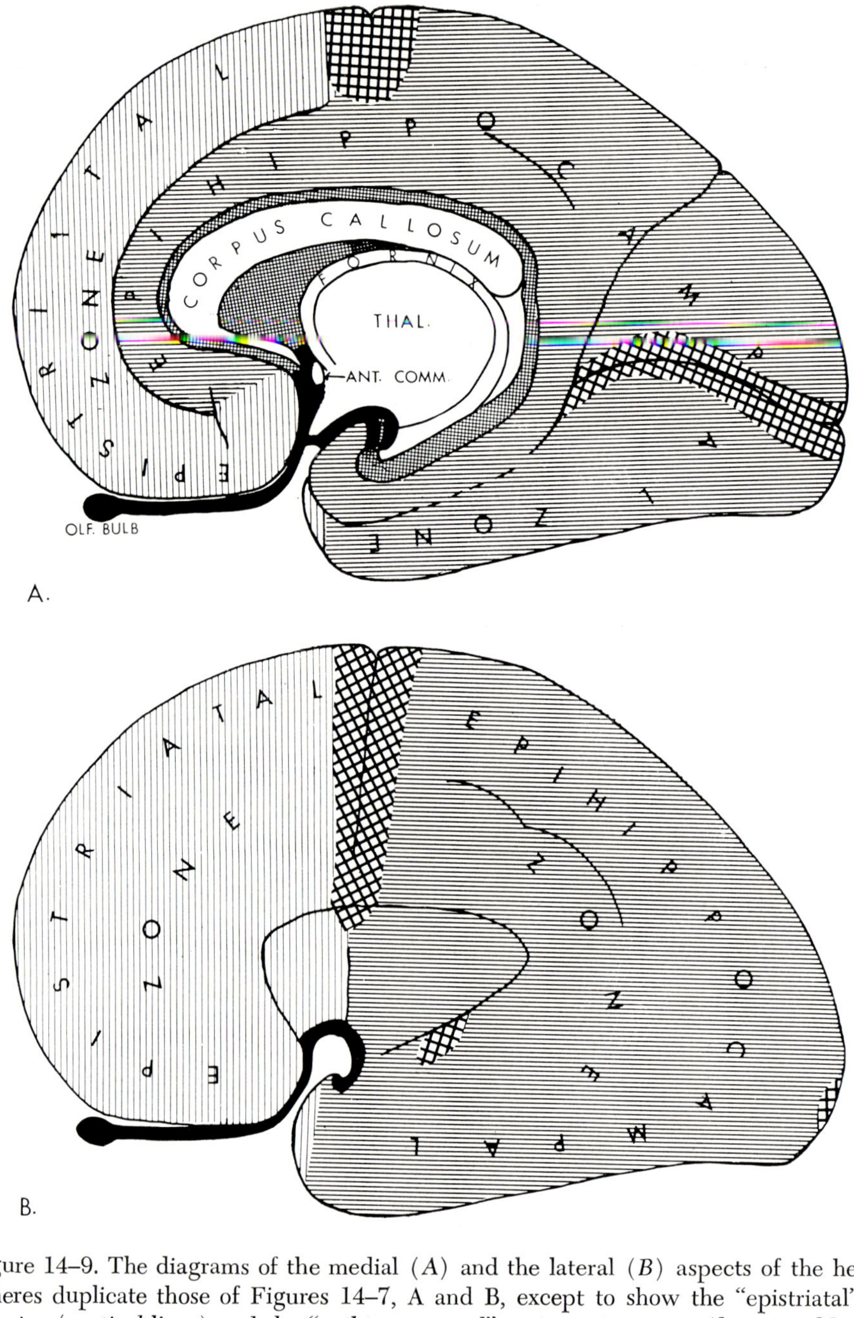

Figure 14–9. The diagrams of the medial (*A*) and the lateral (*B*) aspects of the hemispheres duplicate those of Figures 14–7, A and B, except to show the "epistriatal" or anterior (*vertical* lines) and the "epihippocampal" or posterior zones (*horizontal* lines) of the isocortex. Note that the epihippocampal zone comprises the areas of all "specific thalamocortical projections" (cortical ends of sensory "analyzers") and extends on the medial wall of the hemisphere (A) forward to the septal area and parolfactory lobule (area). The epistriatal part is, in man, nearly athalamic and is the origin of a particularly dense outflow of both short and long corticofugal fibers to the striatum, thalamus and hypothalamus and to the brain stem (system *in parallel,* see section 6). Note that the praecentral (kinesthetic) and the postcentral (somesthetic) "analysor" areas (areas 4, 3, 1, 2 of Brodmann) are interposed between the epistriatal and the epihippocampal zones of the hemispheres.

the manifest nonequipotentiality (dynamic nonsymmetry) of the mechanical levers on the two sides of the plane of the somatic symmetry of the body in the case of the specifically human motility—namely, the manipulation of tools and of objects by means of tools. Such movements are called "voluntary," "intentional," "purposeful," "goal-directed" and "skilled" movements of *dexterity*.[61]

The outstanding common feature of the movements of manipulation of tools and objects of work is that movements of this order are lateralized with a "torque" on the somatic axis to one or the other side of the plane of bilateral symmetry of the body and are skewed in many different planes on the axis of polarization of movements on the object of work (see further, section 5C). The laterality (side) to which the bias of the torque is turned is "preferential"—that is, either hand "will do," yet one is preferred. The preferred side defines the "handedness" of the individual.[61] In early childhood, the "preference" is reversible from one to the other side of the plane of symmetry. Changing handedness becomes more difficult in later life and is uneconomical of energy invested in the handling of tools and objects of the work with the nonpreferred hand. The more exacting the work, the more emphatic is the torque and the less reversible is the handedness. It is a challenging and as yet unexplained fact that in man, in whom the forelimbs are emancipated from the subservience to the needs of locomotion, the torque is turned to one and the same side of the plane of symmetry in more than 80 percent of the species. The side of the statistical prevalence of the preferential handedness is the salient taxonomic attribute of the *Homo erectus faber*. This, the "majority" side, inexorably enough, is called the "right" side, and the bias of the stereodynamic torque is reflected in all products (artifacts) of human thought, language and manufacture (see further, section 5C).

The above empirical facts state clearly that in movements which "mark time"—that is, effect no work outside the body—the somatic antimeres on the two sides of the plane of symmetry are equipotential and isodynamic. However, in movements which effect work, these antimeres are not equipotential and are *anisodynamic* in the manipulation of tools and objects of work. It should follow, then, that in the governance of movements of the body *on the body itself* (such as respiration, mimicry and gesticulation), one hemisphere is functionally equipotential and symmetrical (commensurate) with the other hemisphere (see Note 13). Contrariwise, in the governance of the movements of manipulation of tools and objects—that is, *in the work effected outside the body*—the two hemispheres are not equipotential and are functionally nonsymmetrical, each contributing its own particular share of governance of work, *with a compounded bias* of the torque on the somatic axis to one or the other side of the plane of somatic symmetry of the body and of the skew on the axis of polarization of the action to the object (the end or goal) of work.

The resolution of the apparent conundrum may be sought by defining firstly the *biodynamic* organization of the motility which "marks time" and of the motility which "does work" and, secondly, by enquiring into the principles governing the *topological* organization of the connectivity of the forebrain with the neuraxis proper and effector organs of the body.

5. *The Biodynamic Organization of the Motility*

The organism is a biological action system in constant change and motion. Behavior is movement. All bodily movements

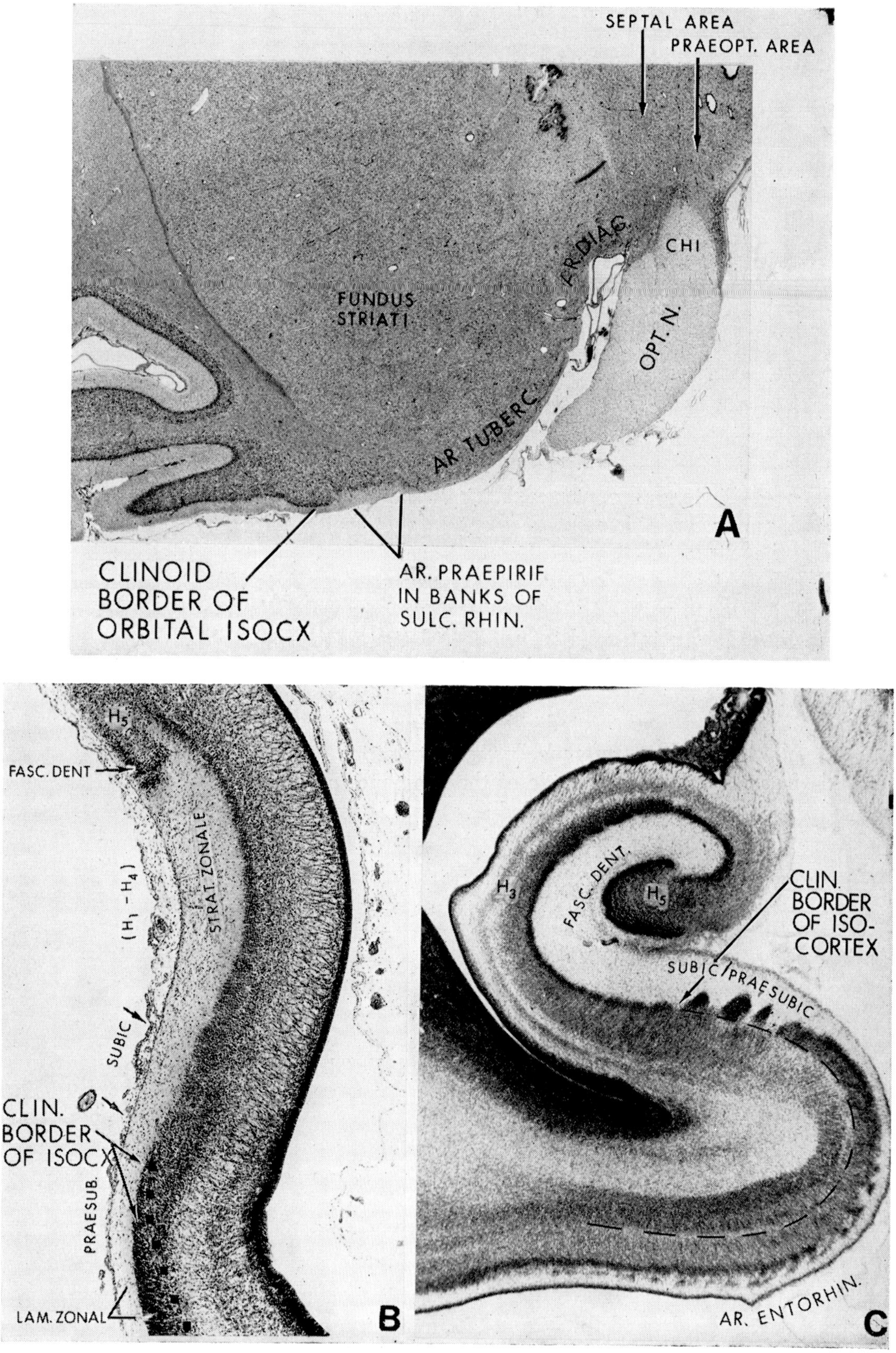
SEPTAL AREA
PRAEOPT. AREA
CHI
AR. DIAG.
FUNDUS STRIATI
OPT. N.
AR. TUBERC.
A
CLINOID BORDER OF ORBITAL ISOCX
AR. PRAEPIRIF IN BANKS OF SULC. RHIN.
H5
FASC. DENT
STRAT. ZONALE
(H1 – H4)
SUBIC
CLIN. BORDER OF ISOCX
PRAESUB.
LAM. ZONAL
B
H3
FASC. DENT.
H5
CLIN. BORDER OF ISO-CORTEX
SUBIC / PRAESUBIC
AR. ENTORHIN.
C

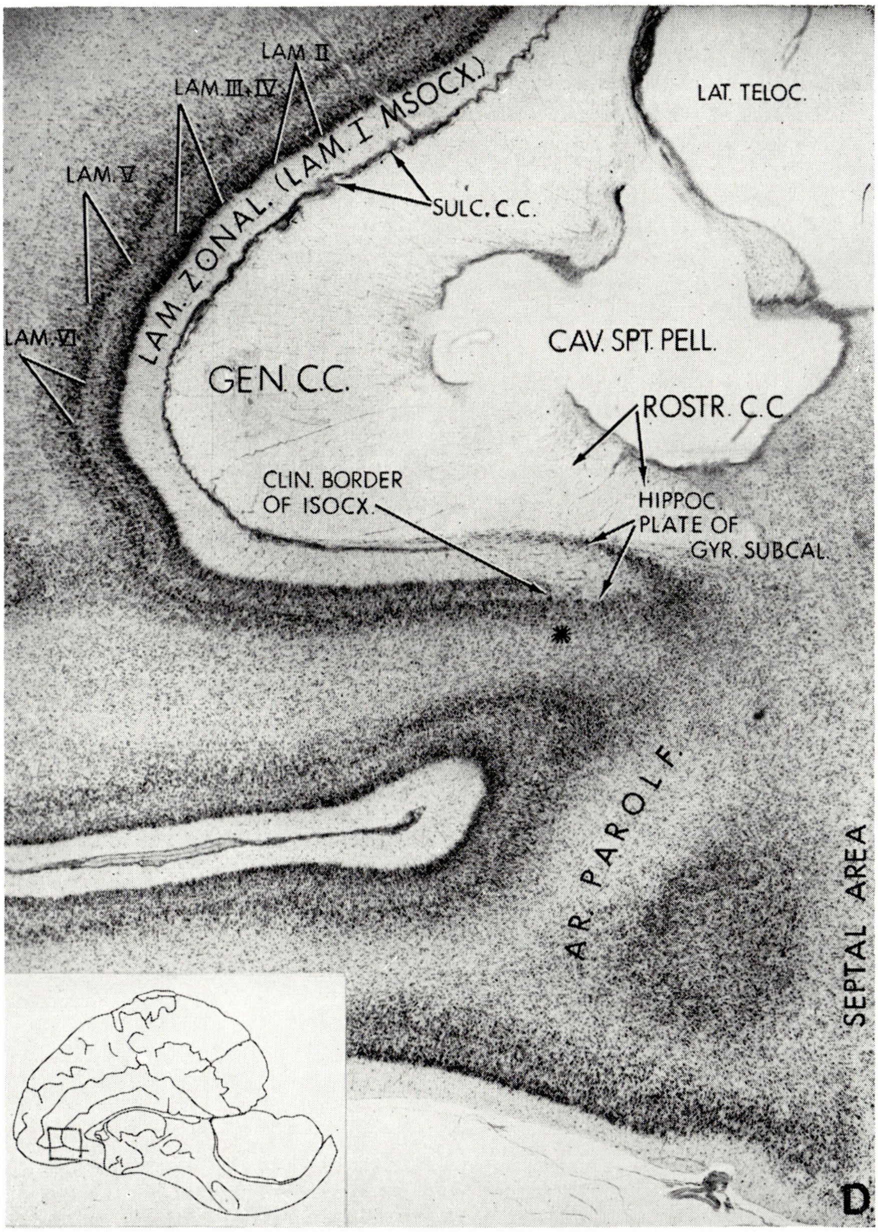

Figure 14–10. (*A*) The clinoid border of the upper laminae of the orbitolimbic isocortex (limes isocorticalis) ends at the bank of the rhinal sulcus (brain of a dolphin, *Tursiops truncatus*), parasagittal section). Note the continuity of the deep laminae (*V* and *VI*) with the reticulate gray matter of the olfactory lobe (paleocortex). (The specimen was prepared and studied in my laboratory and was supplied by M. S. Jacobs and P. J. Morgane, see further in their publication with McFarland.[26] (*B and C*) Clinoid attenuation of the superficial laminae of the heterotypical mesocortex (entorhinal area) which "superlaminates" the subiculum, while the deep laminae and the lamina dissecans are continuous respectively with the hippocampal plate (H 1–4) and with the wide stratum zonale of the Ammon's horn. Human fetus of 5 months. (*D*) The same relationships at the subcallosal gyrus and the rostrum of the corpus callosum in the brain of the fetus of a dolphin (stenella) in parasagittal section. Note the abrupt end of the superficial laminae of the limbic isocortex and the continuity of the deep laminae with the hippocampal plate of the subcallosal gyrus. (The specimen supplied by P. J. Morgane.)

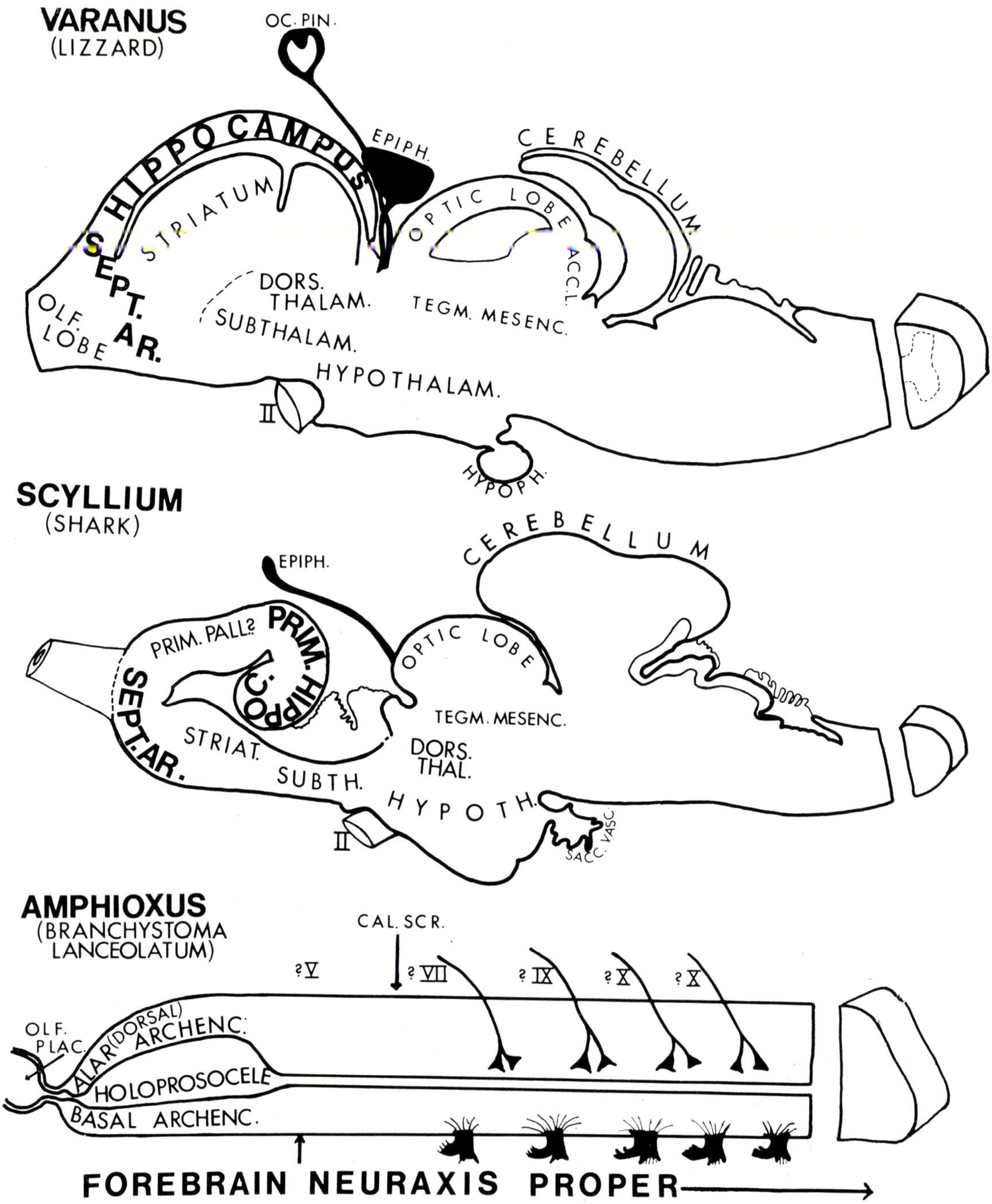

Figure 14–11. Outlines of the forebrain of vertebrates from that of amphioxus to that of man. The intent is to represent the progressive elaboration of the vertebrate forebrain and, especially, of the endbrain, from a holospheric "archencephalon" such as that in the amphioxus and from pedimental olfacto-viscerosomatic telencephalon "impar" (SEPT. AR., PRIM. HIPPOC.) such as in the shark and in the lizard, to the *limbic* isocortex (mesocortex) of the smooth-surfaced and partially paired (semipar)

→

MAN

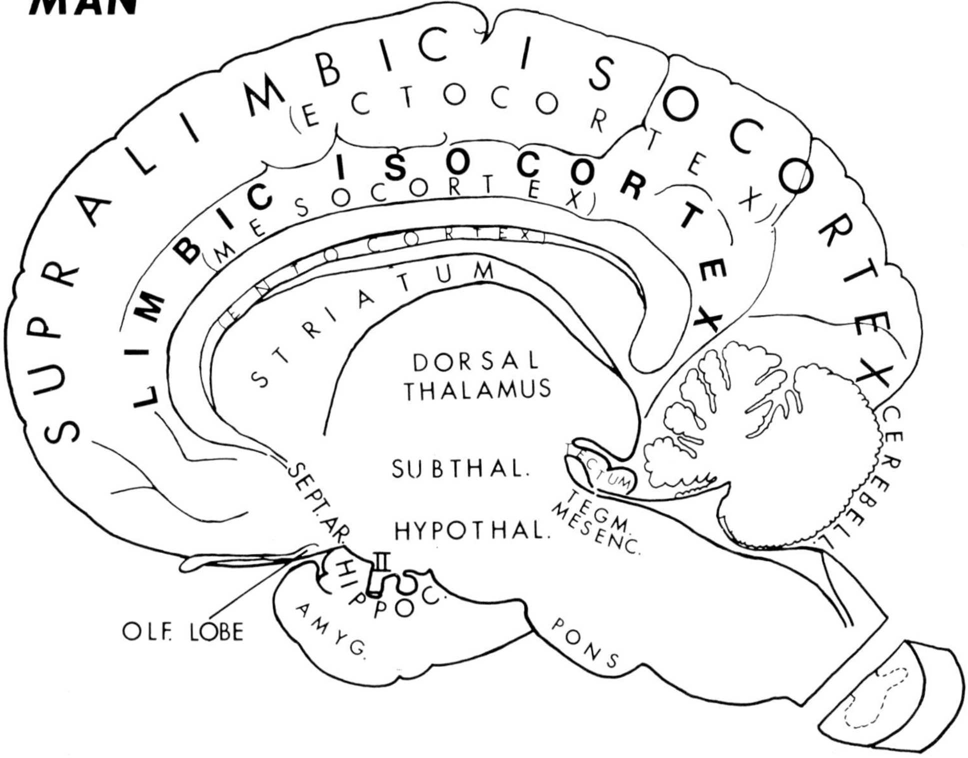

MARSUPIAL
(OPPOSSUM)

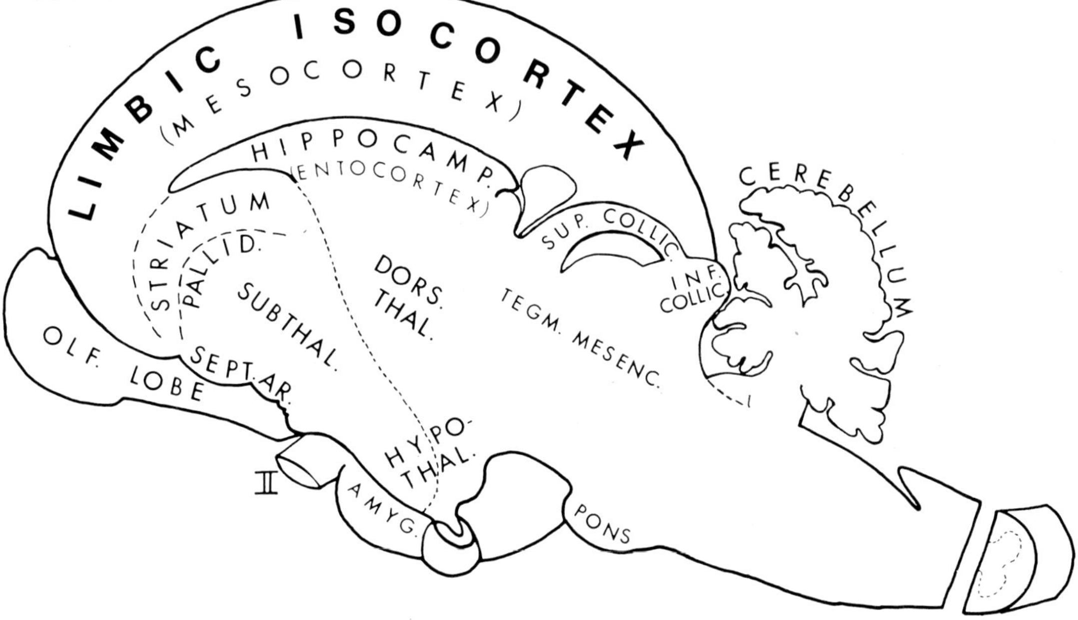

hemispheres, arising upon the striatum and the hippocampus in a marsupial, such as the oppossum. The phyletic palimpsest of structural elaborations of the forebrain becomes overlain in man by the *supralimbic* isocortex (ectocortex) of the intricately folded and totally paired division of the hemispheres. (Redrawn from U. C. Ariëns Kappers': *Tabulae Anatomo-Comparative Cerebri,* edited by Kosmos. Amsterdam, circa 1910. Details omitted, labeling of telencephalic structures modified.)

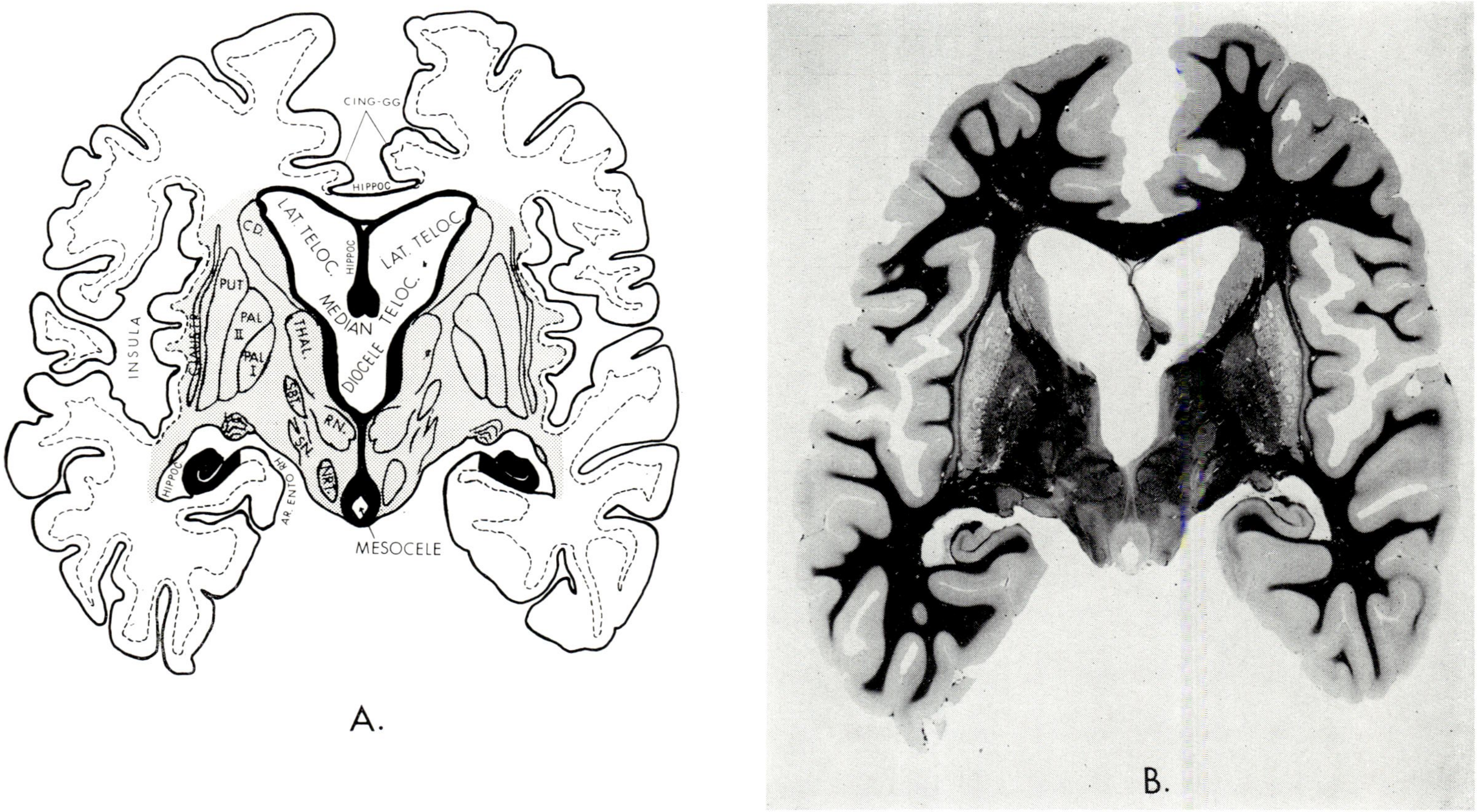

Figure 14–12. Topography of the three neuropils of the forebrain as may be seen in any Weigert- or Nissl-stained (and in unstained) section of an adult's brain. (A) outlines of structures seen in the section shown at (B). The left hemisphere is on the left side of the reader; the plane of section is at nearly a right angle to the plane of the Sylvian cleft (Loyez myelin stain). *Symbols in* (A): *Solid black*—reticulate (deep) neuropil (and the hippocampus or "entocortex"; the "entocortex" of the septal area and olfactory lobes is out of the plane of this section). *Stipple*—nucleate (intermediate) neuropil. The cingulate (CING. GG.), parahippocampal (AR. ENTORH.) gyri and the insula ("mesocortex") represent the superficial neuropil overlaying the nucleated neuropil. Note that outlines of nuclei of this neuropil gradually change from near spherical, for example, red nucleus—R.N., to increasingly laminar (e.g. claustrum) configurations. *White*—stratilaminate (superficial) neuropil (isocortical) plate and white matter of the corona radiata joined by the corpus callosum which traverses the hippocampus in the median telencephalic zone.

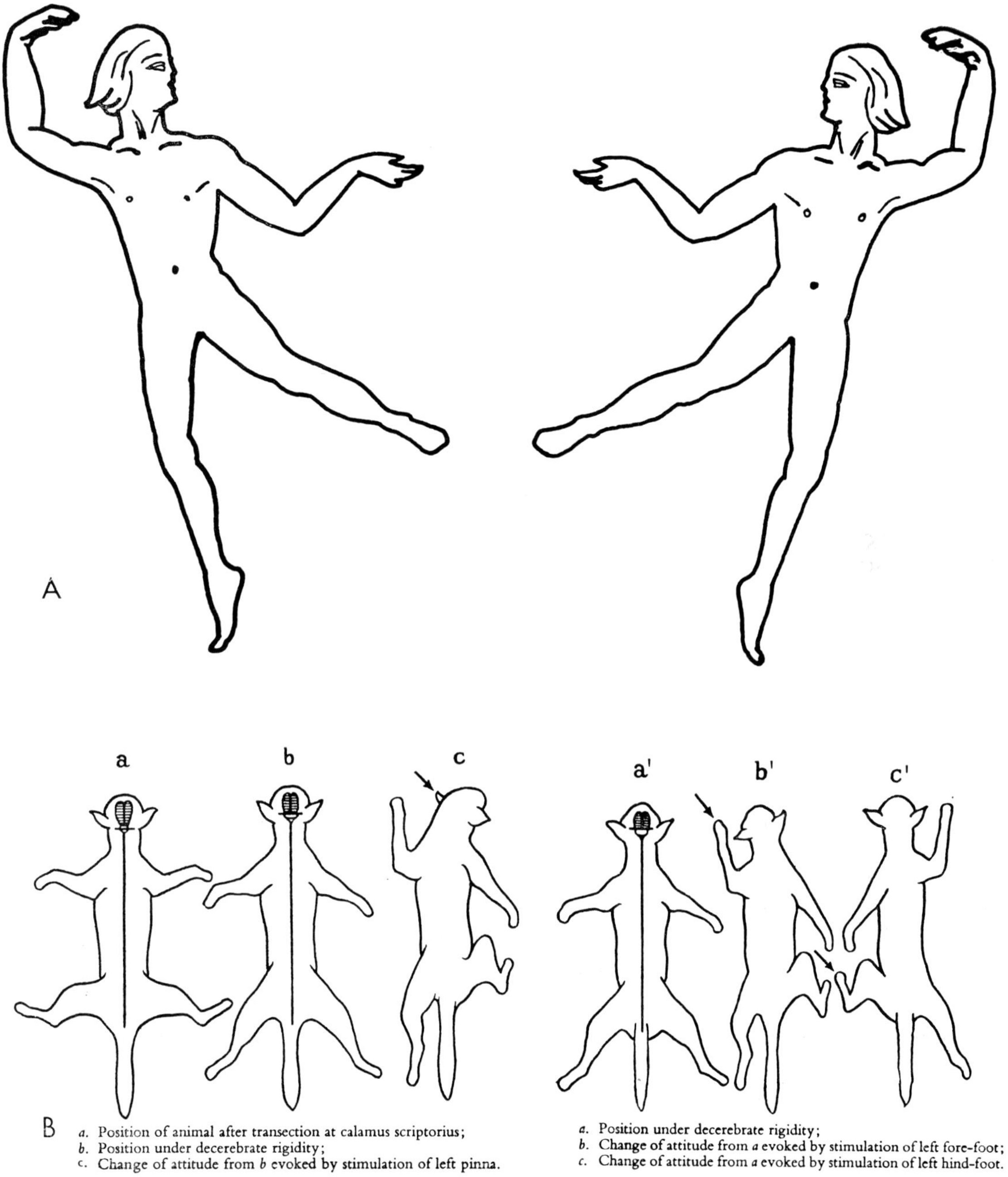

Figure 14–13. (*A*) Mirror-image stereodynamic symmetry of the "left" and "right" isodynamic (equipotential) postural configurations of the body of a ballet dancer. Movements of the body (here of the dancer) on the body itself in the case of an *open* action system (the dancer). (*B*) The "reflex figures" in the case of a "closed" action system represented in a "spinal" (at *a*) and in "decerebrate" (at *b*) preparations and evoked by stimulation of the left *pinna* (at *c*), of the left *fore*foot (at *b'*) and of the left *hind*foot (at *c'*) in the preparation shorn of the forebrain ("decerebrate"). These orderly postural stereotypes are "built into" the neuraxis proper and represent the isodynamic *stereokinetic* (mechanical) fragments of the motility of expression, "organized" in the forebrain into the motility of expression of an *open* action system (*stereodynamic* organization). (Extrapolated from C. S. Sherrington,[47] his Figs. 47 and 48.)

are physiological functions *defined by the biological end that they serve* in the bodily economy.[19-21] The ends are the symmetry and equipoise as the universal *needs* of living. The needs are met by responses of the cells, tissues and organs of the body to the challenges of the *forces* in the environment (see Note 14). These forces are "stimuli" besieging the body with sovereign indifference as to where, when and how they strike. It makes a difference to the organism how it meets the challenge; hence, the hierarchy of the stimuli and responses of the organism—a "corporation" of cells, tissues and organs—according to the exigency of the *need to respond.*

The motility ("behavior") of bilaterally symmetrical vertebrates are movements of three general orders[55,65,66]: the *ablateral* movements of cells, tissues and of visceral organs *on themselves* within the finite (closed) space, bound by the skin; the *bilateral* movements of the body wall and of its parts *on the body itself* within this private, finite, structured and *symmetrical* space; and the *lateralized* movements, "spearheaded" by parts of the body (e.g. hand or tool) and projected with an angular deviation (skew) on the objects and events and on the other "bodies" in the *public,* wide open (nonfinite, boundless) and *dissymmetrical* space.[41]

Bodily activities (behavior) in these three space-referred spheres of motility are responses to the challenge of stimuli (forces) of the three general orders of *priority in the need to respond:* (a) the *un*condition*al* stimuli *physical agents;* (b) the condition*al* stimuli *signals* and *signs*[52] of these agents; and (c) the condition*ed* stimuli *symbols* of the signals and signs of physical agents.

A. Stimuli Physical Agents and Motility of Cells, Tissues and Organs—The Visceration. The stimuli *agents* (light, sound, gravity, heat and the like "forces") are *unconditional* stimuli. They tolerate no compromise and allow no choice in the mode of response. Stimuli of this order are existential events of the present moment, *nonpredictive* in themselves of future events. The responses to the unconditional stimuli physical agents are akin to tropistic (negative or positive) reactions.[52] They fulfill the absolute and universal need of all organisms—the need to *occupy space.* The responses to the need of this order of priority are *autonomous* activities of cells, tissues and organs and are present in "cultures" of individual cells, tissues and whole organs removed from the body. The physiological functions (the ends) of these activities are the cells, tissues and organs themselves. Taken together, they represent the motility of visceration[55] or "endokinesis."[19-21]

B. Stimuli Signals and Motility of Expression—The "Emotions." All stimuli are agents of physical changes (events) propagated in space and reflected in responses as "causes" are reflected in "effects." The radical difference between the unconditional stimuli physical agents as defined above and the conditional stimuli *signals* of these agents is that the latter imply an anatomical system of propagation (transmission) of "messages"—the nervous system, a "decoding device" or analyzer of information—the brain and the "semaphores" or apparatus of signalization—the skeletal musculature of the body wall and extremities.

Stimuli *signals* of physical agents are conditional stimuli "signalling" the bodily needs epitomized in the need of a "constant" internal environment. This intimately private fraction of space occupied by the body ("organic" space) is relentlessly contested by the random, unpredictable forces of the environment and is not "constant." The need for constancy—that is, of symmetry and equipoise—is met by the responses conditioned by chance pairing in repetitive succession of many different agents (random forces), one of the agents becoming the signal *predictive* of events with which it has been paired and rewarded with a response satisfying a homeostatic need (e.g. hunger, thirst, mechanical threat, temperature changes, etcetera).[6] These are imperative needs, ever present, recurring in cycles and predictable. They tolerate a compromise in the time and mode of response within a narrow limit of variation and allow a finite choice of responses. The structural devices (cells, tissues, organs)—that is, "organic means" available to the body (organism) to respond to signals of the homeostatic needs are *species-specific*. The inventory of such devices is limited to the catalog of devices *evolved* by the species. The individual organism *develops* the inventory and in this development (ontogeny) recapitulates the phyletic catalog. It can add nothing new to the devices already evolved by the species and *no longer* in evolution.[39] Hence, the choice of responses to stimuli signals of physical agents within the body is also *finite*.

The symmetrical movements of the bilateral organs of the body wall on the somatic axis of the body (musculature of the face, trunk and extremities), "isodynamic" in their effects on the two sides of the plane of somatic symmetry, are responses to signals of the ablateral, visceral events within the body.[19-21,38] Movements of this order are conditioned by the phyletic responses to the stimuli physical agents "acting" on cells, tissues and organs in the closed (private) body space. The physiological ends (functions) of movements of mimicry, body attitudes, gestures and vocalizations and of speech as a vocalized gesture are *in* the body. All such movements, comparable to the movements of the "arms" of a semaphor or "hands" of a clock, change the external form—that is, surface configuration of the body—and are somatic responses to signals of events within the body. They meet the private, *visceral* needs.

At the same time, the movements of the somatic apparatus of the body wall are public signs of these private needs. When taken together, these symmetrical, isodynamic movements of the body wall and of its parts on the body itself represent the motility of *outward expression* of the internal (visceral) needs of the body or *emotions*.[19-21,55] They uphold the integrity of the body and are always *candid signs* of the state of affairs within the body itself. The body-bound motility of this order, responding to signals of predictable and imperative needs of the body, may be a sign of some gentle and ineffable bliss, or some "sweet sorrow," or it may be a violent expression of dismal woes, excruciating pain, elemental wrath or some orgiastic exaltation. Yet, all these body-bound movements of expression are of the order of a monologue of the body "addressed" to the body itself. As the outward *signs* of the internal states, they "signify" these states, but do nothing else. They "mark time" as do movements of the hands of a clock or the arms of a semaphor. In the states of intense emotional exaltation, they express the state of a homeostatic "panic" within the body. The objects, events and the "other bodies" as the *agents* of the disarray, may be the *targets* of such emotional movements. Yet the biological *ends* of such emotional movements are not these targets absolved from the body, but the imperative needs of the body itself as a corporation of cells, tissues and organs.

It should be clear, then, that the "emotions" are *somatic* expressions (signs) of the intimately private, ineffable and non-shareable internal states, made *public* and shareable in somatic movements of mimicry, gestures, vocalizations and speech, as candid signs of these states. By this definition, we "voice" the emotions, "sound" them in speech and "signal" them by other signs with greater or lesser eloquence and fervor, yet ever in candor.

The candor of emotions is commensurate with the homeostatic visceral equipoise and with the stereodynamic symmetry of its somatic expression. The greater the visceral disarray, the more candid and symmetrical is its somatic expression. Both hands are outstretched in candid protestation and in the embrace of genuine affection. A wry smile is the expression of a *biased* emotion. The vocal cords vibrate in unison with exquisite symmetry in the outcry of pain and in a song of exalted pathos; there is something other than pain and pathos when they do not. A premeditated murder 'in cold blood" is not the same as an impromptu murder of "passion." In brief, speech as vocalized gesture and all symmetrical movements of the somatic apparatus of the body as candid signs of visceral arousal, while being all that, become something other than candid when they breach their isodynamic symmetry and are skewed on the body axis with a torque to one or other side of the plane of symmetry. They become anisodynamic and then serve different biological ends. I will attempt to describe these ends.

C. Stimuli Symbols and Motility of Effectuation—The Work. The stimuli symbols are *representations* of the forces contesting the integrity of the body. The stimuli of this order are words spoken, written or printed, and all the otherwise reproduced emblematic artifacts of language and manufacture. A crucifix, a swastica, a totem pole and the like emblems or symbols represent the physical forces "by proxy." They "move mountains" and make live and destroy by proxy. The words and emblems may be sublime, exalting, prosaic or obscene. As symbols they all have this in common that they are provocative stimuli and carry either a negative (repellent) or positive (appellant) meaning. The stimuli symbols provoke rather than evoke a response. In contrast to stimuli signals of the physical agents (forces) which evoke a monologue of the body addressed to itself, the stimuli symbols are a provocation to a "dialogue" between the body and the forces contesting its integrity.

The stimuli symbols are conditioned by the responses to the conditional stimuli signals of the unconditional and inexorable stimuli physical agents which act within the body. Stimuli symbols are conditioned also by the signs of these forces acting on *other* bodies. The symbols (words, emblematic artifacts) as stimuli are thus the derivatives—that is, secondary products of all these different conditional and unconditional stimuli and responses. They allow an unlimited choice of response and tolerate a compromise. The responses to stimuli symbols may be a revelation of a sublime (exalted) "truth," or they may be a deliberate deception at a calculated risk of an "exposure." Hence, the "imperative" of morality.

The responses to the stimuli symbols are conditioned also by the words and emblematic artifacts to whose symbolic meaning the body has been conditioned by the physical forces and the signals and signs of these forces. The stimuli symbols are abstract models of these forces, signals and signs. As such models they are approximate and ever biased reproductions of these agents.

The symbols are modeled in the

image of the modeler. The symmetry of the upright body in equipoise is the "protomodel" of all representation of the random, ever-changing and unpredictable forces in the nonfinite, dissymmetrical fraction of space external to (i.e. absolved from) the finite and symmetrical body space. It should be clear that the symbols are the representations of realities (forces) and are biased models—a "candid" symbol is a contradiction *in adjecto.* Herein is the cardinal difference between the responses to the stimuli signals of the physical agents acting within the body, and the stimuli symbols of the signals and signs of these agents. The conditioned stimuli symbols represent the societal environment—the *medium* in which the body is *cultivated.* The language and the artifacts (products) of manufacture are *the culture.*

In contrast to the responses to stimuli signals fulfilling the needs of the somatic symmetry and homeostatic equipoise within the body, the responses to stimuli symbols are *motivated* by the needs of the thermodynamic adjustments of the body to the "social" forces in the societal transactions (dialogue) of the body with other bodies absolved from and foreign to the body itself. This is the biological end (function) of all languages and of the symbolic artifacts of human manufacture which represent different "cultures" of the *Homo erectus faber disputans;* hence, the radical difference in the physiological function of *speech* as a system of articulate, vocalized gestures—the semaphores which *communicate* and "mark time"—and the function of *language* and of emblematic artifacts (the "facts") as a system of symbols which *represent* and *do work.*

The somatic apparatus of the body wall, facing both the internal and the external environments, may be regarded as a reversible engine. Muscular contractions use energy and release heat. They contribute powerfully to the maintenance of the thermodynamic homeostasis of the internal medium. At the same time they are the immediate source of the *motive power* for the system of articulated muscular levers. The mechanical work of these levers uses heat and releases energy which is transformed into movements of the body wall and extremities. It should be clear that in releasing heat the thermal energy of muscular contractions is within the body and thus is "private." The thermal energy generated by these same contractions, in supplying power to the muscular levers, is converted into work effected by the body in the external environment—that is, ekphorized and either dissipated or translated into work—*outside* the body. The free energy of work is absolved from the body and thus becomes "public" in the work effected in the external—the societal—environment. In work, the activities of the body, spearheaded by its parts (head, jaws, tail, extremities or whatever part of the body available in the phyletic catalogue of its somatic "hardware"), are guided by the sense organs (the "sentinels")[9] facing the forces of the environment, and are targeted and projected on the objects and events and on the other bodies. In the case of man the somatic apparatus of the body wall is extended by the mechanical tools, be that the shaft of a power drill, the "business end" of a rifle barrel or the 2000-pound Apollo space ship targeted on Mars. The targets constantly shift in position and change in the velocities of their motion. The parts leading the targeted action (bare hands or hands extended by tools) must be projected onto the targets in an infinite number of different planes. The symmetrical levers, isodynamic and equipotential in movements which "mark time," become anisodynamic and nonequipotential in movements which "do work." Hence the *bias* of all the object-bound, *targeted* movements which effect work. Movements of this order represent the motility of *effectuation* [55,58,61] or *telokinesis.*[19-21] In this sphere of motility the physical forces (the objects, events and the other bodies) competing for the space occupied by the body and for the energy upholding its integrity are no longer "sovereign" and inexorable. Through work they become *manageable* forces.

Effective action is consumed in the work of the somatic levers upholding the body erect and in equipoise against the forces contesting its integrity. To free energy in excess of the thermal energy consumed in work is the biological end of *effective* work. The physiological function of the object-bound, targeted motility of effectuation (work) is to *probe* the external environment, to *locate* and to *take* the *measure* of these forces and to *tap* the energy of the forces at its sources in this boundless fraction of the environment. The other bodies are the immediate sources; the minerals and inert bodies (objects) are sources of energy which is mediated by tools. Objects, events and bodies (organisms) other than the body itself are the sources of free energy.

Work is an universal function of all biological action systems (organisms) in the biosphere.[49-51] It fulfills the need of thermodynamic adjustments of the body to the random, *unpredictable* forces of the environment and constantly transforms the biosphere ("geological zone of life")[49] into a new state of energy-matter.[31] In the scope and tempo of these transformations on the planetary scale, man seems to lead all other biological systems. In this sense, man and his motility of effectuation appear to represent the *crest* of evolution—evolution "in the making." [3,39,50]

The distinction between the *evolved* and the *derived* products of evolution is important. In the case of the human motility of effectuation such as language and manufacture, the distinction becomes essential. Erect locomotion, speech and other expressions of internal states (gestures, mimicry) are *evolved* functions and are no longer in evolution. The functions such as symbolized thought, language and manufacture are products *derived* from the *individual* experience of *societal* living and represent the evolution in the making.[3,39,55] These are taxonomic attributes of specifically human behavior and represent the "crest" of evolution.

The management of the unpredictable (random) forces of the environment implies the choice of the targets—that is, of the ends of telokinesis—and of the effective movements—that is, of the means to consume the ends in the products of work. In contrast to the motility of emotional expression fulfilling the imperative and ever predictable needs, the object-bound, targeted motility has as its biological ends the random and unpredictable forces of the environment—the targets *absolved* from the body. The means to consume these ends are nonfinite, they are ever in the making.

The end-products (results) of work are never predictable. The choice of targets (goals) and of the means to consume the ends of telokinesis is made always at a calculated risk. The unpredictable ends (the outcome) may be fatal to the somatic symmetry and homeostatic equipoise of the body. Hence, the need of all biological action systems to keep the option *open*, the need of "survival," and the derived need to extend the inventory of somatic levers (means) to meet the challenge of the unpredictable forces (objects, events and other bodies) in the external fraction of space.

Of these derived needs, the animals have

but little. They live "empirically" (*experimento vivendi*). The *Homo erectus faber disputans* lives "operationally," *ex acto mensurandi, comparandi atque computandi* (by the act of measuring, comparing and computing). The tools of "exact" sciences ("calibrated instruments") spearhead human telokinesis (rather than the spying eye, probing finger and the "bare hand" alone). By means of these products of "industry," all targets—whether a duck in flight or an orbiting planet—are made potentially *equidistant* from the body of "Man, the computer"—that is, they move (change positions and velocities in abstract space) in *parallel* with the body.

The body and the targets are an open system of dynamic *transaction* between the contending forces—the *body* as the source of the thermal energy converted into work and the *targets* as the stimuli agents (forces) acting on the body and consuming the thermal energy of the bodily action (responses)—the work. In such a system of transaction ("body target") the body is represented as a *constant*—that is, "fixed" reference of the bodily action—while the targets are the *variables.* The parts which spearhead the targeted ("goal-directed," "wish-fulfilling," "purposeful," "voluntary") action of the body must be projected onto different targets in an infinite number of different planes. The planes of action are defined by the angular deviation of the axis of polarization of the system "body target" from the somatic axis of the body; hence (a) the *torque* on the somatic axis to one or the other side of the plane of symmetry of the body (which constantly tends towards equipoise and is no longer in equipoise in a targeted action) and (b) the *skew* or angular deviation on the axis of polarization of the movements of spearhead-parts of the somatic apparatus of the body (hand or tool) projected on the targets of work.

The torque is movement of the body on the body itself. It is an evolved function of the action system and implies a deviation from the equipoise and symmetry (i.e. towards *asymmetry*) of the system. Like any evolved function (respiration, locomotion), it can only repeat itself as an ever-ready stereotype of the equipotential mirror-image duplicates "built-into" the neuraxis proper and lateralized on the somatic axis to one or the other side of the plane of bilateral symmetry—a response to stimuli signals within the body, a *closed* system.

The forces challenging the symmetry and equipoise of the body *tend to open* the closed system. The skew on the axis of polarization of the dynamic transaction "body-target" is a function of *the targets.* The axis of polarization and planes of the targeted action change with the targets and are never the same. The targeted action never repeats itself. It is a derived function. Herein lies the contrast in biodynamic organization of the motility of outward expression of internal states—the emotions, a closed system of stereotypes as "old" as the species, and the movements of effectuation which are never exact reproductions of movements executed in the work "done" and are ever "new" in the work "aborning."

The bias of the skew on the axis of polarization of the transaction system: body target is reflected in the bias of all responses to representations (stimuli symbols) projected onto the external fraction of space and onto all the objects, events and other bodies in that space. The "right" and "left" are not discernible in the non-finite, dissymmetrical external fraction of space which has neither an axis nor a plane of symmetry of its own.[53] The notions of what is "right" and "left" are ever disputable representations of the body space projected ever with a bias onto the space of objects, events and on the other bodies. It is not generally appreciated that the adjectival attributes of "right" and "left" lose all meaning as soon as they are *beyond* the range (radius) of the telokinetic motility of the beholder of the objects, events and of other bodies as targets of transaction. Once beyond that range, the representation of the external fraction of space loses all reference to "right" or "left" and becomes to the beholder a structureless, empty, amorphous "space" of Euclidean geometry. The plane of symmetry and equipoise of the beholder is the only reference. The representation (concepts) of right and left reflect the angular deviation of the skew of the axis of polarization from the somatic axis to one or to the "other" side of the plane of symmetry and equipoise in the transaction system: "beholder-target."

There must be some "forces" that turn the torque on the somatic axis in 80 percent of mankind to one and the same side of the plane of bilateral symmetry (and so impose the sense of the bias of the skew on the axis of polarization of telokinetic action. I assume that these forces are the *targets* and, hence, are forces *external* to the body. I assume that the turn of the torque and the sense of bias in the skew to this—the majority side—must be more economical in energy consumed in work. The natural selection and genetic tradition have imposed the laterality of the torque to this—the majority side—which in the case of the *Homo disputans* is the *"right"* side of the symmetry of the erect body in equipoise, whenever the body is aroused to action.

Evidence in support of the above proposition may be found (a) in the principles governing the evolution of the interneuronal connectivity within each of the three neuropils and (b) in the principles of *topological* organization of the connectivities of each neuropil of the forebrain on one hand with the respective telencephalic divisions (impar, semipar and totopar) and, on the other hand, with the neuraxis proper as the penultimate common path of the three neuropils.

6. *Topological Organization of Connectivity of the Forebrain*

A. Principles of Interneuronal Connectivity in the Central Nervous System. The connections between more than two neurons in the centralized nervous system of vertebrates may be reduced to three elementary orders of connectivity: (a) at random, (b) in series and (c) in parallel.[56] The autonomic system and the reticular formation are the nearest approximations to a random, ablateral synaptic nerve-net in the centralized nervous system of vertebrates. A higher order of connectivity would obtain when three (or more) neurons are connected *seriatim.* This is the connectivity represented by the conventional model of the "reflex arc." It implies space commitment of the conduction of impulses and an invariable path of propagation of stimuli from neuron A to B to C, and so forth. Such a principle is ideal for the mechanical precision and efficiency of a finite catalog (repertoire) of stereotyped responses calibrated by the stimuli to fulfill the ever recurrent and predictable needs at the expense of plasticity and adaptive modulation of the responses. A still higher order of connectivity would result when a neuron in the assembly would send collaterals of its axon to many neurons. Such a neuron would assume a "nodal" position relative to the other neurons in the assembly and would be connected *in parallel* to these other neurons.

Collateralization is the leading principle in the evolution of the centralized nervous system of vertebrates. Connectivity *in parallel* increases the range of choice and modulation of the activity of the neuronal assembly, as compared to an assembly *seriatim.* In the phylogeny of the central nervous system, the principle of connectivity seriatim is outspoken in the ganglia of invertebrates and is prominent in the neuromeres of the neuraxis proper of the vertebrates. With the evolution of the pallium of mammals, the principle of connectivity seriatim is preempted by the principle of connectivity *in parallel.* This principle becomes outspoken in the organization of the connectivity of the cerebral cortex of primates and man.

B. Topological Organization of the Connectivity of the Three Neuropils of the Forebrain with the Neuraxis. Three great paths converge onto the neuraxis proper from the three telencephalic divisions of the forebrain: the *fornix,* from the median telencephalon impar; *the cingulum,* from the limbic telencephalon semipar; and the massive outflow of fibers descending mainly via the internal capsule from the supralimbic telencephalon totopar. This latter outflow may collectively be called the great *capsulopeduncular* tract.

The Fornix. The fornix and derivates of the median forebrain bundle, arising in the septal area, olfactory lobes and hippocampus represent collectively the common path of the telencephalon impar. The fibers of the fornix system and of the medial (virtually "median") forebrain bundle (see Note 15) from the telencephalon impar are distributed in the deep neuropil (the reticulate core of the forebrain) and in the brain stem *ablaterally*—that is, without reference to the plane of the aboriginal symmetry of the neuraxis proper and of the body wall. In this sense, they are distributed in this median zone *at random,* for there is no such plane in the forebrain (see section 2). The activities of this ablateral periventricular neuropil (Fig. 14–12) of the forebrain are conveyed via this median common path to the neuraxis proper and via the autonomic and endocrine systems to the cells, tissues and organs developing in the visceral axis of the body. The topological ablaterality of distribution of this phylogenetically old "paleopallial" and "archipallial" fiber system suggests that this innermost neuropil of the forebrain represents the mechanism for the regulation of the ablateral, peristaltic and rhythmic motilities of the cells, tissues and visceral organs on themselves (the motility of visceration) in response to stimuli physical agents acting within the body.

The Cingulum. The cingulum and the system of relays in the intermediate neuropil may be regarded as the great bilateral (direct and crossed), *symmetrically* distributed *limbic* path—a common path of the limbus of each hemisphere.[59,62] The bilateral cingular bundles and the uncinate bundles (which may be regarded as the orbito-insular counterparts of the cingulum), arising in the limbic (semipar) division, are distributed bilaterally and symmetrically from each hemisphere to the paired neuronal aggregates of the nucleated (intermediate) neuropil. The organization of connectivity of this neuropil is characteristic: The nucleated aggregates are interconnected *seriatim* by the multiple overlapping relays (direct and decussating) and in this way reflect the *seriatim* connectivity of the metameric neuromeres which, in turn, reflect in the neuraxis proper the aboriginal bilateral symmetry of the somatomeres of the body wall. However, the ipsilateral (direct) callosoperforant and transcallosal (crossed) and the corticoperforant collaterals (the latter distributed ablaterally in the septal area, septum and hippocampus) of each of the paired cingular bundles[59] *duplicate* the median system of the fornix in the paramedian planes and connect the limbus of each hemisphere to the striatum and to the nucleated aggregates of the intermediate neuropils *in parallel* (Fig. 14–2, collaterals *a*, *b*, *c*, and *ax*, *bx*, *cx*).

Such an organization of connectivity, on one hand between the limbic cortex of the neuronal aggregates of the intermediate neuropil *in parallel* and on the other hand between the nuclei within this neuropil seriatim, is most suitable for the governance of "automatic," body-bound, isodynamic, bilaterally symmetrical movements of the body wall on the body itself in the somatic axis of the body. It may be assumed that the limbic cortex and the intermediate neuropil of the forebrain represent the anatomical mechanisms governing the responses to stimuli signals of the visceral events and the outward *somatic* expression (signs) of these events —the "emotions"—such as movements of respiration and gasping, posture, body attitudes, facial mimicry, gesticulation and grasping, vocalizations and speech as a vocalized gesture.

It is significant that in contrast to the ablateral fornix fibers, the collaterals of the *cingulum* and of the uncinate bundles (orbito-insular cingulum) are distributed not randomly. They are highly organized with reference to the laterality of position in the two hemispheres and location of the cells of their origin in the heterotypical mesocortex (area entorhinalis) in the anteroposterior plane in each hemisphere, and in their widespread, bilateral and symmetrical distribution in the corpora striata, in the paired nuclei of the intermediate neuropil and in the adjacent neocortex and in the hippocampus. This strongly suggests an orderly, three-dimensional somatotopic representation in the limbus and in the striatum of each hemisphere of the movements of head, trunk and extremities. The symmetry of the bilateral distribution of the collaterals of each cingulum in the paramedian planes appears to reflect the cephalocaudal sequence and symmetry of the neuromeres of the neuraxis proper and of the somatomeres of the body wall.

The "Pyramidal" Tracts. The massive outflow of the repeatedly bifurcating, short and long, associational and commissural (callosal) fibers from the *supralimbic* (totopar) division of the paired hemispheres interconnects the apihippocampal parts with the epistrital (anterior) supralimbic zones, and these zones with the limbic (semipar) divisions of each hemisphere, to the corpora striata and to the hippocampus (telencephalon impar) *in parallel.* However, the phylogenetic epitome of the principle of connectivity in parallel is attained in the organization of the projection fibers of the capsulopeduncular tracts to the neuraxis proper, from the special heterotypical cortical areas of the telencephalon totopar. In primates, the fibers of this great tract connect the paired hemispheres *exclusively in parallel* to the striatum and to the nuclei of the intermediate neuropil in the forebrain and to *all the neuromeres of the neuraxis proper.*

This massive outflow of direct (ipsilateral) and decussating (crossed) pyramidal tract fibers from *both* hemispheres is distributed bilaterad in the neuraxis proper and presents an outspoken spiral or helicoid symmetry. The capital hodological fact, which throws light on the apparent conundrum to which I referred above (see section 4), is that the distribution of these longest and, phyletically, the most recent fibers from the supralimbic (totopar) divisions of the paired hemispheres (the *corticospinal tracts*) exhibits a consistent, statistically probable *torque,* skewed on the axis of the double helix to *one or to the other side* of the plane of symmetry of the neuromeres of the *spinal cord.* In approximately 80 percent of individuals the torque is turned to the *right* side of the spinal cord. (Figs 14–2 and 14–14).

The torque in the distribution of the fibers of the pyramidal tracts from both hemispheres to one side of the neuraxis, below their decussation in the medulla, has been statistically confirmed in my laboratory in a study of 309 autopsy specimens of normal fetal (179 specimens) and of adult neuraxes (130 specimens). The evidence of torque was obtained (a) from a comparison of the *priority of the right-of-way* (preempted or conceded) by the decussating (crossed) fibers of each pyramid in crossing the raphe of the medulla (Figs. 14–14A and 14–14B), and (b) from the difference in the sums of cross section areas of both corticospinal tracts on the two sides of the spinal cord at consecutive levels (Figs. 14–14A and 14–14B, see diagrams of the spinal cord).[43,67]

Judging by these two criteria, it was found that the torque was "probable" in 80 percent of the autopsy specimens by inspection of gapless serial sections of the medulla and spinal cord of fetuses and adults. In less than 20 percent of the specimens, a torque was not "probable" (short of individual fiber counts) in the Weigert and Nissl-stained material used in these studies.

Of 130 specimens from adults, 105 specimens were technically adequate for study. The skew of the torque was demonstrable in Weigert preparations in eighty-eight specimens (Fig. 14–14B). The torque was to the right side of the spinal cord in seventy-two cases (80 percent). In sixteen cases (20 percent), the torque was skewed to the left side. However, the torque did not correlate with the clinical records of the *left*-handedness. Of the four specimens in the sample of individuals who were allegedly left-handed, all four presented a torque of the pyramidal tracts skewed below the decussation to the *right* side of the spinal cord (see Note 16).

This last fact is important. It shows that the topo-anatomical (hodological) torque of the pyramidal tracts to the right side of the spinal cord is, as is right-handedness, a statistical (respectively anatomic and anthropometric) *constant,* while the left-handedness and the left torque of the pyramidal tracts are in the order of *incommensurate variables*—that is, are indeterminate statistical "anomalies."

It follows then that the lateralization of the targeted motility of effectuation (telokinesis) preferentially to the right hand in approximately 80 percent of the population is not determined by the "right" torque of the pyramidal tracts. It is imposed by the targets absolved from the body. The "right-handed" management of these forces must be more *economical* of the visceral energy of the human body than the "left-handed" management of these forces. We live in a "right-handed" world of *man's making*—the world of abstract symbols (representations) and of the artifacts of language and manufacture.

7. *Definition of the Limbic System*

In the framework of the tripartite representation of the body and brain, the *limbic system* is the limbus of the paired hemispheres and the intermediate neuropil of the forebrain. The metameric neuraxis (neuromeres of the brain stem and spinal cord) is the penultimate common path of this system to the *somatic* apparatus of the body wall. The "system" governs the move-

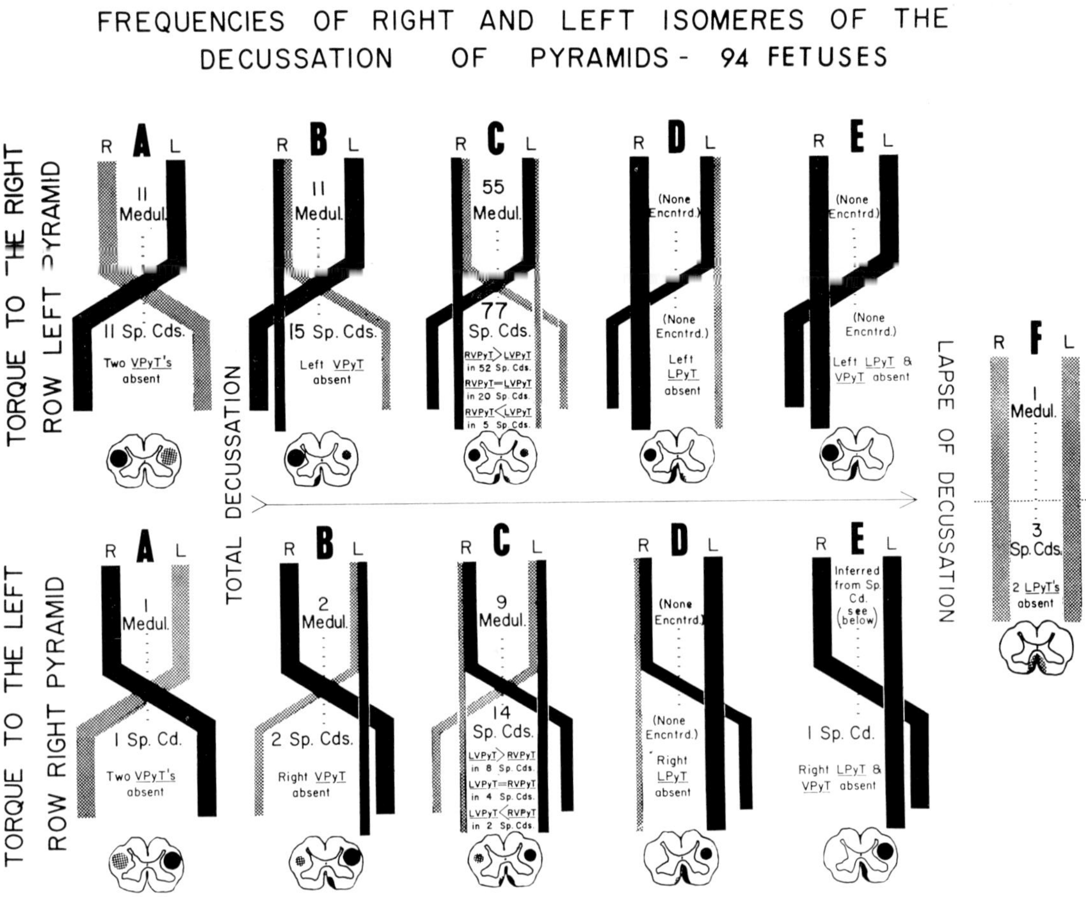

Figure 14–14A. Six a priori possible patterns of Turck's decussation of the bulbar pyramids as seen in 94 fetuses from 5th fetal month to term. Larger crossed and larger direct pyramidal fiber bundles are shown in black. (*Upper row, A* to *E*) Patterns and number of cases in which the crossed fibers of the left pyramid preempted the "right-of-way" (ROW) and crossed first (i.e. at higher levels) and in larger bundles than the crossed fibers of the right pyramid. (*Lower row, A* to *E*) The same for cases in which the crossed fibers of the left pyramid preempted the "right-of-way." Below each pattern are shown diagrams of the relative size of the cross section areas of the lateral ("crossed") and of the ventral ("direct") pyramidal tracts on the two sides of the spinal cord. The *statistical* prevalence ("preference") of the torque in the course and distribution of the pyramidal tracts towards the right side of the spinal cord is evident. Note that pattern C is statistically the prevalent one, patterns B and A are less frequent, and patterns D, E and F (total lapse of decussation of one or both pyramids) are exceptional; the latter three patterns are associated, as a general rule, with other malformations and represent fetal "anomalies."

ments of the body and of its parts on the body itself. These movements maintain the integrity of the body. The function of the limbic system in the biodynamic organization of behavior (see section 4) is the *ekphoresis* of thermal energy released by the motility of visceration. The activities of the limbic system fulfill the need

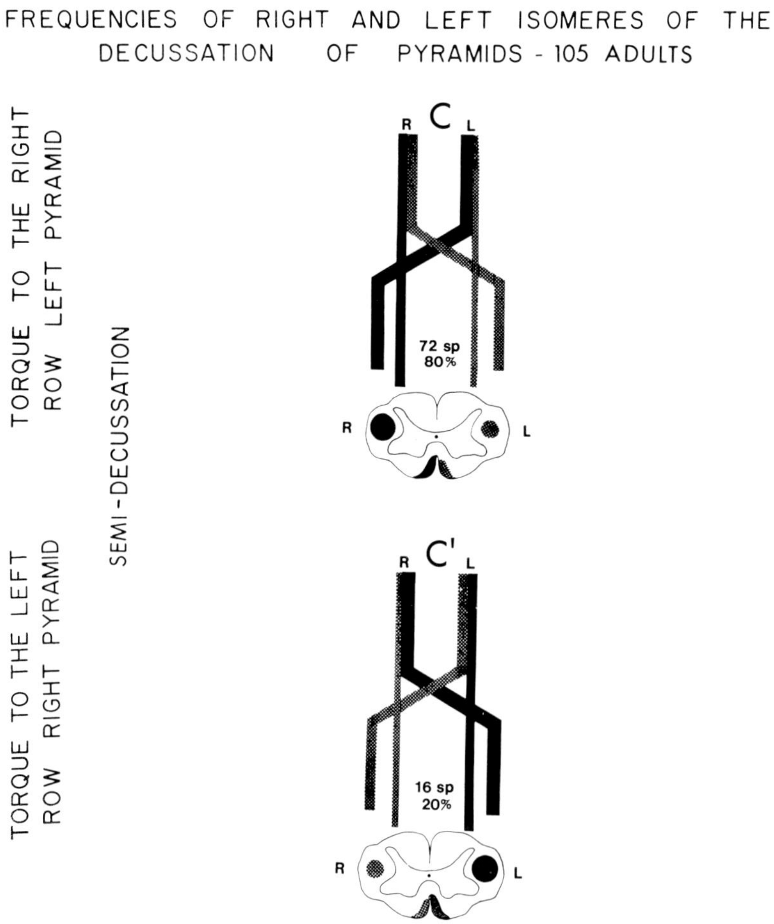

Figure 14–14B. Torque of the pyramidal tracts to the right and to the left sides of the spinal cord verified (probated) in autopsy specimens of the medulla and at least the upper cervical segments of the spinal cords of 105 adults of both sexes without neurological disease. Note that in all these adults, only the pattern C (semidecussation) was encountered (compare with the sample of fetal medullae and spinal cords in A). The torque was not probable, on technical grounds, in 17 out of 105 cases. The diagrams show statistical prevalence of the torque to the right side of the spinal cord in 72 out of 88 cases in whom the "right-of-way" and the difference in cross section areas of the pyramidal tracts on two sides were probable and verified in serial sections of the medulla and cervical spinal cord (detailed report in preparation).

of homeostatic equipoise by bilateral equipotential responses to condition*al* signals of visceral events conditioned by the sovereignly indifferent forces (stimuli physical agents) of the external environment constantly besieging the body.

Thus defined, the limbic system is distinct in structure, connectivity and function from the system of *visceration.*

The system of visceration is represented by the telencephalon impar (septal area, paired olfactory lobes and hippocampus) and deep periventricular neuropil of the forebrain. It is an autonomous system.

This system exercises regulatory influence upon the ablateral activities of cells, tissues and organs, including the cells and tissues of the somatic organs and of the brain itself. These activities are the *source* of the thermal energy (heat) as motive power of all bodily activities (movements) which "go on unbeknownst to us, whether we willst or not."[54] The ablateral functions of the telencephalon impar and of the deep neuropil "arouse" or "suppress" the bilateral functions of the limbic system, and are independent of the latter. The domain of the activities of the telencephalon impar and deep neuropil are *unconditional* responses of the cells, tissues and organs to the inexorable stimuli physical agents which tolerate no compromise and allow no choice in the mode of the response.

The *supralimbic* division of the superficial neuropil develops in phylogeny and ontogeny of primates upon the olfactory lobe (the anterior or "epistriatal" part of the telencephalon totopar) and upon the *hippocampus* ("epihippocampal" part). The epihippocampal part contains all the "analyzers" (specific heterotypical projection areas) of sensory information and is intimately thalamusbound. It may be regarded as the end of all the "private" paths. The *epistriatal* part in man appears to be emancipated from the tutelage of the thalamic activities. It is the origin of the main mass of the efferent fibers of the great capsulopeduncular tract from the telencephalon totopar distributed in parallel to all three neuropils of the forebrain and to all neuromeres of the neuraxis proper. In this sense, the epistriatal part may be said to "innervate the innervation" of all three systems of organs of the body. The capsulopeduncular system of fibers of the telencephalon totopar represents the penultimate common path of the forebrain from all the "private" paths of inherently nonshareable and, therefore, nonmeasurable ("immense") private *sensory experience* of living, to the "final," the *public,* path of the only "common"—that is, shareable and so—the only measurable experience, namely that of *movement.*

We think movement. Language and manufacture are the "fabric" of thought. In the words of Goethe:

> The texture of thought, it is a weaver's fabric.
> A single thrust of shuttle arrays a thousand threads in order.
> Back and forth the shuttles fly;
> The threads unseen, in a pattern come to lie;
> A single stroke, and a thousand bonds are bound together.

This is the function of the supralimbic neuropil of the human forebrain.

GOETHE *

* See note 17.

REFERENCES

1. von Baer, K. E.: *Uber die Entwicklungsgeschicte der Thiere.* Beobachtungen und Reflexion. 1. Teil. Konisberg, Bei den Gebrudern Borntrager, 1928.
2. Bergquist, H., and Källen, B.: Notes on the early histogenesis and morphogenesis of the central nervous system in vertebrates. *J. Comp. Neurol., 100:*627, 1954.
3. Bergson, H.: *L'évolution Créatrice.* Paris, Alcan, 1930.
4. von Bertallanffy, F.: *Das Biologische Weltbild.* Bern, Francke, Erster Band, 1949, pp. 124–126.
5. von Bertallanffy, L.: The theory of open systems in physics and biology. *Science, 111:*23, 1950.
6. Cannon, W. B.: *Bodily Changes in Pain, Hunger, Fear and Rage.* New York, Appleton & Co., 1915.
7. Chatel, M.: *Contribution a l'Etude de l'An-*

arthrie: les Troubles d'Articulation Verbale chez les Aphasiques—Analyse Oscillographique. Thesis Faculty of Medicine and of Pharmacy of Rennes (France), 1968. (Mimeographed copy)

8. Cobb, S.: *Emotions and Clinical Medicine.* New York, Norton, 1950.
9. Cobb, S.: *Foundations of Neuropsychiatry.* Baltimore, Williams & Wilkins, 1952.
10. Dalcq, A.: Recent experimental contributions to brain morphogenesis in amphibians. *Growth, 10 (Suppl. 6)*:85, 1946.
11. Eckstein, G.: *The Body Has a Head.* New York, Harper & Row, 1969.
12. von Economo, C., and Koskinas, G. N.: *Die Cytoarchitektonik der Hirnrinde des Erwachsenen Menschen.* Wien, Springer, 1925.
13. Filimonov, I. N.: The allocortical and periallocortical formation in man and their ontogenesis. *Contrib. Brain Institute* (USSR), *3/4*:15, 1938 (in Russian).
14. Filimonov, I. N.: Cytoarchitectonics. General concepts. Classification of the architectonic formations. In Sarkisov, S. A., Filimonov, I. N, and Preobrajenskaia, N. S. (Eds.): *Cytoarchitectonics of the Cerebral Cortex of Man.* Moscow, Medgiz, 1949 (in Russian).
15. Foster, M., and Balfour, F. M.: *The Elements of Embryology.* London, Macmillan, 1874.
16. Herrick, C. J.: *Neurological Foundations of Animal Behavior.* Henry Holt, 1924. (Reprinted by Hafner, New York, 1962.)
17. Herrick, C. J.: *Brains in Rats and Men. A Survey of the Origin and Biological Significance of the Cerebral Cortex.* Chicago, University of Chicago Press, 1926. (Reprinted by Hafner, New York, 1963.)
18. Herrick, C. J.: *The Brain of the Tiger Salamander (Amblystoma tigrinum).* Chicago, University of Chicago Press, 1948.
19. Hess, W. R.: *Die Funktionelle Organisation des Vegetativen Nervensystems.* Basel, *Schwalbe,* 1948.
20. Hess, W. R.: *Die Zwischenhirn. Syndrome, Lokalisation. Funktionen.* Basel, Schwalbe, 1949.
21. Hess, W. R.: *Psychologie in Biologischer Sicht.* Stuttgart, Thieme, 1962.
22. His, W.: *Die Entwidklung des Menschlichen Gehirns während der Ersten Monate.* Leipzig, Hirzl, 1904.
23. Hochstetter, F.: *Beitrage zur Entwicklungsgeschicte des Menschlichen Gehirns.* Wien and Leipzig, F. Deuticke, 1929.
24. Hopf, A.: Personal communication.
25. Jackson, J. H.: Evolution and Dissolution of the Nervous System. Croonian Lectures, 1884. In Taylor, James (Ed.): *Selected Writings of John Hughlings Jackson.* London, Hodder & Stoughton, 1932, Vol. II, pp. 45–75.
26. Jacobs, M. S., Morgane, P. J., and McFarland, W. L.: The anatomy of the brain of the bottlenose dolphin (*Tursiops truncatus*). Rhinic Lobe (Rhinencephalon). I. The paleocortex. *J. Comp. Neurol., 141:* 205, 1971.
27. Kingsbury, B. F.: The fundamental plan of the vertebrate brain. *J. Comp. Neurol., 34*:461, 1922.
28. Koelliker, A.: Entwicklungsgeschichte des Menschen und der Hoheren Tiere, 2. Aufl. Leipzig, Engelmann, 1876.
29. Kononova, E. P.: The frontal lobe. In Sarkisov, S. A., Filimonov, I. N., and Preobrajenskaja, N. S. (Eds.): *Cytoarchitectonics of the Cerebral Cortex of Man.* Moscow, Medgiz, 1949 (in Russian).
30. Lehmann, F. E.: Regionale Verschiedenheiten des Organisators von Triton, insbesonders in der Vorderen und Hinteren Kopfregion, nachzuweisen durch Phasenspezifische Erzeugung von Histaminbedingten und Operativ Bewirkten Regionaldefekten. *Arch. Entw. Mech., 138*:106, 1938.
31. Le Roy, E.: *L'Exigence Idéaliste et le Fait d'Evolution.* Paris, Boivin, 1927.
32. Lorenz, K.: The objectivistic theory of instincts. In Grasse, P. P. (Ed.): *L'Instinct dans le Comportement des Animaux et de l'Homme.* Symposium, Fondation Singer-Polignac. Paris, Masson, 1956.
33. MacLean, P. D.: Psychosomatic disease and the "visceral" brain. Recent developments bearing on the Papez theory of emotions. *Psychosom. Med., 9*:338, 1950.
34. MacLean, P. D.: The limbic system and its hippocampal formation. Studies in animals and their possible application to man. *J. Neurosurg., 11*:29, 1954.
35. MacLean, P. D.: The limbic system with respect to self-preservation of the species. *J. Nerv. Ment. Dis., 127*:1, 1958.

36. MacLean, P. D.: Contrasting functions of the limbic and neocortical systems of the brain and their relevance to physiological aspects of medicine. *Amer. J. Med., 25:* 611, 1958.
37. MacLean, P. D.: The triune brain, emotion, and scientific bias. In *The Neurosciences: Second Study Program.* Schmitt, F. O. (Ed.): New York, The Rockefeller University Press, 1970, pp. 336–349.
38. von Monakow, C.: Gefühl, Gesittung und Gehirn. (Reprinted from Arb. a.d. Hirnanat. Inst. Zurich. Heft X, pp. 115–213, 1916.)
39. von Monakow, C., and Mourgue, R.: *Introduction Biologique a l'Etude de la Neurologie et de la Psychopathologie: Intégration et Désintégration de la Fonction,* Paris, Alcan, 1928.
40. Papez, J. W.: A proposed mechanism of emotion. *Arch. Neurol. Psychiat., 38:*725, 1937.
41. Pasteur, L.: La dissymétrie moléculaire. Conference at the Chemical Society of Paris, December 22, 1883. In Vallery-Radot, Pasteur (Ed.): *Oeuvres de Pasteur.* Paris, Masson, 1922, Vol. I, pp. 369–380.
42. Pernkopf, E.: Topographische anatomie des menschen. 2. Aufl. Bd. 1/1. *Der Bauplan des Menschlichen Körpers (Promorphologie).* Wien, Urban & Schwarzenberg, 1943, pp. 15–16.
43. Poliakov, G. I.: Sturctural organization of the cerebral cortex of man in the light of its ontogenetic development. In Sarkisov, S. A., Filimonov, I. N., and Preobrajenskaia, N. S. (Eds.): *Cytoarchitectonics of the Cerebral Cortex of Man.* Moscow, Medgz, 1949 (in Russian).
44. Sabouraud, O., Gagnepain, J., and Chatel, M.: Qu'est-ce que l'Anarthrie? *La Presse Med., 79:*675, 1971.
45. Sanides, F., and Krishnamurti, A.: Cytoarchitectonic subdivision of sensory-motor and prefrontal regions of the bordering insular and limbic fields in slow horis (*Nycticabus coucang coucang*). *J. Hirnforschung., 9:*225, 1967.
46. Sanides, F.: Functional architecture of motor and sensory cortices in primates in the light of a new concept of neocortex evolution in the primate brain. In Noback, C. R., and Montagna, W. (Eds.): *Advances in Primatology.* New York, Appleton-Century-Crofts, 1970, Vol. I, pp. 137–208.
47. Sherrington, C. S.: *The Integrative Action of the Nervous System.* New York, Charles Scribner's Sons, 1906. (Reprinted by Yale University Press, New Haven, 1948.)
48. Sholl, D. A.: *The Organization of the Cerebral Cortex.* London, Methuen, and New York, John Wiley & Sons, 1956.
49. Vernadsky, W. I.: *La Biosphere.* Paris, Alcan, 1930.
50. Vernadsky, W. I.: Problems of biogeochemistry, II. *Trans. Conn. Acad. Arts Sci., 35:*483, 1944.
51. Vernadsky, W. I.: The biosphère and the noosphere. *Amer. Sci., 33:*1, 1945.
52. Viaud, G.: Taxies et tropismes dans le comportement instinctive. In Grassé, P. P. (Ed.): *L'Instinct dans le Comportement des Animaux et de l'Homme.* Paris, Masson, 1956, pp. 5–49.
53. Weyl. H.: *Symmetry.* Princeton, Princeton University Press, 1952.
54. Willis, Th.: *Cerebri Anatome, Nervorumque Descriptio & Usus.* In Blasius G. (Ed.): *Thomae Willis, Med. Doct. Opera Omnia.* Amsterdam, Henricus Wetstenius, 1662, Chap. XV, pp. 50–52.
55. Yakovlev, P. I.: Motility, behavior and the brain. Stereodynamic organization and neural co-ordinates of behavior. *J. Nerv. Ment. Dis., 107:*313, 1948.
56. Yakovlev, P. I.: Patterns of neuronal assemblies and the anatomical substratum of epileptic seizures. *Epilepsia (3rd series), 1:*51, 1952.
57. Yakovlev, P. I.: Pathoarchitectonic studies of cerebral malformations. III. Arrhinencephalies (holotelencephalies). *J. Exp. Neurol., 18:*22, 1959.
58. Yakovlev, P. I.: Anatomy of the brain and the problem of mental retardation. In Bowman, P. W., and Mauthner, H. V. (Eds.): *Mental Retardation.* New York, Grune & Stratton, 1960, pp. 1–43.
59. Yakovlev, P. I., and Locke, S.: Limbic nuclei of thalamus and connections of limbic cortex. III. Corticocortical connections of the anterior cingulate gyrus, the cingulum, and the subcallosal bundle in monkey. *Arch. Neurol., 5:*364, 1961.
60. Yakovlev, P. I.: The traditional and the new

in Pavlov's theory of "higher nervous activity." In Wortis, J. (Eds.): *Recent Advances in Biological Psychiatry.* New York, Plenum Press, 1962, Vol. 4, pp. 24–28.

61. Yakovlev, P. I.: Telokinesis and handedness (An empirical generalization). In Wortis, J. (Ed.): *Recent Advances in Biological Psychiatry.* New York, Plenum Press, 1963, Vol. VI, pp. 21–30.
62. Yakovlev, P. I., Locke, S., and Angevine, J. B., Jr.: The limbus of the cerebral hemisphere, limbic nuclei of the thalamus and the cingulum bundle. In Purpura, B. P., and Yahr, M. D. (Eds.): *Thalamic Integration of Sensory and Motor Activities. Columbia Symposium.* New York, Columbia University Press, 1966.
63. Yakovlev, P. I., and Rakić, P.: Patterns of decussation of bulbar pyramids and distribution of the pyramidal tracts on the two sides of the spinal cord. *Trans. Amer. Neurol. Assoc.*, pp. 366–367, 1966.
64. Yakovlev, P. I.: Development of the nuclei of the dorsal thalamus and of the cerebral cortex. Morphogenetic and tectogenetic correlation. In Locke, S. (Ed.): *Modern Neurology.* Boston, Little, Brown, & Co. 1969, pp. 15–53.
65. Yakovlev, P. I.: Telencephalon "impar," "semipar" and "totopar." Morphogenetic, tectogenetic and architectonic definitions. *Int. J. Neurol.*, *6*:245, 1968.
66. Yakovlev, P. I.: The structural and functional "trinity" of the body, brain and behavior. In Wycis, H. T. (Ed.): *Current Research in Neurosciences. Topical Probl. Psychiat. Neurol.*, *10*:197, 1970.
67. Yakovlev, P. I., Kertecz, A., and Rakic, P.: In preparation.

ACKNOWLEDGMENTS

I wish to acknowledge my gratitude for support I have received in the form of grants of the National Institutes of Health, NINDS 00152 and 03190.

I am grateful to Dr. Elizabeth Dooling, for her help in tidying the grammar and tightening the syntax of my manuscript and in labeling the illustrations.

I thank also Dr. Zvonimir Djordjevic, for drawing most of the diagrams from my sketches; Mr. Edward DiRamio, for photography; Mrs. Olga Aire, for histotechnical help; Miss Gayanne DeVry, for labeling illustrations; and Miss Fritzi Zohn and Miss Elizabeth Ellis, for typing the innumerable scrap notes and drafts of this "open-ended" paper.

NOTES

1. The *centrum semiovale* of the cerebral hemisphere is the layer of white and gray matter adjacent to the lateral ventricles, is best seen in coronal sections at the level of the lenticular nuclei (Fig. 14–8). It is demarcated from the *corona radiata* by the external sagittal stratum of fibers ("specific" thalamocortical projections).
2. The term "pallium" is often used to designate the gray matter covering the *entire* endbrain (telencephalon) and its subdivisions: *paleo*pallium (syn.: "praepiriform cortex," "paleocortex," "olfactory cortex"), *archi*pallium (syn.: "archicortex," i.e. fascia dentata + hippocampus + subiculum), *neo*pallium (syn.: "neocortex," "homogenetic" cortex, "isocortex"). Here the term "pallium" is used to designate exclusively the gray matter covering the hemispheres proper (the neo- or *iso*cortex).
3. The *corona radiata* is the subcortical layer of white matter outside the centrum semiovale. It consists mainly of radially disposed projection fibers and commissural (callosal) fibers (hence, "radiate").
4. The *cingular* and *parahippocampal* gyri, and the parietal, occipital and temporal lobes overlying these limbic gyri, develop posterior

to the plane of the sulcus of Rolando, upon the hippocampus as their pediment, hence, "epihippocampal."

5. The paraolfactory lobule of Broca, the insula with the claustrum and the frontal lobe, including the frontal and orbital opercula, develop anterior to the plane of the sulcus of Rolando upon the olfactory lobe, anterolateral and above the corpus striatum as their "pediment" (hence, "epistriatal") and are demarcated from the olfactory lobe in all mammals by the rhinal sulcus (Fig. 14–5).[65]
6. The clinoid border ("limes duplex" of Filimonov) of the isocortex (neocortex) is found throughout the circumference of the border of the hemisphere which it defines and in most sectors is demonstrable in the adult brain. It is present in the brain of fetal and adult man and monkey and is particularly conspicuous in cetacea (*Tursiops truncatus*) (Figs. 14–10, A and D). (Personal observations with M. S. Jacobs and P. J. Morgane.[26])
7. I have used, in an earlier paper,[55] the terms "entocortex," "mesocortex" and "ectocortex" to designate respectively the olfactory lobe and hippocampus (entocortex), the limbic division of the hemisphere proper (mesocortex) and the supralimbic division of the hemisphere (ectocortex). The terms emphasizing the topographic sequence of the innermost (ento), intermediate (meso) and the outermost (ecto) divisions of the endbrain.
8. The term "holosphere" is justified on teratogenetic evidence.[57, 58] In typical malformations such as "cyclopia," the paired optic, hemispheric and olfactory vescicles fail to evaginate. The entire *prosencephalon* remains a single vesicle—a "holoprosencephaly" results. In the less profound (but far more common) malformation of the same type known as "arrhinencephaly," the olfactory and the hemispheric vesicles fail to evaginate from the single median *telencephalic* vesicle and a "holo*telen*cephaly" results. All transitions between the two types may occur. The precise meaning of the prefixes holo*tel*- and holo*pros*- in the designations of these two distinct types of the same malformation has been, most unfortunately, confused in the recent literature.
9. Prof. Adolf Hopf has made a tentative and interesting suggestion that the ratio of brain size to the length of the spinal cord may be a more reliable index of encephalization in mammals than the other parameters used for comparison.[24] Should this prove to be true, then, in my opinion, it should be expected that in the case of man the index should be high, particularly for the ratio of the telencephalon totopar/*neuraxis proper* (as here defined).
10. The activities of microorganisms and of green vegetation are the major factor in physical transformations of the biosphere in a geological time scale. Among animals the activities of man are apparently next in order of magnitude and are increasing in tempo with each generation (Vernadsky).[49, 50]
11. From Greek, to *set* to arrange *around* some reference point or line—for example, circular and longitudinal smooth muscles "arranged round" the lumen of the intestinal tract in the visceral axis of the body.
12. From Greek, to *set apart,* to *distinguish* with regard to some reference (a line, plane or interval of time). In the present context, to distinguish movements of articulated parts of the body wall on the somatic axis of the body with reference to the plane of their symmetry, such as respiration, vocalization, mimicry, gesticulation and the like symmetrical movements, either towards or away from the plane of symmetry.
13. A contralateral paralysis or convulsion following a lesion (or stimulation) of one hemisphere is the pragmatic appodict of clinical experience. It localizes *symptoms* of a lesion (locus of "pathology") in the brain. It does not either localize or define *functions*—that is, activities of the intact brain as an organ. These activities and their anatomical substrates are products of evolution. Their localization in the structures of the brain is "chronogenic." [30]
14. The notion of "force" has become accepted in natural sciences as the agent (cause) of events only since the time of "Renascimento." Vermadsky credits to Boskovic, a Croatian scholar of the eighteenth century, the empirical generalization that the force which moves the arrow to its target is the force of tension of the bow-string rather than the force of the archer. It seems that when Archimedes looked for a "lever" that would "lift the World off its hinges," he meant that his own force would unhinge the world and not the force of the

action (work) of some mechanical lever as a tool. No one would mean in our time that it was the force (power) of Einstein, Oppenheimer or Fermi that blew the Island of Bikini off the face of the Pacific Ocean. The atomic "fusion" did it.

15. The *basal* forebrain bundle of Edinger is conventionally subdivided in comparative anatomical literature into "medial" (median, nonpaired) and "lateral" (paramedian and paired) *forebrain bundles.* The *stria semicircularis* and *fornix* may be regarded as the products of phyletic and ontogenetic segregation of these fiber systems from the ablateral (median) basal forebrain bundle. The fornix and the cingulum bundles segregate in human embryo from the originally common mass of median longitudinal fiber bundle in the floor and banks of the median groove (*sulcus medianus telencephali medii* of the primitive hippocampus). The fornix fibers remain in the sulcus medianus. This bundle bifurcates dorsad and posteriorly with the bifurcation of the hippocampus (Ammon's horns) attendant on the growth of the hemispheres bilaterad from it. The *cinqulum* fibers become separated from the fornix by the growth of the massive corpus callosum which perforates the primitive hippocampus and the fornix.
16. I owe thanks to Dr. Andrew Kertecz, now of London, Ontario, and to Dr. Norman Geschwind, Professor of Neurology and Chief of the Harvard-Boston City Hospital Neurological Unit, for making available to me the autopsy specimens of 153 adults and for information on handedness culled by Dr. Kertecz from the clinical records. A detailed report of anatomical observations of this (and of fetal material collected in cooperation with the NIH Institute of Neurological Disease and Stroke) is in preparation (Projects NS-03190 and NS-00152).
17. A quotation (in German—my translation) from Goethe's *Faust,* on the frontispiece of D. A. Sholl's monograph.[48]

Index